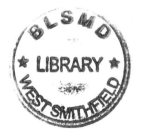

ESSENTIALS IN OPHTHALMOLOGY: **Cataract and Refractive Surgery.**
T. Kohnen · D. D. Koch (Eds.)

ESSENTIALS IN OPHTHALMOLOGY

G. K. Krieglstein · R. N. Weinreb
Series Editors

Glaucoma

Cataract and Refractive Surgery

Uveitis and Immunological Disorders

Vitreo-retinal Surgery

Medical Retina

Oculoplastics and Orbit

Paediatric Ophthalmology,
Neuro-ophthalmology, Genetics

Cornea and External Eye Disease

Editors Thomas Kohnen
Douglas D. Koch

Cataract and Refractive Surgery

With 126 Figures, Mostly in Colour,
and 37 Tables

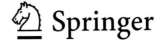 Springer

Series Editors

GÜNTHER K. KRIEGLSTEIN, MD
Professor and Chairman
Department of Ophthalmology
University of Cologne
Joseph-Stelzmann-Straße 9
50931 Cologne
Germany

ROBERT N. WEINREB, MD
Professor and Director
Hamilton Glaucoma Center
Department of Ophthalmology – 0946
University of California at San Diego
9500 Gilman Drive
La Jolla, CA 92093-0946
USA

Volume Editors

THOMAS KOHNEN, MD
Professor of Ophthalmology
Johann-Wolfgang-Goethe Universität
Klinik für Augenheilkunde
Theodor-Stern-Kai 7
60590 Frankfurt
Germany

DOUGLAS D. KOCH, MD
Professor and the Allen, Mosbacher,
and Law Chair in Ophthalmology
Baylor College of Medicine
Cullen Eye Institute
6565 Fannin, Suite NC 205
Houston, TX 77030
USA

ISBN 3-540-20046-0
Springer Verlag Berlin Heidelberg New York

ISSN 1612-3212

Library of Congress Control Number: 2004105920

Springer is a part of Springer Science + Business Media

springeronline.com

© Springer-Verlag Berlin Heidelberg 2005
Printed in Germany

Cover picture "Cataract and Refractive Surgery" from Kampik A, Grehn F (eds) Augenärztliche Therapie. Georg Thieme Verlag Stuttgart, with permission.

Editor: Marion Philipp, Heidelberg
Desk editor: Martina Himberger, Heidelberg
Production: ProEdit GmbH, Heidelberg
Cover design: Erich Kirchner, Heidelberg
Typesetting and reproduction of the figures:
AM-productions GmbH, Wiesloch
Printing: Saladruck GmbH, Berlin
Binding: Stein & Lehmann, Berlin

Printed on acid-free paper
24/3150beu-göh   5 4 3 2 1 0

Foreword

Essentials in Ophthalmology is a new review series covering all of ophthalmology categorized in eight subspecialties. It will be published quarterly; thus each subspecialty will be reviewed biannually.

Given the multiplicity of medical publications already available, why is a new series needed? Consider that the half-life of medical knowledge is estimated to be around 5 years. Moreover, it can be as long as 8 years between the description of a medical innovation in a peer-reviewed scientific journal and publication in a medical textbook. A series that narrows this time span between journal and textbook would provide a more rapid and efficient transfer of medical knowledge into clinical practice, and enhance care of our patients.

For the series, each subspecialty volume comprises 10–20 chapters selected by two distinguished editors and written by internationally renowned specialists. The selection of these contributions is based more on recent and note-worthy advances in the subspecialty than on systematic completeness. Each article is structured in a standardized format and length, with citations for additional reading and an appropriate number of illustrations to enhance important points. Since every subspecialty volume is issued in a recurring sequence during the 2-year cycle, the reader has the opportunity to focus on the progress in a particular subspecialty or to be updated on the whole field. The clinical relevance of all material presented will be well established, so application to clinical practice can be made with confidence.

This new series will earn space on the bookshelves of those ophthalmologists who seek to maintain the timeliness and relevance of their clinical practice.

G. K. KRIEGLSTEIN
R. N. WEINREB
Series Editors

Preface

This second volume in the *Essentials in Ophthalmology* series provides detailed and concise updates of the major topics in cataract and refractive surgery. Because of the remarkable growth of these two subspecialties, our challenge was to highlight new advances, with the primary emphasis on clinical applications.

The section on cataracts calls attention to recent progress in surgical techniques and the management of complications. Topics include new anaesthesia and small incision techniques, new devices (ophthalmic viscosurgical devices and intraocular lenses), prevention and management of complications and the treatment of difficult cases, such as mature, uveitic and paediatric cataracts.

As refractive surgery now encompasses an increasing array of procedures, the book covers excimer laser surface and lamellar procedures, incisional corneal surgery and the use of intraocular implants to correct refractive errors. Particular emphasis is placed on topics related to quality of vision, such as wavefront technology, measuring quality of vision and issues in pupil measurement. We believe that these issues will be of growing importance as refractive surgical techniques are refined. Interestingly, many of the topics in this section are also pertinent to cataract surgery, reflecting the merging of technologies that is occurring in these two major ophthalmic subspecialties.

The goal of the editors of this book has been to provide up-to-date, clinically relevant overviews in these fields and to highlight the most interesting areas of research and controversy. This was only possible with the support of our many outstanding authors. We truly appreciate the thought, time and care they put into their chapters. We would also like to thank the series editors for giving us the opportunity to do the book, Springer for its excellent work on all aspects of preparing it and our wives, Eva-Maria and Marcia, for their wonderful support during its realization.

THOMAS KOHNEN
DOUGLAS D. KOCH

Contents

Cataract Surgery

CHAPTER 5
"Accommodative" IOLs
OLIVER FINDL

CHAPTER 4
Foldable Intraocular Lenses
LILIANA WERNER, NICK MAMALIS

CHAPTER 6
Prevention of Posterior Capsule Opacification
RUPERT M. MENAPACE

CHAPTER 7
Management of the Mature Cataract
SAMUEL MASKET

CHAPTER 8
The Treatment of Uveitic Cataract
ARND HEILIGENHAUS, CARSTEN HEINZ,
MATTHIAS BECKER

Refractive Surgery

Contributors

ARSHINOFF, STEVE A., MD, FRCSC
York Finch Eye Associates
The University of Toronto
2115 Finch Avenue W. #316
Toronto, Ontario, M3 N 2V6, Canada

AZAR, DIMITRI T., MD
Professor of Ophthalmology
Harvard Medical School
Director of Cornea and Refractive Surgery
Massachusetts Eye and Ear Infirmary
243 Charles Street
Boston, MA 02114, USA

BECKER, MATTHIAS, MD
Department of Ophthalmology
University of Heidelberg
69121 Heidelberg, Germany

BEHRENS-BAUMANN, WOLFGANG, MD
Professor of Ophthalmology
Universitäts-Augenklinik
Leipziger Str. 44
39120 Magdeburg, Germany

BELLUCCI, ROBERTO, MD
Chief of Ophthalmological Unit
Hospital of Verona
Sede Legale P. le A. Stefani, 1
37126 Verona, Italy

BÜHREN, JENS, MD
Department of Ophthalmology
Johann Wolfgang Goethe-University
Theodor-Stern-Kai 7
60590 Frankfurt am Main, Germany

CHEN, CHUN CHEN, MD
Taipei Municipal Jen-Ai Hospital
10, Sec 4, Jen-Ai Road
National Yang-Ming University,
Taipei, Taiwan

FINDL, OLIVER, MD
Professor of Ophthalmology
Department of Ophthalmology
Vienna University
Waehringer Guertel 18–20
1090 Vienna, Austria

Fine, I. Howard, MD
1550 Oak Street, #5
Eugene, OR 97401-7701, USA

GRIS, OSCAR, MD
Instituto Microcirugia Ocular de Barcelona
c. Munner 10, 08022 Barcelona, Spain

GÜELL, JOSE LUIS, MD, PhD
Associate Professor of Ophthalmology
Autonoma University of Barcelona
Director of Cornea and Refractive Surgery Unit
Instituto Microcirugia Ocular de Barcelona
c. Munner 10, 08022 Barcelona, Spain

HARDTEN, DAVID R., MD
Minnesota Eye Consultants
Department of Ophthalmology
University of Minnesota
Minneapolis, MN 55404, USA

HEILIGENHAUS, ARND, MD
Professor of Ophthalmology
Department of Ophthalmology
St. Franziskus Hospital
Hohenzollernring 74
48145 Muenster, Germany

HEINZ, CARSTEN, MD
Department of Ophthalmology
St. Franziskus Hospital
Hohenzollernring 74
48145 Muenster, Germany

HOFFMAN, RICHARD S., MD
1550 Oak Street, #5
Eugene, OR 97401-7701, USA

KASPER, THOMAS, MD
Department of Ophthalmology
Johann Wolfgang Goethe-University
Theodor-Stern-Kai 7
60590 Frankfurt am Main, Germany

KNORZ, MICHAEL C., Professor Dr.
FreeVis LASIK
Zentrum Universitätsklinikum Mannheim
Theodor Kutzer Ufer 1–3
68167 Mannheim, Germany

KOCH, DOUGLAS D., MD
Professor and the Allen, Mosbacher,
and Law Chair in Ophthalmology
Baylor College of Medicine
6565 Fannin NC 205
Houston, TX 77030-2703, USA

KOHNEN, THOMAS, MD
Professor of Ophthalmology
Department of Ophthalmology
Johann Wolfgang Goethe-University
Theodor-Stern-Kai 7
60590 Frankfurt am Main, Germany

KOO, JACQUELINE T., MD
Minnesota Eye Consultants
Department of Ophthalmology
University of Minnesota
Minneapolis, MN 55404, USA

LINDSTROM, RICHARD L., MD
Minnesota Eye Consultants
Department of Ophthalmology
University of Minnesota
Minneapolis, MN 55404, USA

LINEBARGER, ERIC J., MD
Assistant Professor
University of California, San Diego
Shiley Eye Center, 0946
La Jolla, CA 92093, USA

LU, DENNIS C., MD
Minnesota Eye Consultants
Department of Ophthalmology
University of Minnesota
Minneapolis, MN 55404, USA

MAMALIS, NICK, MD
Professor of Ophthalmology
John A. Moran Eye Center
University of Utah
50 North Medical Drive
Salt Lake City, UT 84132, USA

MANERO, FELICIDAD, MD
Instituto Microcirugia Ocular de Barcelona
c. Munner 10, 08022 Barcelona, Spain

MASKET, SAMUEL, MD
Jules Stein Eye Institute, UCLA
Los Angeles, CA 90048, USA

MENAPACE, RUPERT M., MD
Professor of Ophthalmology
Department of Ophthalmology
University of Vienna Medical School
Vienna General Hospital
Waehringer Guertel 18–20
1090 Vienna, Austria

MORSELLI, SIMONETTA, MD
Department of Ophthalmology
Hospital of Verona
Sede Legale P. le A. Stefani, 1
37126 Verona, Italy

PACKER, MARK, MD
1550 Oak Street, #5
Eugene, OR 97401-7701, USA

ROSEN, EMANUEL, MD
FRCSE FRCOphth FRPS
"Rosen Eye Clinic", Harbour City
Salford, Manchester M3 4DY, UK

SANDOVAL, NANCY, MD
Fellowship in Cornea and Refractive Surgery
Autonoma University of Barcelona
Instituto de Microcirugia Ocular de Barcelona
c. Munner 10, 08022 Barcelona, Spain

TERZI, EVDOXIA, MD
Department of Ophthalmology
Johann Wolfgang Goethe-University
Theodor-Stern-Kai 7
60590 Frankfurt am Main, Germany

WANG, LI, MD, PhD
Cullen Eye Institute
Baylor College of Medicine
6565 Fannin, NC 205
Houston, TX 77030, USA

WEIKERT, MITCHELL P., MD, MS
Baylor College of Medicine
6565 Fannin NC 205
Houston, TX 77030-2703, USA

WERNER, LILIANA, MD, PhD
Assistant Professor
John A. Moran Eye Center, University of Utah
50 North Medical Drive
Salt Lake City, UT 84132, USA

ZETTERSTRÖM, CHARLOTTA, MD
Professor of Ophthalmology
Ophthalmology, St. Eriks Eye Hospital
11282 Stockholm, Sweden

Topical and Intracameral Anaesthesia for Cataract Surgery

Roberto Bellucci, Simonetta Morselli

Core Messages

- Topical anaesthesia consists in blocking the production and not the transmission of pain sensation
- It is suitable for cataract surgery because akinesia is not required by phacoemulsification
- Treatments proven to be safe and effective include: repeated eyedrop instillations, gel application, use of drug-soaked sponge, intracameral injection of drug dilutions or of anaesthetic viscoelastic substance
- Ester-bound compounds like tetracaine and benoxinate have faster and shorter action than amide-bound compounds like lidocaine and ropivacaine
- Different anaesthetic drugs give similar results
- The authors' preferred schedule includes 4% unpreserved lidocaine eyedrops, with or without 1% intracameral injection
- Patient selection or intravenous sedation are less employed with experience
- Side effects of topical anaesthesia consist in immediate and postoperative ocular dryness, that can last up to a few weeks
- Intracameral anaesthesia has been proven safe for intraocular structures, although its necessity remains controversial

1.1 Introduction

1.1.1 Foreword

Topical and intracameral drug administration is now the preferred method for anaesthesia in cataract surgery [47], and an increasingly preferred method for anaesthesia in anterior and posterior segment surgery. Despite its universal use, standards have never been established and many variations in the technique are currently employed, while many studies about new drugs or protocols continue to appear. In this chapter we will review the current knowledge about topical and intracameral anaesthesia, examining both pharmacological and clinical aspects. In addition, we will discuss recent advances in order to formulate some recommendations for clinical practice.

1.1.2 History

Topical anaesthesia for cataract surgery is not new. First introduced in Europe at the end of the 19th century when cocaine was widely available to ophthalmologists [44], it almost fell out of use in favour of retrobulbar injections following the introduction of newer and less toxic anaesthetic agents such as procaine [6]. Surgical technique modifications in cataract extraction with the advent of small incision surgery and of phacoemulsification, and the continuous report of severe complications due to retrobulbar needle injections prompted surgeons to look for gentler and safer methods of anaesthesia. Davis and Mandel proposed peribulbar injections in 1986 [19], Smith published a work on subconjunctival injections in 1990 [73], and 2 years later the sub-Tenon approach by a plastic cannula was proposed by Greenbaum [29].

Modern topical anaesthesia in cataract surgery began in 1991, when Fichman performed a series of phacoemulsifications under topical anaesthesia using 0.5% tetracaine [22]. This technique spread rapidly, and other drugs like lidocaine were tested, lidocaine eventually becoming the most used drug. Intraocular irrigations of anaesthetic agents to improve analgesia were postulated in 1993 [26], and the first results on a large series of patients were published in 1997 [27, 41].

1.1.3
Definitions

For a number of years, many anaesthetic techniques without periocular needle injections have been named "topical". Variations include use of oral or IV sedation, administration of lid block, use of subconjunctival injections or sub-Tenon irrigations, intraocular irrigations and more. At present we consider "topical anaesthesia" only the use of anaesthetic eyedrops without sedation, and "intracameral anaesthesia" the use of anaesthetic irrigation of the anterior chamber at any step of surgery.

1.2
Bases of Topical/Intracameral Anaesthesia in Cataract Surgery

1.2.1
Physiological Bases

Ocular sensitivity is based on terminations of the 5th cranial nerve, especially distributed to the cornea and to the ciliary body in the anterior part of the eye. These fibres are generally non-myelinated, types A-delta and C. They are able to carry sensation of pain, temperature and touch, and are blocked by lower concentrations of drugs in comparison with motor fibres. Clin-ically, the order of loss of nerve function is as follows: pain, temperature, touch, proprioception, and skeletal muscle tone. However, the cornea has very little temperature sensation, while the conjunctiva and the iris have more. As it can be expected, ocular sensitivity is decreased by low temperatures, and decreases with age. Because pain sensation reflects more the amount of involved nerves than the tissue deepness of the injury, corneal abrasions are by far more painful than corneal penetrations.

1.2.2
Pharmacological Bases

Sensitive nerves have to be blocked by anaesthetic agents to suppress pain. The block can take place along the nerve itself, or at its sensory terminations. Nerve block is commonly achieved in local anaesthesia by drug injection. The anaesthetic agent has to come in touch with the sensory nerve, exerting its activity on non-myelinated fibres or on Ranvier nodes of myelinated fibres. To suppress impulse propagation, three to five nodes of Ranvier must be blocked, for a length of 3–7 mm [36]. This relatively long length of portion could explain the variability we find in the level of anaesthesia after peribulbar injections.

Sensory termination block is the most important feature of topical anaesthesia. It involves the inhibition of sodium channels at nerve endings or receptors by the anaesthetic agents, thus blocking the production (and not the transmission) of nervous impulse.

According to these considerations, anaesthetics topically applied to the eye could act directly on the corneal epithelium and stroma, and the part of drug penetrating into the anterior chamber could suppress iris and ciliary body pain. The amount of anaesthetic coming in touch with deeply settled structures can be increased by repeating eyedrop applications before surgery starts, or by adding some drug after first surgical incisions: additional eyedrops after conjunctival incision, or intracameral injection after opening the anterior chamber.

The duration of the effect of topically applied anaesthetics depends on the properties of the employed drug. Usually it lasts up to 15–20 min for the commonly used agents, but eyedrop instillations or intracameral irrigations can be repeated during surgery, if needed.

If proper concentrations are achieved, motor fibres are also blocked. In cataract surgery, intraocular muscles are affected by topical/intracameral anaesthesia, but the akinesia of the eyeball we obtain by retrobulbar or peribulbar injections cannot be achieved in any way.

1.2.3
Surgical Bases

In cataract surgery, the absence of ocular akinesia makes small incision surgery with phacoemulsification mandatory. Usually two incisions are made, allowing the surgeon to stabilise and to direct the eye with two instruments. Not only is akinesia no longer needed, but the retained ocular motility can be of help in some passages of surgery if the patient follows surgeon's instructions. The reduced length of the incisions makes them less painful, as lower numbers of nerves are cut compared with wider incisions. During surgery, instruments are moved as levers through the incisions thus preventing fluid leakage and excessive intraocular pressure variations, a possible cause of ciliary pain. Careful hydrodissection prevents excessive ciliary body stimulation by zonular fibres during nucleus rotation. During surgery, a decrease of ocular sensitivity is provided by the frequent use of cold irrigation solution. In addition, there are no painful manoeuvres typical of extracapsular surgery like muscle sutures, conjunctival incisions, iris manipulations, tissue sutures. The advantages of topical anaesthesia over periocular injections include not only a higher safety level, but also better consistency of analgesia during surgery and lower intraocular pressure. Moreover, the limited amount of drug employed inhibits the general side effects commonly observed with local anaesthesia. The return of sensitivity soon after surgery makes it possible to immediately detect any unexpected ocular pain suggestive of complications.

Summary for the clinician:

- Topical anaesthesia consists of analgesia
- Motor, thermal and tactile fibres are not suppressed
- The production and not the transmission of nervous impulse is blocked
- Phacoemulsification surgery does not require akinesia

1.3
Drugs Employed

1.3.1
Topical Anaesthetic Drugs

The chemical compounds employed for ophthalmic topical anaesthesia are tertiary amines composed of an aromatic hydrophobic ring – usually benzene – and an amidic hydrophilic group, with an ester (proparacaine, tetracaine, benoxinate) or an amidic (lidocaine, etidocaine, mepivacaine, ropivacaine) intermediate chain. The pharmacological properties of the drugs (potency, onset and duration of action, selectivity) are determined by the chemical configuration of the two ends of the molecule. The anaesthetic agents useful in clinical practice are unstable in their amine form, and insoluble in water. Therefore, they are prepared as salts that are stable in solution at relatively acid pH. The low pH of commercially available solutions is the main cause of the burning sensations perceived on the first eyedrop application. After topical application in the conjunctival sac, the compounds have to make the non-dissociated form cross the tear film and the cornea, and return to the dissociated form at nerve endings or axons to exert the anaesthetic activity. The chemistry of body fluids and the activity of tissue enzymes favour these passages. The ester compounds are rapidly hydrolysed by plasmatic esterases, and to a lesser extent by tissue esterases. The amide compounds are degraded more slowly, and mainly outside the eye in the liver, and therefore are endowed with longer duration of action. Table 1.1 reports a summary of the chemical characters of commonly employed topical anaesthetic agents [18].

Table 1.1. Anaesthetic agents most used for topical applications in ophthalmic surgery

Agent	pH[a] (25°C)	pKa[b] (pH 7.4)	% Base (eyedrops)	Concentration (%)	Action onset (min)	Action duration (min)
Ester compounds						
Tetracaine	4.5–6.5	8.5	≈15	0.5%	0.5	10–15
Proparacaine	5.0–6.0	3.7	≈75	0.5%	0.25	5–10
Benoxinate	5.0–6.0	2.2	≈80	0.4%	0.25	5–10
Amide compounds						
Lidocaine	6.0–6.5	7.9	≈25	4.0%	2–5	15–20
Bupivacaine	4.5–6.0	8.1	≈15	0.5–2%	5–10	20–30
Ropivacaine	5.0–6.5	8.1	≈15	1.0%	2–5	15–20
Mepivacaine	5.5–6.0	7.6	≈40	2%	1–3	10–15

[a] The low pH of the instilled solution is associated with subjective burning on application.
[b] If the pKa is high, the molecule is more dissociated at physiologic pH (low % base at pH 7.4) with higher surface activity but poorer corneal penetration.

1.3.2
Ester-Bound Compounds

1.3.2.1
Tetracaine

Tetracaine was the first anaesthetic employed topically for cataract surgery [23], but at present it is less used because of its short duration of action and because of the esterase deficiency that can lead to toxic reactions in some patients. It is available in some countries at concentrations between 1% and 2%. After eyedrop application its action begins within 1 min and lasts for 10–15 min. Tetracaine is considered more toxic than other agents for the corneal epithelium.

1.3.2.2
Proparacaine

Proparacaine is not degraded to para-aminobenzoic acid, and therefore is considered safer than other ester-bound compounds. It is less irritating and less painful on instillation than benoxinate, and does not show bacteriostatic properties. It is available in some countries at the 0.5% concentration for topical use. The onset of action is a matter of seconds, but the duration is usually shorter than 10 min.

1.3.2.3
Benoxinate

Benoxinate is available at 0.4% concentration as a widely used anaesthetic for office examinations in ophthalmology. Its instillation is painful, and its corneal epithelium toxicity is also high. It has bacteriostatic properties. After touching the cornea, the anaesthetic action takes place in seconds, and lasts up to 10 min. Being rapidly degraded by ocular esterases, its activity on intraocular structures is less strong than other compounds.

1.3.3
Amide-Bound Compounds

1.3.3.1
Lidocaine

Currently, lidocaine may be the most employed topical anaesthetic in cataract surgery, and it is the most employed for intracameral irrigations [47]. It is available in concentrations of 1%–4%, the unpreserved preparation being preferred for the better local tolerability. Instillation is rather painful because the pH of the solution is usually below 6. At the corneal surface, the onset of anaesthesia is slower than with ester compounds.

After eyedrop application, lidocaine crosses rapidly the corneal epithelium and stroma, exerting its sodium channel blockade on the cornea by first. As a result, temporary epithelial and stromal swelling can sometimes be observed even with unpreserved preparations. Lidocaine is not degraded within the eye, and therefore it can exert its anaesthetic effect on anterior chamber structures for a long period, up to 20 min.

1.3.3.2
Bupivacaine

Bupivacaine has been extensively used as local anaesthetic because of its potency and long duration of action, and despite the relatively slow onset of activity [36]. It has been employed at the 0.50%, 0.75% and 2% concentrations as topical anaesthetic for cataract surgery [17, 45, 52], showing low corneal epithelium toxicity. The intraocular penetration is good because bupivacaine is extremely liposoluble. The duration of the effect is about 10 min longer than with other amide agents.

1.3.3.3
Ropivacaine

Ropivacaine is a long-lasting anaesthetic agent that provides up to 12 h of postoperative analgesia. The onset of action is rather slow as it happens with bupivacaine, but ropivacaine has lower cardiac and central nervous system toxicity. It has been employed topically at 1% concentration, assuring good analgesic activity lasting more than 20 min [56].

1.3.3.4
Mepivacaine

Mepivacaine is an amide anaesthetic with rapid onset of activity. Because of its poor corneal penetration, its use in cataract surgery has been mainly limited to intraocular injections in patients showing pain after topical anaesthesia with 2% bupivacaine [52]. In that study, intraocular irrigation with 0.4 ml of unpreserved 2% mepivacaine solution proved to be effective in relieving pain and safe for the corneal endothelium [52].

Summary for the Clinician

- Ester anaesthetics are better employed for surface anaesthesia because of their fast onset of action and poor penetration
- Amide anaesthetics have slower onset of action but better intraocular penetration
- Lidocaine is the most employed topical drug for phacoemulsification surgery
- Bupivacaine is the most liposoluble among topical anaesthetics

1.3.4
Influence of Formulation

1.3.4.1
pH

The available dilutions of anaesthetic drugs for ocular use often contain sodium chloride or other salts to make them isotonic. This frequently results in a pH between 5 and 7, that contributes to the burning sensation on the first eyedrop application. The pH of these solutions can be raised by further diluting the drugs in BSS or BSS plus, approaching the physiologic normal of 7.2–7.4. However, some anaesthetic agents could be unstable in solutions at pH above 7 at certain concentrations: this is especially true for bupivacaine and mepivacaine, while lidocaine can be buffered to 7.4 without precipitating even at the 4% concentration.

1.3.4.2
Preservatives

The presence of preservatives in drug solutions improves stability and sterility, but the chemical agents employed can be toxic for the ocular structures. Corneal epithelial swelling has been frequently observed with preserved formulations of lidocaine, and the intraocular safety of preservatives remains even more controversial. Although some preservatives – like benzalkonium chloride – increase corneal penetration, we recommend the use of unpreserved formulations of anaesthetic agents both for topical application and for intraocular irrigation [27].

1.3.4.3
Temperature

Temperature influences the stability of solutions. A warm solution is probably more stable, better tolerated by patients and therefore more active. Therefore ampoules should not be refrigerated immediately before use.

Summary for the Clinician

- Low pH means burning on instillation
- Only unpreserved drugs should be used
- Drugs should not be refrigerated

1.4
Routes of Administration

1.4.1
Eyedrop Instillations

Many different instillation schedules have been proposed for topical anaesthesia in cataract surgery. Common features include bilateral instillation, number of applied eyedrops, intervals between instillations.

1.4.1.1
Bilateral Instillation

Usually the anaesthetic agent is applied to both eyes, to prevent blinking and Bell's phenomenon elicited by the non-operated eye. This practice allows the patient to keep both eyes open without effort during surgery. However, because of corneal epithelial toxicity of the drugs and lack of hydration, some vision impairment in the non-operated eye for the first postoperative week has to be anticipated in the patient.

1.4.1.2
Number of Instillations

Unpreserved eyedrops of the selected drug are instilled in the 10–60 min preceding surgery, according to the local protocol. When topical anaesthesia is employed alone, we prefer six instillations of 4% lidocaine at 10-min intervals, that assure steady analgesia for 15–20 min. When intracameral irrigation of an anaesthetic agent is planned, the number of eyedrops can be reduced to three. Usually the gained lack of any sensitivity to instillation is considered a sign of obtained anaesthesia. The great variations in instillation schedule probably reflect more the characters of the local population than the precision of the surgical technique.

1.4.1.3
Intraocular Penetration of Drugs

Only a few studies about intraocular penetration of topically applied anaesthetic drugs have been carried out (Table 1.2). For 4% lidocaine eyedrops, Zehetmayer et al. [84] found high dependence on the solution pH, as expected from chemical properties. Behndig and Linden [11] measured the lowest aqueous humour levels among published investigations. Higher levels were found in our study [13] following instillations at 10-min intervals, probably because the damage to the corneal surface favoured penetration. In this study, pain sensations during surgery were higher when the intraocular level of lidocaine was <12 µg/ml. This correlation between lidocaine levels in aqueous humour and pain scores was not found by Bardocci et al. [8].

Intraocular penetration of topically applied bupivacaine has been studied by Lagnado et al. [45]. Following three or six instillations, they found the number of instillations was not related to the intraocular level of bupivacaine or pain scores.

1.4.1.4
Side Effects and Toxicity

General Side Effects

Anaesthetic agents of the ester group cannot have general side effects at commonly employed doses, as they are rapidly degraded by tissue and plasma esterases. Anaesthetics of the amide type are metabolised in the liver, and some concern arose about possible general effects. For topically applied 4% lidocaine, blood levels found after 1 h from the last instillation were 0.009 ± 0.001 µg/ml following three instillations, and 0.12 ± 0.02 µg/ml following six instillations [13]. For topically applied 0.75% bupivacaine,

Table 1.2. Aqueous humour concentration of topically applied anaesthetics

Reference	Drug	Concentration	pH	Drops (n)	Installation (n)	Interval (min)	Level (µg/ml)
[84]	Lidocaine	4%	5.2	3	3	3	4.75±3.5
		4%	7.2	3	3	3	15.06±8.2
[11]	Lidocaine	4%	NR	1	3	1.5	1.4±0.5
		4%	NR	1	6	1.5	4.2±1.5
[13]	Lidocaine	4%	6.0	1	3	10	8.7±2.4
		4%	6.0	1	6	10	23.2±8.9
[8]	Lidocaine	4%	6.0	0.5 ml	3	5	12.7±5.8
	Lidocaine gel	2%	NR	0.5 ml	2	15	27.1±13.8
[45]	Bupivacaine	0.75%	NR	1	3	10	5.9±4.3
				1	6	10	5.7±4.0

NR, not reported.

less than 1 µg/ml were measured in plasma [45]. These amounts are too low to cause systemic problems even in diseased patients, and are much lower than the 2.13 µg/ml found by Salomon et al. [71] after periocular injections. In all the performed studies, no differences were found in pulse rate, blood pressure and oxygen saturation following topical anaesthesia [8, 12, 45].

Local Side Effects

With topical anaesthesia the potential risks of needle injections are avoided, but still local side effects can occur. Apart from burning sensation, the instillation of an anaesthetic agent into the conjunctival sac impairs the tear film because of dilution and because of the pH of applied solutions. Especially in older patients with low tear secretion, the inhibition of cellular sodium channels causes some swelling of the corneal epithelium, with the possibility of superficial punctate keratitis [74]. Epithelial toxicity is even more pronounced when preservatives are added to the solution [53]. This local toxicity is increased by the anaesthetic interruption of the blinking reflex and pushes to have patient's eyes closed after bilateral instillation. These epithelial side effects can impair visibility during surgery, and are an argument favouring the reduction of eye drops instillation and the adjunct of

intracameral anaesthetic irrigation. A part of this toxicity can last a few days after surgery, slightly affecting vision often in both eyes following bilateral instillation. Some of our patients reported dry eye sensations lasting 8–12 weeks after surgery, that they did not experience following retrobulbar block in the contralateral eye.

1.4.2
Gel Application

Gel formulations of anaesthetic agents have been employed to prolong the contact between the drug and ocular surfaces. A single application of lidocaine 2% gel into the conjunctival sac has been found as effective as repeated eyedrop instillation in providing anaesthesia for cataract surgery [5, 8, 9, 31, 42], with more elevated intraocular drug level [8]. Tetracaine is the other anaesthetic agent that has been employed as gel [85]. Improvements over eyedrop instillations include less burning on application and less corneal dehydration. Lidocaine gel seems to be an efficacious alternative to eye drops instillation, with the advantage of simplicity.

1.4.3
Drug-Soaked Sponges

Sponges soaked with an anaesthetic agent in contact with ocular surfaces to obtain analgesia were proposed in 1995 [15, 70]. Bloomberg and Pellican developed a ring-shaped sponge soaked in anaesthetic, that was left in place for 10 min before surgery and during surgery itself, if no contraindication emerged [15]. Since then similar devices appeared sometimes in literature, employing different anaesthetic agents [46, 67], but they weren't widely used. The advantages of sponges could be a lesser amount of drug in contact with corneal epithelium, although the effects on ocular surface have never been compared to that of eyedrop instillation.

| Summary for the Clinician |

- Intraocular penetration of drugs depends on lipophilicity
- General side-effects are negligible
- Local side effects on ocular surfaces can occur
- Gels and sponges seem to reduce these effects

1.4.4
Intracameral Irrigations

1.4.4.1
Modalities

Intracameral irrigation with anaesthetics as an adjunct to topical anaesthesia was first proposed by Gills et al. [27], and then widely adopted to suppress pain coming from intraocular structures [12, 26, 41]. Currently intracameral irrigations are employed by over 80 % of surgeons adopting topical anaesthesia [47]. The most employed drug is lidocaine at 1 % concentration, probably because of simplicity in preparation. Lidocaine 1 % is mainly prepared at surgery from 4 % solutions by diluting in BSS or BSS plus, with obtained pH of 6.39 and 7.11, respectively [13]. Other drugs tested for intracameral irrigation are bupivacaine [3, 48] and mepiva-

caine [52], that also proved to be effective and safe in published studies.

After being delivered into the anterior chamber, a part of the anaesthetic drug is rapidly absorbed by iris, ciliary body and cornea, while the drug still present in solution is removed by subsequent anterior chamber irrigations, thus limiting tissue exposure [4]. With the commonly used irrigation of 1 % unpreserved lidocaine, anterior chamber levels of the drug are 100 times more elevated than after eye drop application: Behndig and Linden found $341.8\pm151.6\,\mu g/mL$ in their study [11], a study from Wirbelauer et al. [81] gave similar results.

The intraocular irrigation of diluted anaesthetics is usually performed either immediately after the first corneal incision, or at hydrodissection. The first method requires a lower amount of anaesthetic eyedrops, but adds one passage to surgery; the second method looks somewhat simpler, but capsulorhexis has to be performed under topical anaesthesia alone. The intraocular irrigation can be repeated in prolonged or complicated surgeries, because lidocaine is rapidly removed from ocular tissues by irrigating BSS [4]. Every surgeon should check the pH and the osmolarity of injected solutions.

1.4.4.2
Safety

The safety of intracameral irrigations with lidocaine and other anaesthetic agents has been extensively studied starting from the amaurosis encountered in some patients after posterior capsule rupture [33]. Experimental studies on rabbits showed the lack of toxicity of common preparations both for corneal endothelium [37, 38, 40, 79] and for the retina [48]. Reversible cellular swelling could be observed when the concentration was at least 1 % [40], with permanent damage only at 2 % [38]. Clinical and experimental studies on human corneas confirmed these results, at least for lidocaine [21, 25, 40, 43, 54, 55] and mepivacaine [52]. Other compounds, like bupivacaine, seem more toxic [3]. A study on retinal and optic nerve function in patients who received intracameral irrigation by 2 % lidocaine showed no differences in electroretinograms or in visually evoked potentials as compared with controls [64].

Following the sensation of some amaurosis during uncomplicated surgery, Hoh et al. [34] investigated the speed of visual recovery after phacoemulsification with intracameral lidocaine: he found prompt return to normal vision after 4 h.

1.4.5
Viscoelastic-Borne Anaesthesia

Solutions combining ophthalmic viscosurgical devices with lidocaine have recently been developed. The purpose was to avoid the additional step of irrigating the anterior chamber with lidocaine solution, and to prolong anaesthesia time to cover little delays in the completion of surgery. One system is based on methylcellulose [35], while a second system is based on sodium hyaluronate [76]. This system is commercially available in some countries and includes a prepared syringe with viscoanaesthetic mixture and two ampoules of jelly eyedrops to be applied before surgery to minimise corneal epithelial toxicity. Available data collected on experimental settings indicates viscoanaesthesia is safe for corneal endothelium [76], with no evidence of any postoperative reaction after phacoemulsification [50], and no impairment of the mechanical properties of the viscoelastic device [63]. Early clinical data indicates good efficacy [35].

Summary for the Clinician

- Intracameral irrigations with anaesthetics are safe and effective
- Lidocaine 1% unpreserved solution is currently the most employed drug
- Viscoelastic-bound anaesthetic also proved safe and effective

1.5
Preferred Procedures

1.5.1
Patient Selection and Counselling

Topical/intracameral anaesthesia was not appreciated immediately as an universal procedure, but as a procedure requiring patient selection. Grabow [28] was one of the first addressing difficulties in applying topical anaesthesia to some patients, like foreigners and those affected by deafness, dementia and uncontrolled eye movements. In addition, patients unable to cooperate during tonometries or A-scan measurements were not considered good candidates for topical anaesthesia [24]. At present topical and intracameral anaesthesia are considered the standard technique for cataract surgery. Some of the old contraindications remain, but the most part have been overcome by the confidence both of surgeons and of patients.

As patients now expect to be operated under topical anaesthesia, little instructions have to be given before surgery. On the contrary, too much dialogue could increase patient anxiety. We tell patients simply that anaesthesia will be present, but with no needle injection; that anaesthesia can be increased at any time during surgery should they perceive pain; that the lack of burning sensation on eyedrop application is the proof of achieved anaesthesia; and that eye movement will not affect surgery.

1.5.2
Surgery Adaptation

A few adaptations have to be made to adjust cataract surgery for topical anaesthesia. Usually surgeons appreciate the lower posterior vitreous pressure as compared with peribulbar injections, due to the lower pressure in the orbit. However, the corneal surface rapidly dries during surgery, and must be frequently irrigated. The microscope light frequently causes patient discomfort, especially with subcapsular posterior cataracts and in young patients, and sometimes it must be reduced during the first phases of surgery. Toothed forceps are more likely to cause discomfort than notched forceps. Corneal tunnels without conjunctival incisions or diathermy are likely to be better tolerated than scleral incisions. Additional eyedrop instillation after any conjunctival opening and before further manipulation must be considered. The eye can be better stabilised by a second instrument within the side port incision than grasping the sclera. Cataract extraction should be made with phacoemulsification, because the manoeuvres required for manual fragmentation could be more traumatising for the eye. IOL implantation should not stretch the incision, as at that point analgesia is lower than at the beginning of the procedure. The lids must remain free from trauma because they are not anaesthetised, a condition evident on draping removal.

1.5.3
Management of Complications

The short duration of topical and intracameral anaesthesia points out the necessity to repeat instillations and/or irrigations in prolonged surgeries. Even repeated iris touch are painless if sufficient amount of drug is present in the anterior chamber. Topical anaesthesia has not been associated with a higher complication rate in published studies, but complications can nevertheless occur, as with peribulbar anaesthesia, and have to be managed safely and efficiently. Even suprachoroidal haemorrhages have been reported [10]. Posterior capsule rupture and anterior vitrectomy typically cause little or no additional pain. Scleral fixation of the intraocular lens can be achieved with intraocular irrigation of unpreserved lidocaine [12], but profound amaurosis has to be expected. Probably, the only manoeuvres requiring either subconjunctival or peribulbar injection of anaesthetic agents – to block the eye – is a pars plana incision or incisional enlargement to convert to extracapsular extraction.

1.5.4
Postoperative Instructions

One of the advantages of topical anaesthesia is the rapid recovery of sensation. Patients should be aware that ocular burning will be perceived by most of them, but ocular pain should not appear in uncomplicated cases. As most surgery is now performed on an ambulatory basis, operated patients should be instructed to report any unexpected pain, ocular hypertension being the most common cause. Burning sensation and vision impairment can be perceived also in the fellow eye, if the anaesthetic agent was applied bilaterally. Following intraocular anaesthetic irrigation, vision in the operated eye is usually low at the end of surgery, but it takes only a few hours to improve [34].

Summary for the Clinician

- Topical anaesthesia can be adapted to almost all adult patients
- Phacoemulsification procedures require only minor adaptations: non-toothed forceps, no iris touch, no conjunctival touch
- Complications can be managed by repeating anaesthesia administration
- Postoperative pain is not masked by persisting anaesthesia

1.6
Clinical Experience

1.6.1
Topical Anaesthesia

1.6.1.1
Validity of the Procedure

The first clinical reports about the feasibility of phacoemulsification with topical anaesthesia appeared in 1993 [28, 39, 80]. Although preliminary in many aspects, those early works already pointed out the most important features of topical anaesthesia: the efficacy of the obtained analgesia; the possible decrease of corneal transparency during surgery; the steady rate of surgical complications as compared with peribulbar injections; the good acceptance from patients' point of view; the early recovery of vision; the obvious lack of risks typical of needle injections. Since then countless papers on topical anaesthesia appeared, underlining many different aspects of the procedure. Large field studies proved it effective and safe from a population-based perspective [14, 59], other investigations found eyedrop instillation [61] and the placement of the IV cannula [57] as the most painful part of the procedure [58]. Topical anaesthesia has been demonstrated suitable for inexperienced surgeons [57].

Despite this wide demonstration of validity, many variations of the treatment schedule have been proposed to answer local needs and opinions of patients and of surgeons. In some instances topical anaesthesia was augmented by sub-conjunctival or periocular injections [2, 51], mainly reflecting some difficulties in changing surgeon's mentality and in establishing new relations with the patient in the operating room [65, 66].

Not surprisingly, patients were delighted by topical anaesthesia. All the published studies report as anecdotal the preference for needle injections, the most feared part of cataract surgery itself. This preference of topical anaesthesia occurs despite the occasionally reported greater discomfort during surgery and in the postoperative period as compared with peribulbar injections [60]. At present there is a push from patients towards topical anaesthesia, which is now regarded as the standard technique in many countries. This change in mentality will probably further increase success rates and will extend topical anaesthesia to other procedures on the anterior and posterior segment [78, 82].

1.6.1.2
Different Anaesthetics

While many studies have been devoted to investigating the activity of single drugs, comparisons of two topical anaesthetics are scant in the literature. The availability of the new drug ropivacaine stimulated two comparisons with lidocaine [49, 56]. Ropivacaine was tested at 1% concentration, and lidocaine at 4% concentration.

The studies found both drugs effective and safe, with better results for ropivacaine regarding endothelial cell count [56] and need for further drug administration [49].

A comparison of lidocaine 2% gel vs. bupivacaine 0.5% plus benoxinate 1% eyedrops was also performed on a limited number of patients, reporting similar results in relation to analgesic effect. Should these comparisons continue, they will probably confirm that almost all the anaesthetic drugs employed for local anaesthesia can be employed as topical agents in cataract surgery, with some minor differences among them.

1.6.1.3
Sedation

Oral or IV sedation is present in the protocol of many surgeons, especially during transition or when comparison studies were carried out [65, 69, 77, 83]. In other studies sedation was used only in selected cases, demonstrating the feasibility of topical anaesthesia in almost 100% of patients [20]. The current approach to no sedation surgery was opened by studies demonstrating that in peribulbar cases sedation was necessary more for needle anaesthesia delivery than for surgery itself [64, 72], and by studies finding that patients' objective anxiety for the surgical procedure was very low [23]. More recently self-administered sedation during surgery has been studied, comparing patients receiving fentanyl after pressing a button with patients receiving saline [7]. Better comfort both for the patient and for the surgeon was found associated with general sedation in that study. Other surgeons think that sedation diminishes patient co-operation during surgery, and could lead to unwanted ocular movements that could increase surgical difficulties.

1.6.2
Intracameral Anaesthesia

1.6.2.1
Efficacy and Safety

Proposing intracameral irrigation with unpreserved 1% lidocaine, Gills and Koch [26, 41] helped change surgeons' mentality. With intracameral irrigation, intraocular levels of drug are about 100 times the level after topical instillations [11], completely eliminating pain and discomfort coming from intraocular structures. In his study on 1000 subjects, Koch [41] had only four failures. In our study spanning the first 2 years of use [12], we had 14 partial failures (after surgery patients preferred peribulbar injections because of the high intra-operative discomfort perceived with topical anaesthesia) and 11 total failures (peribulbar injection selected by the surgeon before or during surgery) out of 1442 operations, a percentage of 1.7%.

Recent studies continue to underline the safety of intracameral anaesthesia. Heuermann et al. [32] demonstrated that long-term endothelial cell loss was similar to peribulbar: 12.55% vs. 11.11%. Pang et al. [64] showed intracameral anaesthesia to be as safe as topical anaesthesia for the retina, while Roberts and Boytell [68] found no statistical difference in topical anaesthesia as regards systolic blood pressure, pulse rate and oxygen saturation.

1.6.2.2
Topical vs. Topical Plus Intracameral

Although more than 80% of surgeons adopting topical anaesthesia for phacoemulsification also employ intracameral irrigation [47], its necessity in phacoemulsification surgery remains controversial [43]. At first many studies were demonstrating better analgesia and better patient comfort with intracameral irrigations [25, 54, 55], but thereafter other studies failed to confirm the need for intracameral drug delivery, showing no significant relationship between the use of intracameral lidocaine and the intraoperative or postoperative pain scores [33, 64, 68, 75]. In most cases intraocular irrigations probably offer little advantage after proper topical anaesthetic instillation, particularly in uncomplicated cases performed by experienced surgeons. However, also in these circumstances it adds to our surgery the confidence not to cause pain even with sudden or unwanted movements. Intracameral anaesthesia can also increase pupillary dilation.

Based on our review of the literature and clinical experience, it could be an option to keep the in-

tracameral irrigation ready, and to use it only if necessary or in selected cases. With this approach, intraocular irrigation was employed in 22% [52] and in 14% [56] in two published studies.

Summary for the Clinician

- Topical anaesthesia is now the standard for phacoemulsification surgery
- Intracameral anaesthesia could not be required in most uncomplicated cases

1.7
No Anaesthesia Cataract Surgery

After the first experience in India by Argawal et al. [1], some reports of cataract surgery with no anaesthesia has appeared in various countries in recent years [30]. In a prospective randomised study, Pandey et al. [62] found similar pain scores in patients operated under topical BSS, topical lidocaine and topical plus intracameral lidocaine, although surgeon anxiety was increased. The authors conclude that cataract surgery can be performed with no anaesthesia, at least in older patients with lower corneal sensitivity, and probably with some racial differences. Other important features of no anaesthesia cataract surgery are pupil dilation with cycloplegic eyedrops, the use of cold eyedrops and solutions, the low level of microscope lights, the avoidance of forceps, and especially the confidence of the surgeon. At present cataract surgery with no anaesthesia is not growing in popularity among ophthalmic surgeons, but its feasibility could be of interest in very selected cases.

1.8
Current Recommendations

1.8.1
Treatment Schedule

A useful scheme for topical and intracameral anaesthesia for phacoemulsification surgery could be the following (see also Table 1.3):

Table 1.3. Schedule for topical/intracameral anaesthesia for phacoemulsification

1. Base drug	Lidocaina 4% monodose Alfa-Intes, Casoria, Naples Single-dose sterile units 0.5 ml without preservatives
2. Topical instillations	One drop in both eyes every 5 min at times –15, –10, –5 min
3. Intracameral irrigation	1% Lidocaine obtained adding 1.5 ml of BSS to 0.5 ml of the 4% solution (pH 6.4) Approximately 1–1.5 ml used to obtain hydrodissection
4. Topical repeated	In case of conjunctival manipulation
5. Intracameral repeated	In case of prolonged surgery/complications

1. Excessive eyedrop instillation should be avoided, to minimise unwanted effects on ocular surfaces
2. Intracameral irrigation with anaesthetics could be used routinely to achieve standard anaesthesia and to reduce surgeon anxiety
3. Repeated instillations or intracameral irrigations in the case of pain sensation did not cause evidence of problems in some of our patients
4. Pain in the case of conjunctival or scleral manipulation at the end of surgery (e.g. suture apposition) should be expected
5. Patients should be made aware of possible postoperative mild discomfort due to dry eye, lasting up to 8 weeks

1.8.2
Drug Selection

At present, the selection of the preferred anaesthetic drug is probably conditioned by a number of factors that can address or limit surgeon's choice.

1.8.2.1
Tolerance

Ester-bound compounds frequently cause some allergic reactions due to their metabolite para-aminobenzoic acid, proparacaine being a notable exception [36]. Therefore they are not preferred as default drugs in favour of the amide lidocaine.

1.8.2.2
Speed of Action

Ester-bound compounds exert their anaesthetic activity immediately after administration. Therefore they should be preferred when instant analgesic effect is required, as in the case of pain during surgery. The combination of different anaesthetic drugs in the same eyes did not lead to relevant complications in published reports [16, 52]. Amide compounds, especially bupivacaine and ropivacaine, require a longer time to act and therefore they should be administered beginning 10–15 min before surgery. If used intra-operatively, surgery should be stopped for at least 1 min to allow analgesia. For this reason Malecaze et al. [52] used intraocular mepivacaine to control intra-operative pain after topical anaesthesia with bupivacaine eyedrops.

1.8.2.3
Duration of the Effect

Amide compounds have a longer lasting effect than ester compounds. Any of them covers the entire duration of uncomplicated cataract surgery, although bupivacaine and ropivacaine have longer lasting activity.

1.8.2.4
Drug Availability

Sterile vials of the selected unpreserved drug must be available to prepare dilutions for topical and intracameral use. As the most available in the different countries is lidocaine, this is now the standard drug for topical and intracameral anaesthesia in phacoemulsification surgery [12, 47]. Ampoules should be checked for pH both before and after dilution preparation, at least at the beginning of use and at intervals thereafter.

1.9
Conclusions

Topical drug administration is rapidly becoming the preferred method of anaesthesia for phacoemulsification in all countries for reasons of simplicity, safety and cost. Although there are some drawbacks, the advantages by far exceed the disadvantages. In addition to the mentioned efficacy and safety, the saving of complex preoperative evaluations of the general health of patients should be underlined. Intraocular irrigation of unpreserved lidocaine is probably not required in every case, although widely accepted as standard. It has induced many uncertain surgeons to abandon peribulbar injections, and helped reduce the number of instillations and therefore their toxicity for the ocular structures. Intracameral anaesthesia will probably be used for a long time if signs of intraocular side effects do not emerge. The feasibility of intraocular irrigation with anaesthetics is prompting surgeons to perform other types of anterior and posterior segment procedures, such as glaucoma and vitreoretinal surgery, under topical/intracameral anaesthesia. Once again, cataract surgery is leading innovation in ophthalmic surgery.

References

1. Agarwal A, Agarwal A, Agarwal S (2000) No anaesthesia cataract surgery with karate chop technique. In: Agarwal S, Agarwal At, Sachdev MS, Metha KR, Fine IH, Agarwal Am (eds) Phacoemulsification, 2nd edn. Jaypee, New Delhi, Thorofare (NJ), pp 195–203
2. Anderson CJ (1996) Circumferential perilimbal anesthesia. J Cataract Refract Surg 22:1009–1012
3. Anderson NJ, Nath R, Anderson CJ, Edelhauser HF (1999) Comparison of preservative-free bupivacaine vs. lidocaine for intracameral anesthesia: a randomized clinical trial and in vitro analysis. Am J Ophthalmol 127:393–402
4. Anderson NJ, Woods WD, Kim T, Rudnick DE, Edelhauser HF (1999) Intracameral anesthesia: in vitro iris and corneal uptake and washout of 1% lidocaine hydrochloride. Arch Ophthalmol 117:225–232
5. Assia EI, Pras E, Yehezkel M, Rotenstreich Y, Jager-Roshu S (1999) Topical anesthesia using lidocaine gel for cataract surgery. J Cataract Refract Surg 25:635–639
6. Atkinson WS (1948) Local anesthesia in ophthalmology. Am J Ophthalmol 31:1607–1618
7. Aydin ON, Kir E, Ozkan SB, Gursoy F (2002) Patient-controlled analgesia and sedation with fentanyl in phacoemulsification under topical anesthesia. J Cataract Refract Surg 28:1968–1972
8. Bardocci A, Lofoco G, Perdicaro S, Ciucci F, Manna L (2003) Lidocaine 2% gel versus lidocaine 4% unpreserved drops for topical anesthesia in cataract surgery: a randomized controlled trial. Ophthalmology 110:144–149
9. Barequet IS, Soriano ES, Green WR, O'Brien TP (1999) Provision of anesthesia with single application of lidocaine 2% gel. J Cataract Refract Surg 25:626–631
10. Basti S, Hu Dj, Goren MB, Tanna AP (2003) Acute suprachoroidal hemorrhage during clear corneal phacoemulsification using topical and intracameral anesthesia. J Cataract Refract Surg 29:588–591
11. Behndig A, Linden C (1998) Aqueous humor lidocaine concentrations in topical and intracameral anaesthesia. J Cataract Refract Surg 24:1598–1601
12. Bellucci R (2002) Topical anaesthesia for small incision cataract surgery. Dev Ophthalmol 34: 1–12
13. Bellucci R, Morselli S (1998) In defence of topical anaesthesia. 16th Congress of the ESCRS, Nice
14. Bellucci R, Morselli S, Pucci V, Zordan R, Magnolfi G (1999) Intraocular penetration of topical lidocaine. J Cataract Refract Surg 25:643–647
15. Bloomberg LB, Pellican KJ (1995) Topical anesthesia using the Bloomberg SuperNumb anesthetic ring. J Cataract Refract Surg 21:16–20
16. Carino NS, Slomovic AR, Chung F, Marcovich AL (1998) Topical tetracaine versus topical tetracaine plus intracameral lidocaine for cataract surgery. J Cataract Refract Surg 24:1602–1608
17. Carruthers JDA, Sanmugasunderan S, Mills K, Bagaric D (1995) The efficacy of corneal topical anesthesia with 0.5% bupivacaine eyedrops. Can J Ophthalmol 30:264–266
18. Covino BG (1986) Pharmacology of local anaesthetic agents. Br J Anaesth 58:701–716
19. Davis DB, Mandel MR (1986) Posterior peribulbar anesthesia: an alternative to retrobulbar anesthesia. J Cataract Refract Surg 12:182–184

20. Dinsmore SC (1996) Approaching a 100% success rate using topical anesthesia with mild intravenous sedation in phacoemulsification procedures. Ophthalmic Surg Lasers 27:935–938

21. Elvira JC, Hueso JR, Martinez-Toldos J, Mengual E, Artola A (1999) Induced endothelial cell loss in phacoemulsification using topical anesthesia plus intracameral lidocaine. J Cataract Refract Surg 25:640–642

22. Fichman RA (1993) Topical anaesthesia. In: Gills JP, Hustead RF, Sanders DR (eds) Ophthalmic anesthesia. Thorofare, NJ, Slack Inc, pp 166–171

23. Fichman RA (1996) Use of topical anesthesia alone in cataract surgery. J Cataract Refract Surg 22:612–614

24. Fraser SG, Siriwadena D, Jamieson H, Girault J, Bryan SJ (1997) Indicators of patient suitability for topical anesthesia. J Cataract Refract Surg 23:781–783

25. Garcia A, Loureiro F, Limao A, Sampaio AM, Ilharco JF (1998) Preservative-free lidocaine 1% anterior chamber irrigation as an adjunct to topical anesthesia. J Cataract Refract Surg 24:403–406

26. Gills JP, Hustead RF, Sanders DR (1993) Editors' comments. In: Gills JP, Hustead RF, Sanders DR (eds) Ophthalmic anesthesia. Slack, Thorofare, NJ, p 183

27. Gills JP, Cherchio M, Raanan MG (1997) Unpreserved lidocaine to control discomfort during cataract surgery using topical anesthesia. J Cataract Refract Surg 23:545–550

28. Grabow HB (1993) Topical anaesthesia for cataract surgery. Eur J Implant Refract Surg 5:20–24

29. Greenbaum S (1992) Parabulbar anaesthesia. Am J Ophthalmol 114:776

30. Gutierrez-Carmona FJ (2000) Phacoemulsification with cryoanalgesia: a new approach for cataract surgery. In: Agarwal S, Agarwal At, Sachdev MS, Metha KR, Fine IH, Agarwal Am (eds) Phacoemulsification, 2nd edn. Jaypee, New Delhi, Thorofare, pp 226–229

31. Harman DR (2000) Combined sedation and topical anesthesia for cataract surgery. J Cataract Refract Surg 26:109–113

32. Heuermann T, Hartmann C, Anders N (2002) Long-term endothelial cell loss after phacoemulsification: peribulbar anesthesia versus intracameral lidocaine 1%: prospective randomized clinical trial. J Cataract Refract Surg 28:639–643

33. Hoffman RS, Fine IH (1997) Transient no light perception visual acuity after intracameral lidocaine injection. J Cataract Refract Surg 23:957–958

34. Hoh HB, Bourne R, Baer R (1998) Visual recovery after phacoemulsification using topical anesthesia. J Cataract Refract Surg 24:1385–1389

35. Hosny M, Eldin SG, Hosny H (2002) Combined lidocaine 1% and hydroxypropyl methylcellulose 2.25% as a single anesthetic/viscoelastic agent in phacoemulsification. J Cataract Refract Surg 28:834–836

36. Hustead RF, Hamilton RC (1993) Pharmacology. In: Gills JP, Hustead RF, Sanders DR (eds) Ophthalmic anesthesia. Slack, Thorofare, NJ, pp 69–102

37. Judge AJ, Najafi K, Lee DA, Miller KM (1997) Corneal endothelial toxicity of topical anesthesia. Ophthalmology 104:1373–1379

38. Kadonosono K, Ito N, Yazama F, Nishide T, Sugita M, Sawada H, Ohno S (1998) Effect of intracameral anesthesia on corneal endothelium. J Cataract Refract Surg 24:1377–1381

39. Kershner RM (1993) Topical anesthesia for small incision self-sealing surgery; a prospective evaluation of the first 100 patients. J Cataract Refract Surg 19:290–292

40. Kim T, Holley GP, Lee JH, Broocker G, Edelhauser HF (1998) The effects of intraocular lidocaine on the corneal endothelium. Ophthalmology 105:125–130

41. Koch PS (1997) Anterior chamber irrigation with unpreserved lidocaine 1% for anesthesia during cataract surgery. J Cataract Refract Surg 23:551–554

42. Koch PS (1999) Efficacy of lidocaine 2% jelly as a topical agent in cataract surgery. J Cataract Refract Surg 25:632–634

43. Kohnen T (1999) Is intracameral anesthetic application the final solution to topical anesthesia for cataract surgery? J Cataract Refract Surg 25:601–602 (editorial)

44. Koller K (1884) Über die Verwendung des Cocaïn zur Anästhesierung am Auge. Wien Med Wochenschr 43:1309–1311

45. Lagnado R, Tan J, Cole R, Sampath R (2003) Aqueous humor levels of topically applied bupivacaine 0.75% in cataract surgery. J Cataract Refract Surg 29:1767–1770

46. Lanzetta P, Virgili G, Crovato S, Bandello F, Menchini U (2000) Perilimbal topical anesthesia for clear corneal phacoemulsification. J Cataract Refract Surg 26:1642–1646

47. Leaming DV (2002) Practice styles and preferences of ASCRS members – 2001 survey. J Cataract Refract Surg 28:1681–1688

48. Liang C, Peyman GA, Sun G (1998) Toxicity of intraocular lidocaine and bupivacaine. Am J Ophthalmol 125:191–196

49. LoMartire N, Savastano S, Rossini L, Pinchera L, Caracciolo F, Savastano MC, Rossini P, Panariti R, Mondello E, Epifanio A (2002) Topical anesthesia for cataract surgery with phacoemulsification: lidocaine 2% vs ropivacaine 1%. Preliminary results. Minerva Anestesiol 68:529–535

50. Macky TA, Werner L Apple DJ, Izak AM, Pandey SK, Trivedi RH (2003) Viscoanesthesia. 2. Toxicity to intraocular structures after phacoemulsification in a rabbit model. J Cataract Refract Surg 29:556–562

51. Maclean H, Burton T, Murray A (1997) Patient comfort during cataract surgery with modified topical and peribulbar anesthesia. J Cataract Refract Surg 23:277–283

52. Malecaze FA, Deneuville SF, Julia BJ, Daurin JG, Chapotot EM, Grandjean HMC, Arnè JL, Rascol O (2000) Pain relief with intracameral mepivacaine during phacoemulsification. Br J Ophthalmol 84:171–174

53. Marr MG, Wood R, Senterfit L, Sigelman S (1957) Effect of topical anesthetics on regeneration of corneal epithelium. Am J Ophthalmol 43:606–610

54. Martin RG, Miller JD, Cox CC, Ferrel SC, Raanan MG (1998) Safety and efficacy of intracameral injections of unpreserved lidocaine to reduce intraocular sensation. J Cataract Refract Surg 24:961–963

55. Martini E, Cavallini GM, Campi L, Lugli N, Neri G, Molinari P (2002) Lidocaine versus ropivacaine for topical anesthesia in cataract surgery. J Cataract Refract Surg 28:1018–1022

56. Masket S, Gokmen F (1998) Efficacy and safety of intracameral lidocaine as a supplement to topical anesthesia. J Cataract Refract Surg 24:956–960

57. Mathew MR, Webb LA, Hill R (2002) Surgeon experience and patient comfort during clear corneal phacoemulsification under topical local anesthesia. J Cataract Refract Surg 28:1977–1981

58. Mathew MR, Williams A, Esakowitz L, Webb LA, Murray SB, Bennett HG (2003) Patient comfort during clear corneal phacoemulsification with sub-Tenon's local anesthesia. J Cataract Refract Surg 29:1132–1136

59. Monestam E, Kuusik E, Wachtmeister L (2001) Topical anesthesia for cataract surgery: a population-based perspective. J Cataract Refract Surg 27:445–451

60. Nielsen PJ, Allerød CW (1998) Evaluation of local anesthesia techniques for small incision cataract surgery. J Cataract Refract Surg 24:1136–1144

61. O Brien PD, Fulcher T, Wallace D, Power P (2001) Patient pain during different stages of phacoemulsification using topical anesthesia. J Cataract Refract Surg 27:880–883

62. Pandey SK, Werner L, Apple DJ, Agarwal A, Agarwal A, Agarwal S (2001) No-anesthesia clear corneal phacoemulsification versus topical and topical plus intracameral anesthesia. Randomized clinical trial. J Cataract Refract Surg 27: 1643–1650

63. Pandey SK, Werner L, Apple DJ, Izak AM, Trivedi RH, Macky TA (2003) Viscoanesthesia. 3. Removal time of OVD/viscoanesthetic solutions from the capsular bag of postmortem human eyes. J Cataract Refract Surg 29:563–567

64. Pang MP, Fujimoto DK Wilkens LR (2001) Pain, photophobia, and retinal and optic nerve function after phacoemulsification with intracameral lidocaine. Ophthalmology 108:2018–2025

65. Patel BCK, Burns TA, Crandall A, Shomaker ST, Pace NL, van Eerd A, Clinch T (1996) A comparison of topical and retrobulbar anesthesia for cataract surgery. Ophthalmology 103:1196–1203

66. Patel BCK, Clinch TE, Burns TA, Shomaker ST, Jessen R, Crandall AS (1998) Prospective evaluation of topical versus retrobulbar anesthesia: a converting surgeon's experience. J Cataract Refract Surg 24:853–860

67. Pham DT, Scherer V, Wollensak J (1996) Superficial sponge anesthesia in cataract surgery (with scleral tunnel incision). Klin Monatsbl Augenheilkd 209:347–353

68. Roberts T, Boytell K (2002) A comparison of cataract surgery under topical anaesthesia with and without intracameral lignocaine. Clin Experiment Ophthalmol 30:19–22

69. Roman S, Auclin F, Ullern M (1996) Topical versus peribulbar anaesthesia in cataract surgery. J Cataract Refract Surg 22:1121–1124

70. Rosenthal K (1995) Deep, topical, nerve-block anesthesia. J Cataract Refract Surg 21:499–503

71. Salomon F, Körprich R, Biscoping J, Bitterich A, Hempelmann G (1986) Plasmaspiegel von Lokalanesthetika nach örtlicher Betäubung am Auge. Fortschr Ophthalmol 83:335–337

72. Shammas HJ, Milkie M, Yeo R (1997) Topical and subconjunctival anesthesia for phacoemulsification: prospective study. J Cataract Refract Surg 23:1577–1580

73. Smith R (1990) Cataract extraction without retrobulbar injection. Br J Ophthalmol 74:205–207

74. Sun R, Hamilton RC, Gimbel HV (1999) Comparison of 4 topical anesthetic agents for effect and corneal toxicity in rabbits. J Cataract Refract Surg 25:1232–1236

75. Tan JHY, Burton RL (2000) Does preservative-free lignocaine 1% for hydrodissection reduce pain during phacoemulsification? J Cataract Refract Surg 26:733–735

76. Trivedi RH, Werner L, Apple DJ, Izak AM, Pandey SK, Macky TA (2003) Viscoanesthesia. 1. Toxicity to corneal endothelial cells in a rabbit model. J Cataract Refract Surg 29:550–555

77. Uusitalo RJ, Manuksela EL, Paloheimo M, Kallio H, Laatikainen L (1999) Converting to topical anesthesia in cataract surgery. J Cataract Refract Surg 25:432–440

78. Vicary D, McLennan S, Sun XY (1998) Topical plus subconjunctival anaesthesia for phacotrabeculectomy: one year follow-up. J Cataract Refract Surg 24:1247–1251

79. Werner LP, Legeais JM, Obsler C, Durand J, Renard G (1998) Toxicity of Xylocaine to rabbit corneal endothelium. J Cataract Refract Surg 24:1371–1376

80. Williamson CH (1993) Clear corneal incision with topical anesthesia. In: Gills JP, Hustead RF, Sanders DR (eds) Ophthalmic anesthesia. Slack, Thorofare, NJ, pp 176–186

81. Wirbelauer C, Iven H, Bastian C, Laqua H (1999) Systemic levels of lidocaine after intracameral injection during cataract surgery. J Cataract Refract Surg 25:648–651

82. Yepez J, Cedeno de Yepez J, Arevalo JF (1999) Topical anesthesia for phacoemulsification, intraocular lens implantation, and posterior vitrectomy. J Cataract Refract Surg 25:1161–1164

83. Zehetmayer M, Radax U, Skorpik C, Menapace R, Schemper M, Weghaupt H, Scholz U (1996) Topical versus peribulbar anesthesia in clear cornea cataract surgery. J Cataract Refract Surg 22:480–484

84. Zehetmayer M, Rainer G, Turnheim K, Skorpik C, Menapace R (1997) Topical anesthesia with pH-adjusted versus standard lidocaine 4% for clear cornea cataract surgery. J Cataract Refract Surg 23:1390–1393

85. Zink T, Babl J, Kampik A, Schönfeld CL (2003) Oberflächenanästhesie mit Tetracain 1%: Tropfen – Gel. CI Congress Deutsche Ophthalmologische Gesellschaft, Berlin

Core Messages

- An incremental yet inexorable reduction in incision size and related morbidity has marked the recent history of cataract surgery
- Continuous curvilinear capsulorhexis has improved stability and centration of intraocular lenses, helped to reduce posterior capsular opacification and spurred the development of endolenticular nucleofractics techniques
- Cortical cleaving hydrodissection has reduced the need for irrigation and aspiration of cortical material and the rate of posterior capsular opacification
- Chop techniques substitute mechanical forces for ultrasound energy to disassemble the nucleus, utilize high vacuum as an extractive technique to remove nuclear material and facilitate the achievement of minimally invasive surgery and rapid visual rehabilitation
- The promise of bimanual, ultra-small incision cataract surgery and companion IOL technology is today becoming a reality, through both laser and new ultrasound power modulations

2.1
Introduction

Phacoemulsification (phaco) means disassembly and removal of the crystalline lens. From its introduction in the late 1960s to the present, phaco has evolved into a highly effective method of cataract extraction. Incremental advances in surgical technique and the simultaneous redesign and modification of technology have permitted increasing safety and efficiency.

Among the advances that have shaped modern phaco are incision construction, continuous curvilinear capsulorhexis, cortical cleaving hydrodissection, hydrodelineation, and nucleofractis techniques. The refinement of cataract removal through a small incision has improved phaco and permitted rapid visual rehabilitation and excellent ocular structural stability. Perhaps the most outstanding characteristic of this era of phaco is the unrelenting quest for excellence that continues to challenge the innovative spirit of cataract surgeons.

2.2
Wound Construction and Architecture

The availability of foldable intraocular lenses which can be inserted through small unsutured phacoemulsification incisions [13] has created a trend away from scleral tunnel incisions to clear corneal incisions [41]. Among the disadvantages of scleral tunnels are the need to perform conjunctival incisions and scleral dissections, and the need for cautery to prevent operating in the presence of blood. In addition, there is increased difficulty with oarlocking of the phaco tip and distortion of the cornea because of the length of scleral tunnels.

Kratz is generally credited as the first surgeon to move from the limbus posteriorly to the sclera in order to increase appositional surfaces, thus enhancing wound healing and reducing surgically induced astigmatism [8, 43]. Girard and Hoffman were the first to name the posterior incision a "scleral tunnel incision" and were, along with Kratz, the first to make a point of entering the anterior chamber through the cornea, creating a corneal shelf [32]. This corneal shelf was designed to prevent iris prolapse. In 1989, McFarland used this incision architecture and recognized that these incisions allowed for the phacoemulsification and implantation of lenses without the need for suturing [44]. Maloney, who was a fellow of Kratz', advocated a corneal shelf to his incisions which he described as strong and waterproof [42]. Ernest recognized that McFarland's long scleral tunnel incision terminated in a decidedly corneal entrance. He hypothesized that the posterior "corneal lip" of the incision acted as a one-way valve thus explaining the mechanism for self sealability (as postulated by Ernest in a presentation to the Department of Ophthalmology, Wayne State University School of Medicine, Detroit, MI, on February 28, 1990). In April of 1992, Fine presented his self-sealing temporal clear corneal incision at the annual meeting of the American Society of Cataract and Refractive Surgery [5].

There have been surgeons who have favoured corneal incisions for cataract surgery prior to their recent popularization. In 1968, Charles Kelman stated that the best approach for performing cataract surgery was with phacoemulsification through a clear corneal incision utilizing a triangular-tear capsulotomy and a grooving and cracking technique in the posterior chamber [37]. Harms and Mackenson in Germany published an intracapsular technique using a corneal incision in 1967 [33]. Troutman was an early advocate of controlling surgically induced astigmatism at the time of cataract surgery by means of the corneal incision approach [12]. Arnott in England utilized clear corneal incisions and a diamond keratome for phacoemulsification although he had to enlarge the incision for introducing an IOL [4]. Galand in Belgium utilized clear corneal incisions for extracapsular cataract extraction in his envelope technique [24] and Stegman of South Africa has a long history of having utilized the cornea as the site for incisions for extracapsular cataract extraction (R. Stegmann, personal communication, December 3, 1992). Finally, perhaps the leading proponent of clear corneal incisions for modern era phacoemulsification was Kimiya Shimizu of Japan [53].

In 1992, Fine began routinely utilizing clear corneal cataract incisions with closure by a tangential suture modelled after Shepherd's technique [51]. Within a very short period, the suture was abandoned in favour of self-sealing corneal incisions [17]. Through the demonstrated safety and increased utilization of these incisions by pioneers in the United States, including Williamson, Shepherd, Martin, and Grabow [61], these incisions became increasingly popular and utilized on an international basis.

Rosen demonstrated by topographical analysis that clear corneal incisions of 3 mm or less in width do not induce astigmatism [49]. This finding led to increasing interest because of better predictability of T-cuts, arcuate cuts, and limbal relaxing incisions for managing pre-existing astigmatism at the time of cataract surgery. Surgeons recognized many other advantages of the temporal clear corneal incision, including better preservation of pre-existing filtering blebs [47] and options for future filtering surgery, increased stability of refractive results because of decreased effects from lid blink and gravity, ease of approach, elimination of the bridle suture and iatrogenic ptosis, and improved drainage from the surgical field via the lateral canthal angle.

Single plane incisions, as first described by Fine [15], utilized a 3.0-mm diamond knife. After pressurizing the eye with viscoelastic through a paracentesis, the surgeon placed the blade on the eye so that it completely applanated the eye with the point of the blade positioned at the leading edge of the anterior vascular arcade. The knife was advanced in the plane of the cornea until the shoulders, 2 mm posterior to the point of the knife, touched the external edge of the incision. Then the point of the blade was directed posteriorly to initiate the cut through

Descemet's membrane in a manoeuvre known as the dimple-down technique. After the tip entered the anterior chamber, the initial plane of the incision was re-established to cut through Descemet's in a straight-line configuration.

Williamson was the first to utilize a shallow 300–400 µm grooved clear corneal incision [21]. He believed that the thicker external edge to the roof of the tunnel reduced the likelihood of tearing. Langerman later described the single hinge incision, in which the initial groove measured 90% of the depth of the cornea anterior to the edge of the conjunctiva [40]. Initially he utilized a depth of 600 µm and subsequently made the tunnel itself superficially in that groove, believing that this led to enhanced resistance of the incision to external deformation.

Surgeons employed adjunctive techniques to combine incisional keratorefractive surgery with clear corneal cataract incisions. Fine used the temporal location for the cataract incision and added one or two T-cuts made by the Feaster Knife with a 7-mm ocular zone for the management of pre-existing astigmatism. Others, including Lindstrom and Rosen, rotated the location of the incision to the steep axis. Kershner used the temporal incision by starting with a nearly full thickness T-cut through which he then made his corneal tunnel incision. For large amounts of astigmatism he used a paired T-cut in the opposite side of the same meridian [38]. Finally, the popularization of limbal relaxing incisions by Gills [25] and Nichamin [46], added an additional means of reducing pre existing astigmatism.

The 3-D Blade (Rhein Medical, Tampa, FL) improved incision construction with differentially sloped bevels on its anterior and posterior surfaces. This design allowed the surgeon to touch the eye at the site of the external incision location and advance the blade in the plane of the cornea without dimpling down. The differential slopes allowed the forces of tissue resistance to create an incision characterized by a linear external incision, a 2-mm tunnel, and a linear internal incision [18]. The trapezoidal 3-D Blade also allowed enlargement of the incision up to 3.5 mm for IOL insertion without altering incision architecture.

Following phacoemulsification, lens implantation, and removal of residual viscoelastic, stromal hydration of the clear corneal incision can be performed in order to help seal the incision [16]. Stromal hydration is performed by gently irrigating balanced salt solution into the stroma at both edges of the incision with a 26- or 27-gauge cannula. Once apposition takes place, the hydrostatic forces of the endothelial pump help seal the incision. In those rare instances of questionable wound integrity, a single 10–0 nylon or Vicryl suture is placed to ensure a tight seal.

Clear corneal incisions, by nature of their architecture and location, have some unique complications associated with them. If one incidentally incises the conjunctiva at the time of the clear corneal incision, ballooning of the conjunctiva can develop which may compromise visualization of anterior structures. In this case, a suction catheter may be used to aid exposure. Early entry into the anterior chamber may result in an incision of insufficient length to be self-sealing. In addition, incisions that are too short or improperly constructed can result in an increased tendency for iris prolapse. A single suture may be required in order to assure a secure wound at the conclusion of the procedure. On the other hand, a late entry may result in a corneal tunnel so long that the phaco tip creates striae in the cornea and compromises the view of the anterior chamber.

Manipulation of the phacoemulsification handpiece intraoperatively may result in tearing of the roof of the tunnel, especially at the edges, resulting in compromise of the incision's self-sealability. Tearing of the internal lip can also occur, resulting in compromised self-sealability or, rarely, small detachments or scrolling of Descemet's membrane in the anterior edge of the incision.

Of greater concern has been the potential for incisional burns [19]. When incisional burns develop in clear corneal incisions there may be a loss of self-sealability. Closure of the wound may induce excessive amounts of astigmatism. In addition, manipulation of the incision can result in an epithelial abrasion, which can compromise self-sealability because of the lack of a fluid barrier by an intact epithelium. Without an intact epithelial layer, the corneal endothelium does not have the ability to help appose the roof and floor of the incision through hydrostatic forces.

In a large survey performed for the American Society of Cataract and Refractive Surgery by Masket [56] there was a slightly increased incidence of endophthalmitis in clear corneal cataract surgery compared to scleral tunnel surgery. However, the survey failed to note the incision sizes in those cases where endophthalmitis in clear corneal incisions had occurred. Masket described several generally accepted techniques of prophylaxis, including preoperative topical antibiotics, 5% povidone-iodine prep and draped eyelashes

Colleaux and Hamilton [7] found no significant difference in the rate of endophthalmitis with respect to clear corneal versus scleral tunnel incisions in a retrospective review of 13,886 consecutive cataract operations. They reported a significant prophylactic effect of subconjunctival antibiotic injection, but found no benefit to preoperative antibiotic drops. In an evidence-based update, Ciulla, Starr and Masket found that current literature most strongly supports the use of preoperative povidone-iodine antisepsis [6]. They found little change in the risk of endophthalmitis in the United States over time, from 0.12% in 1984 to 0.13% in 1994.

Clear corneal cataract incisions are becoming a more popular option for cataract extraction and intraocular lens implantation throughout the world. With clear corneal incisions we have achieved minimally invasive surgery with immediate visual rehabilitation. Clear corneal incisions have had a proven record of safety with relative astigmatic neutrality. In addition, clear corneal incisions result in an excellent cosmetic outcome. We expect that they will continue to increase in popularity, especially as newer modalities, such as non-thermal bimanual phaco, become the standard of care.

Summary for the Clinician

- Increased operating efficiency, improved control of astigmatism and foldable intraocular lens technology have led to increasing utilization of self-sealing, clear corneal incisions for cataract surgery

- Pre-existing corneal astigmatism may be effectively treated at the time of cataract surgery by means of incisional keratorefractive techniques
- Successful clear corneal incisions require attention to detail in order to avoid unique complications associated with them

2.3
Continuous Curvilinear Capsulorhexis

Implantation of the IOL in an intact capsular bag facilitates the permanent rehabilitative benefit of cataract surgery. For many years, surgeons considered a "can-opener" capsulotomy satisfactory for both planned extracapsular cataract extraction and phaco. Problems related to malposition and decentration of implanted posterior chamber IOLs were later recognized. In 1991, Wasserman and associates [59] performed a postmortem study that showed that the extension of one or more V-shaped tears towards the equator of the capsule produced instability of the IOL and resulted in IOL malposition.

We are fortunate to have benefited from the work of Calvin Fercho, who developed continuous tear capsulotomy (as presented in "Continuous circular tear anterior capsulotomy," Welsh Cataract Congress, on 9th September, 1986) and Gimbel and Neuhann, who popularized continuous curvilinear capsulorhexis (CCC) [28, 29, 45].

The technique of CCC is not difficult to learn if certain basic principles are observed:
1. The continuous capsular tear should be performed in a deep, stable anterior chamber. We advocate using a viscoelastic substance that deepens the anterior chamber and stretches the anterior capsule. The use of a viscoelastic material accomplishes two important goals:
   a) It creates space for safe instrumentation in the anterior chamber
   b) By making the anterior capsule taut and pushing the lens posteriorly it resists the action of posterior pressure, which tends to cause the capsular tear to move peripherally

2. The tear is started at the centre of the capsule. This way the origin of the tear is included within the termination of the tear. Starting in the centre of the capsule generates a flap with a peripheral edge that is smooth and continuous

3. Once the initial flap is mobilized, it is inverted to permit a smooth tearing action, such as would be achieved in tearing a piece of paper with one half held stable while the inverted half is torn to the desired configuration. This principle is the same whether a cystotome/bent needle or forceps is used to create the capsulotomy

4. The continuous tear proceeds either clockwise or counter-clockwise in a controlled and deliberate fashion, the surgeon regrasping with the forceps or repositioning the point of the cystotome/bent needle on the inverted flap to control the vector of the tear. Upon completion of the CCC, it is essential that the origin of the peripheral portion of the CCC be included within the circumference of the tear

As we have indicated, it is essential to control the course of the capsular tear. A tear that begins moving peripherally or in a radial fashion is a signal that a condition exists that requires immediate attention. The first thing the surgeon must do is to recognize the situation. Further progress of the tear should be stopped and the depth of the anterior chamber assessed. Frequently the cause of the peripheral course of the tear is shallowing of the anterior chamber and the effect of posterior pressure on the lens and anterior capsule. Adding more viscoelastic to deepen the anterior chamber opposes the posterior pressure, makes the lens capsule taut, widens the pupil, and permits inspection of the capsule to see whether zonular extension onto the anterior capsule is responsible for the misdirection of the tear. Generally, the tear can be redirected and continued.

If the tear has extended peripherally and cannot be safely redirected, one option is to create a small tangential incision at the origin of the CCC with Vannas scissors and to direct the tear in the opposite direction to include the peripheral extension. If this manoeuvre cannot be

accomplished and the discontinuity in the CCC remains, it is probably wisest to make several other small incisions in the capsular rim so that the peripheral force is distributed evenly, reducing the likelihood that a tear will extend around the lens equator.

A similar situation may occur upon completion of the CCC. Again, at this point it is essential that the origin of the peripheral portion of the CCC be included within the circumference of the tear. If this manoeuvre is performed correctly, it will result in a totally blended edge or it will form a small centripetally peaked area (cardioid). If the end of the CCC results in a V-shaped *centrifugally* oriented peak, however, this peak acts as a discontinuity in the anterior capsular opening and may extend peripherally, with the attendant consequences mentioned above. The surgeon must convert this area to a smooth tear by either regrasping an edge to include the V-shaped tear or by making a small incision with a Vannas scissors to create a segmental secondary CCC.

The use of a vital dye to stain the anterior capsule in the absence of a good red reflex constitutes an important adjunctive technique for capsulorhexis construction. The surgeon makes the sideport incision and then fills the anterior chamber with air. The dye, either indocyanine green or trypan blue, is injected into the chamber. The air and residual dye is then exchanged for viscoelastic. Despite the absence of a red reflex the capsule is now easy to see.

The technique of CCC has provided important advantages both for cataract surgery and IOL implantation. Because endolenticular or in situ phaco must be performed in the presence of an intact continuous capsulotomy opening, the capsulorhexis has also served as a stimulus for modification of phaco techniques.

Summary for the Clinician

- Critical elements of technique for the construction of continuous curvilinear capsulorhexis include operating in a deep and stable chamber, initiating the tear in the centre of the capsule and regrasping the flap to maintain control of the vector of the tear at all times

- The use of vital dyes has extended the application of continuous curvilinear capsulorhexis to cases with a reduced or absent red reflex

2.4
Hydrodissection and Hydrodelineation

Hydrodissection of the nucleus in cataract surgery has traditionally been perceived as the injection of fluid into the cortical layer of the lens under the lens capsule to separate the lens nucleus from the cortex and capsule [48]. With increased use of continuous curvilinear capsulorhexis and phacoemulsification in cataract surgery, hydrodissection became a very important step to mobilize the nucleus within the capsule for disassembly and removal [10, 14, 26, 52]. Following nuclear removal, cortical cleanup proceeded as a separate step, using an irrigation and aspiration handpiece.

Fine first described cortical cleaving hydrodissection, which is a hydrodissection technique designed to cleave the cortex from the lens capsule and thus leave the cortex attached to the epinucleus [17]. Cortical cleaving hydrodissection usually eliminates the need for cortical cleanup as a separate step in cataract surgery, thereby eliminating the risk of capsular rupture during cortical cleanup.

2.4.1
Cortical Cleaving Hydrodissection

A small capsulorhexis, of 5–5.5 mm, optimizes the procedure. The large anterior capsular flap makes this type of hydrodissection easier to perform. The anterior capsular flap is elevated away from the cortical material with a 26-gauge blunt cannula (e.g. Katena Instruments No. K7–5150) prior to hydrodissection. The cannula maintains the anterior capsule in a tented-up position at the injection site near the lens equator. Irrigation prior to elevation of the anterior capsule should be avoided because it will result in transmission of a fluid wave circumferentially within the cortical layer, hydrating the cortex and creating a path of least resistance that will

disallow later cortical cleaving hydrodissection. Once the cannula is properly placed and the anterior capsule is elevated, gentle, continuous irrigation results in a fluid wave that passes circumferentially in the zone just under the capsule, cleaving the cortex from the posterior capsule in most locations. When the fluid wave has passed around the posterior aspect of the lens, the entire lens bulges forward because the fluid is trapped by the firm equatorial cortical-capsular connections. The procedure creates, in effect, a temporary intraoperative version of capsular block syndrome as seen by enlargement of the diameter of the capsulorhexis. At this point, if fluid injection is continued, a portion of the lens prolapses through the capsulorhexis. However, if prior to prolapse the capsule is decompressed by depressing the central portion of the lens with the side of the cannula in a way that forces fluid to come around the lens equator from behind, the cortical-capsular connections in the capsular fornix and under the anterior capsular flap are cleaved. The cleavage of cortex from the capsule equatorially and anteriorly allows fluid to exit from the capsular bag via the capsulorhexis, which constricts to its original size, and mobilizes the lens in such a way that it can spin freely within the capsular bag. Repeating the hydrodissection and capsular decompression starting in the opposite distal quadrant may be helpful. Adequate hydrodissection at this point is demonstrable by the ease with which the nuclear-cortical complex can be rotated by the cannula.

2.4.2
Hydrodelineation

Hydrodelineation is a term first used by Anis to describe the act of separating an outer epinuclear shell or multiple shells from the central compact mass of inner nuclear material, the endonucleus, by the forceful irrigation of fluid (balanced salt solution) into the mass of the nucleus [3].

The 26-gauge cannula is placed in the nucleus, off centre to either side, and directed at an angle downward and forward towards the central plane of the nucleus. When the nucleus starts to move, the endonucleus has been rea-ched. It is not penetrated by the cannula. At this point, the cannula is directed tangentially to the endonucleus, and a to-and-fro movement of the cannula is used to create a tract within the nucleus. The cannula is backed out of the tract approximately halfway, and a gentle but steady pressure on the syringe allows fluid to enter the distal tract without resistance. Driven by the hydraulic force of the syringe, the fluid will find the path of least resistance, which is the junction between the endonucleus and the epinucleus, and flow circumferentially in this contour. Most frequently, a circumferential golden ring will be seen outlining the cleavage between the epinucleus and the endonucleus. Sometimes the ring will appear as a dark circle rather than a golden ring.

Occasionally, an arc will result and surround approximately one quadrant of the endonucleus. In this instance, creating another tract the same depth as the first but ending at one end of the arc, and injecting into the middle of the second tract, will extend that arc (usually another full quadrant). This procedure can be repeated until a golden or dark ring verifies circumferential division of the nucleus.

For very soft nuclei, the placement of the cannula allows creation of an epinuclear shell of any thickness. The cannula may pass through the entire nucleus if it is soft enough, so the placement of the tract and the location of the injection allow an epinuclear shell to be fashioned as desired. In very firm nuclei, one appears to be injecting into the cortex on the anterior surface of the nucleus, and the golden ring will not be seen. However, a thin, hard epinuclear shell is achieved even in the most brunescent nuclei. That shell will offer the same protection as a thicker epinucleus in a softer cataract.

Hydrodelineation circumferentially divides the nucleus and has many advantages. Circumferential division reduces the volume of the central portion of nucleus removed by phacoemulsification by up to 50 %. This allows less deep and less peripheral grooving and smaller, more easily mobilized quadrants after cracking or chopping. The epinucleus acts as a protective cushion within which all of the chopping, cracking and phacoemulsification forces can be confined. In addition, the epinucleus keeps the bag on stretch throughout the procedure, making it unlikely that a knuckle of capsule will come forward, occlude the phaco tip, and rupture.

Summary for the Clinician

- Critical steps of cortical cleaving hydrodissection include injection of balanced salt solution under the anterior capsule such that a fluid wave traverses the posterior aspect of the lens and decompression of the capsule by depression of the central portion of the lens
- Hydrodelineation means separation of the epinucleus from the endonucleus in order to allow the epinucleus to serve as a protective cushion during manipulation and extraction of the endonucleus

2.5
Nucleofractis Techniques

The evolution of phaco from the initial procedure as described by Kelman [10] in the late 1960s to the techniques that we currently practice is nothing less than remarkable. The contributions of talented ophthalmic surgeons who persevered throughout these years should be commended, since they laid the groundwork for our present methods.

The major distinction between the phaco techniques practised today and the earlier techniques is that modern methods have facilitated phaco of dense cataracts within the capsular bag, allowing the central endonucleus to be removed before the epinucleus is encountered. With previous techniques, we worked from the peripheral portion of the epinucleus/nucleus complex toward the centre. This change was influenced by the recognition that the nuclear mass of firm and hard lenses could be divided into smaller pieces for controlled removal within the protective layer of the epinucleus and that a capsular opening produced by a CCC would withstand the forces involved in nuclear cracking. Retention of an intact CCC opening also required sequential microsurgical removal of the contents of the capsular bag, best achieved by performing phaco in the central and deepest portion of the anterior chamber.

2.5.1
Divide and Conquer Technique

Divide and conquer nucleofractis phaco, described by Gimbel [26], was the first nucleofractis (two-instrument) cracking technique developed. After adequate hydrodissection, a deep crater is sculpted into the centre of the nucleus, leaving a dense peripheral rim that can later be fractured into multiple sections. It is important that the crater include the posterior plate of the nucleus; otherwise, fracturing of the rim will be much more difficult. A shaving action is used to sculpt away the central nuclear material. When the central material is no longer accessible to the phaco probe, the lens should be rotated and additional central phaco performed to enlarge and deepen the crater. The size of the central crater should be expanded for progressively denser nuclei. Enough of the dense material must be left in place, however, to allow the phaco probe and second instrument to engage the rim and fracture the lens into sections.

The surgeon uses his experience as a guide to determine how deeply the central crater should be sculpted. The peripheral nuclear rim stretches the entire capsular bag and acts as a safety mechanism to prevent the posterior capsule from suddenly moving anteriorly and being cut by the phaco probe. For harder nuclei, small sections should be fractured from the rim. Rather than emulsify the sections as they are broken away, the sections should be left in place within the rim to maintain the circular rim and the tension on the capsule. Leaving the sections in place also facilitates rotation and the progressive fracturing of the remaining rim. It is sometimes advisable to initially remove one small section to allow space for fracturing of the other segments of the remaining rim. If only a small fragment is removed, the remaining segments can maintain capsular stretch and help to avoid rupture of the capsule. After the rim is fractured around the entirety of its circumference, each segment can then be brought to the centre of the capsule for safe emulsification. One must be more cautious at this point because as more segments are removed, less lens material is available to expand the capsule and the capsule will have a greater tendency to be aspirated into the phaco tip, especially if high aspiration flow rates are used.

2.5.2
Phaco Fracture Technique

In phaco fracture, a widely used nucleofractis technique described by Shepherd [53], the surgeon sculpts a groove from the 12- to 6-o'clock position after performing hydrodissection and hydrodelineation. The width of the groove should be one and a half to two times the diameter of the phaco tip. Using the phaco handpiece and a second instrument, the surgeon rotates the nucleus 90°. A second groove is sculpted perpendicular to the first, in the form of a cross. Sculpting continues until the red reflex is seen at the bottom of the grooves. Additional rotations and removal of nuclear material is often necessary to accomplish adequate grooving. Care should be taken to avoid sculpting completely through to the cortex peripherally, since this puts the equatorial and posterior capsule at increased risk of damage. A bimanual cracking technique is used to create a fracture through the nuclear rim in the plane of one of the grooves. The nucleus is then rotated 90°, and additional fractures are made until four separate quadrants are isolated. The segments are then tumbled toward the centre of the capsule for safe emulsification. A short burst of phaco power is used to embed the phaco tip into the bulk of the isolated quadrant, and then with the use of aspiration, the quadrant is gently pulled into the centre for emulsification. Alternatively, the second instrument can be used to elevate the apex of the wedge to facilitate mobilization of the nuclear quadrant to the capsule's centre.

2.5.3
Chip and Flip Technique

Introduced by Fine [14] and useful for softer grades of nuclei, this procedure relies on a nucleus that rotates freely within the capsular bag. Initially a central bowl is sculpted in the nucleus until a thin central plate remains. The second instrument introduced through the side port incision engages the subincisional nuclear rim to move the inferior nuclear rim to toward the centre of the capsule bag. Then clock-hour pieces of the rim are carefully emulsified as the nucleus is rotated. Once the entire rim is removed, the second instrument is used to elevate the remaining central thinned nuclear plate (the chip), which is then emulsified. The epinucleus is engaged at the 6-o'clock position with aspiration alone. As the phaco tip is moved superiorly, the second instrument pushes the epinucleus toward the 6-o'clock position, thereby tumbling the epinuclear bowl and permitting it to be aspirated (the flip).

2.5.4
Crack and Flip Technique

Fine and colleagues modified Shepherd's phaco fracture technique by adding hydrodelineation, resulting in the crack and flip technique [22]. Sculpting two deep grooves at right angles to each other that extend to the golden ring permits bimanual nucleus cracking. Only the endonucleus cracks, since the epinucleus is separated from it by hydro-delineation. Each quadrant is then sequentially removed with the use of pulsed phaco and moderate aspiration. The second instrument elevates the apices of each quadrant so that the tip of the phaco needle can be totally occluded to aid in aspiration. Once the nucleus is removed, the epinucleus is aspirated as with the chip and flip technique.

There are several helpful tips in using the crack and flip technique or a modification of this method. The sculpting portion of the procedure is performed with minimal vacuum, relatively low aspiration flow, and low phaco power. The forward passes of the phaco needle only shave the nuclear material to ultimately sculpt a groove. The phaco tip is never totally occluded during this phase of the operation. Rather, only a portion of the phaco needle contacts the nucleus to remove controlled amounts of lens material. This process is continued until the grooves are deep. The appropriate depth can be assessed by a brightening of the red reflex, which suggests that the denser portion of the nucleus has been emulsified on the region of the grooves.

To achieve nuclear cracking, two instruments are placed deeply in the grooves and moved down and outward. The phaco needle and a second instrument introduced through the side port, paracentesis, or incision will crack the nucleus if the grooves are sufficiently deep and the instruments placed in the depth of the grooves. If cracking does not readily occur, additional deepening of the grooves is warranted. Phaco energy is not required during this step. The limit of the grooves is the golden ring, which represents the perimeter of the endonucleus. The loosened quadrants of the endonucleus remain within the cushion of the surrounding epinucleus.

Removing the nuclear fragments requires a change in the parameters for phaco. For this step, it is desirable to have lens material in contact with the phaco needle. Increasing the aspiration flow slightly directs lens material to the phaco tip, while increasing the vacuum encourages the nuclear fragments to be aspirated with application of only a minimum of phaco power. These parameters will be influenced by the density of the nucleus, but in principle, these settings will result in successful nucleus removal. A second instrument guides the control of nuclear fragments.

Removing the epinucleus is accomplished as described in Sect. 2.5.3. The parameters can be modified such that: (1) the aspiration flow is slightly reduced from the setting used in nuclear fragment removal, and (2) pulsed phaco power is used. If cortical cleaving hydrodissection is successful, the cortex is removed along with the epinucleus during this step of the procedure.

2.5.5
Phaco Chop

The phaco chop technique was initially introduced by Nagahara, who used the natural fault
lines in the lens nucleus to create cracks without
creating prior grooves (as presented by K. Nagahara, at the American Society of Cataract and
Refractive Surgery film festival, in 1993). The
phaco tip is embedded in the centre of the nucleus after the superficial cortex is aspirated. A
second instrument, the phaco chopper, is then
passed to the equator of the nucleus, beneath
the anterior capsule, and drawn to the phaco tip
to fracture the nucleus. The two instruments are
separated to widen the crack. This procedure is
repeated until several small fragments are created, which are then emulsified.

Koch and Katzen [39] modified this procedure because they encountered difficulty in mobilizing the nuclear fragments. They created a
central groove or central crater, depending on
the density of the nucleus. This modification
permits ease of removing the nuclear fragments
liberated by the phaco chop technique.

Advocates of these nucleus-dividing techniques have suggested that high levels of vacuum help to remove the nuclear fragments and
minimize the need for ultrasound energy. With
some of the newer phaco instruments, higher
vacuum power can be applied with minimal
risk of anterior chamber collapse.

2.5.6
Choo Choo Chop and Flip

Fine described the "choo-choo chop and flip"
technique in 1998 [20]. Subsequently, Fine,
Packer and Hoffman correlated the reduction of
ultrasound energy with this technique to improvement in uncorrected post-operative day
one visual acuity [23]. A 30° standard bevel
down tip is used throughout endonuclear removal. After aspirating the epinucleus uncov-
ered by the capsulorhexis, a Fine/Nagahara
chopper (Rhein Medical, Tampa, FL) is placed in
the golden ring by touching the centre of the nucleus with the tip and pushing it peripherally so

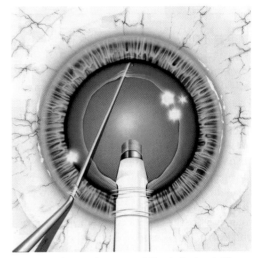

Fig. 2.1. The nucleus is stabilized during lollipop-
ping for the initial chop

that it reflects the capsulorhexis. The chopper is
used to stabilize the nucleus by lifting and
pulling toward the incision slightly, after which
the phaco tip lollipops the nucleus in either
pulse mode at two pulses/s or 80-ms burst mode
(Fig. 2.1). Burst mode is a power modulation that
utilizes a fixed per cent power (panel control), a
programmable burst width (duration of power),
and a *linear interval* between bursts. As one enters foot position 3, the interval between bursts
is 2 s; with increasing depressions of the foot
pedal in foot position 3 the interval shortens until at the bottom of foot position 3 there is continuous phaco. In pulse mode, there is *linear
power* (%) but a *fixed interval between pulses*,
resulting at two pulses/s in a 250-ms pulse (linear power) followed by a 250-ms pause in power followed by a 250-ms pulse, etc. However, in
both of these modulations with tip occlusion,
vacuum is continuous throughout the pulse and
pause intervals. With the energy delivered in
this way, ultrasound energy into the eye is min-
imized and hold on the nucleus is maximized as
vacuum builds between pulses or bursts. Because of the decrease in cavitational energy
around the tip at this low pulse rate or in burst
mode, the tunnel in the nucleus in which the tip
is embedded fits the needle very tightly and
gives us an excellent hold on the nucleus, thus

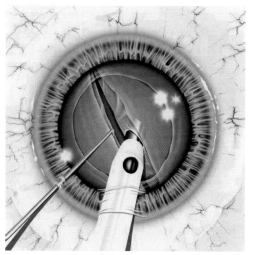

Fig. 2.2. The initial chop is completed

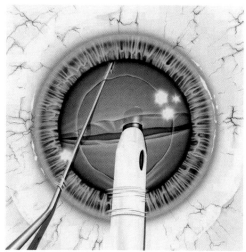

Fig. 2.3. The nucleus is stabilized before the second chop is commenced

maximizing control of the nucleus as it is scored and chopped in foot position 2 (Fig. 2.2).

The Fine/Nagahara chop instrument is grooved on the horizontal arm close to the vertical "chop" element with the groove parallel to the direction of the sharp edge of the vertical element. In scoring the nucleus, the instrument is always moved in the direction the sharp edge of the wedge-shaped vertical element is facing (as indicated by the groove on the instrument), thus facilitating scoring. The nucleus is scored by bringing the chop instrument to the side of the phaco needle. It is chopped in half by pulling the chopper to the left and slightly down while moving the phaco needle, still in foot position 2, to the right and slightly up. Then the nuclear complex is rotated. The chop instrument is again brought into the golden ring (Fig. 2.3), the nucleus is again lollipopped, scored, and chopped with the resulting pie-shaped segment now lollipopped on the phaco tip (Fig. 2.4). The segment is then evacuated utilizing high vacuum and short bursts or pulse mode phaco at two pulses/s (Fig. 2.5). The nucleus is continually rotated so that pie-shaped segments can be scored, chopped, and removed essentially by the high vacuum assisted by short bursts or pulses of phaco. The short bursts or pulses of ultrasound energy continuously reshape the pie-

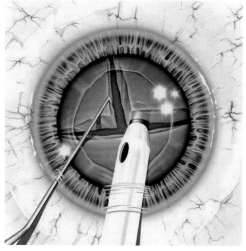

Fig. 2.4. A pie-shaped segment adheres to the phaco tip after the second chop is completed

shaped segments which are kept at the tip, allowing for occlusion and extraction by the vacuum. The size of the pie-shaped segments is customized to the density of the nucleus with smaller segments for denser nuclei. Phaco in burst mode or at this low pulse rate sounds like "choo-choo-choo-choo", ergo the name of this technique. With burst mode or the low pulse

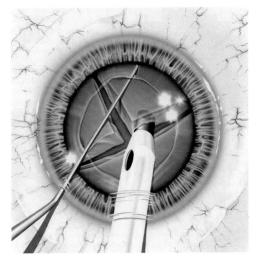

Fig. 2.5. The first pie-shaped segment is mobilized

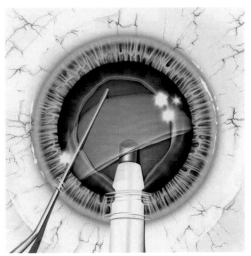

Fig. 2.6. The second heminucleus is scored

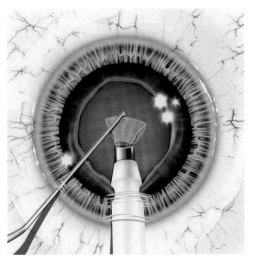

Fig. 2.7. The final quadrant is mobilized

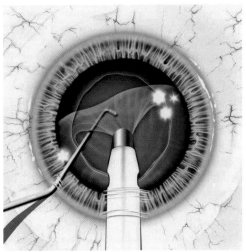

Fig. 2.8. The epinuclear shell is rotated for trimming

rate, the nuclear material tends to stay at the tip rather than chatter as vacuum holds between pulses. The chop instrument is utilized to stuff the segment into the tip or keep it down in the epinuclear shell.

After evacuation of the first hemi-nucleus, the second hemi-nucleus is rotated to the distal portion of the bag and the chop instrument stabilizes it while it is lollipopped. It is then scored and chopped (Fig. 2.6). The pie-shaped seg-

ments can be chopped a second time to reduce their size if they appear too large to easily evacuate (Fig. 2.7).

There is little tendency for nuclear material to come up into the anterior chamber with this technique. Usually it stays down within the epinuclear shell, but the chop instrument can control the position of the endonuclear material. The 30° bevel-down tip facilitates occlusion, as the angle of approach of the phaco tip to the

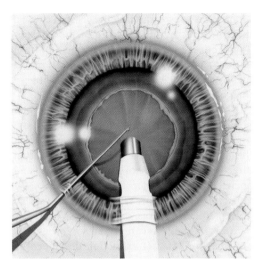

Fig. 2.9. The epinucleus is flipped

endonucleus through a clear corneal incision is approximately 30°. This allows full vacuum to be quickly reached which facilitates embedding the tip into the nucleus for chopping and allows mobilization of pie-shaped segments from above rather than necessitating going deeper into the endolenticular space as is necessary with a bevel-up tip. In addition, the cavitational energy is directed downward toward the nucleus rather than up toward the endothelium.

After evacuation of all endonuclear material, the epinuclear rim is trimmed in each of the three quadrants, mobilizing cortex as well in the following way (Fig. 2.8). As each quadrant of the epinuclear rim is rotated to the distal position in the capsule and trimmed, the cortex in the adjacent capsular fornix flows over the floor of the epinucleus and into the phaco tip. Then the floor is pushed back to keep the bag on stretch until three of the four quadrants of the epinuclear rim and forniceal cortex have been evacuated. It is important not to allow the epinucleus to flip too early, thus avoiding a large amount of residual cortex remaining after evacuation of the epinucleus.

The epinuclear rim of the fourth quadrant is then used as a handle to flip the epinucleus (Fig. 2.9). As the remaining portion of the epinuclear floor and rim is evacuated from the eye, most of the time the entire cortex is evacuated

with it. Downsized phaco tips with their increased resistance to flow are less capable of mobilizing the cortex because of the decreased minisurge accompanying the clearance of the tip when going from foot position 2 to foot position 3 in trimming of the epinucleus.

After the intraocular lens is inserted, these strands and any residual viscoelastic material are removed using the irrigation-aspiration tip, leaving a clean capsular bag.

If there is cortex remaining following removal of all the nucleus and epinucleus, there are three options. The phacoemulsification handpiece can be left high in the anterior chamber while the second handpiece strokes the cortex-filled capsular fornices. Frequently, this results in floating up of the cortical shell as a single piece and its exit through the phacoemulsification tip (in foot position two) because cortical cleaving hydrodissection has cleaved most of the cortical capsular adhesions.

Alternatively, if one wishes to complete cortical cleanup with the irrigation-aspiration handpiece prior to lens implantation, the residual cortex can almost always be mobilized as a separate and discrete shell (reminiscent of the epinucleus) and removed without ever turning the aspiration port down to face the posterior capsule.

The third option is to viscodissect the residual cortex by injecting the viscoelastic through the posterior cortex onto the posterior capsule. We prefer the dispersive viscoelastic device chondroitin sulfate-hyaluronate (Viscoat, Alcon Surgical, Fort Worth, TX). The viscoelastic material spreads horizontally, elevating the posterior cortex and draping it over the anterior capsular flap. At the same time the peripheral cortex is forced into the capsular fornix. The posterior capsule is then deepened with a cohesive viscoelastic device and the IOL is implanted through the capsulorhexis, leaving the anterior extension of the residual cortex anterior to the IOL. Removal of residual viscoelastic material accompanies mobilization and aspiration of residual cortex anterior to the IOL, which protects the posterior capsule, leaving a clean capsular bag.

Chop techniques substitute mechanical forces (chopping) for ultrasound energy (grooving) to disassemble the nucleus. High vacuum is utilized as an extractive technique to remove nuclear material rather than utilizing ultrasound energy to convert the nucleus to an emulsate that is evacuated by aspiration. These techniques maximize safety, control and efficiency, allowing phaco of harder nuclei, even in the presence of a compromised endothelium. Chop techniques facilitate the achievement of two goals: minimally invasive cataract surgery and maximally rapid visual rehabilitation.

2.5.7
Laser Phacoemulsification

Cataract extraction modalities employing laser energy currently include the Erbium:YAG Phacolase (Carl Zeiss Meditec, Jena, Germany), the Neodymium:YAG Photon Laser PhacoLysis System (Paradigm Medical, Salt Lake City) and the Dodick Q-switched Neodymium:YAG laser (ARC GmbH, Jona, Switzerland). Several potential advantages over ultrasound have maintained interest in laser, including relative reduction in the energy requirement for cataract extraction, the absence of any potential for thermal injury, and improved protection of corneal endothelial cells.

The erbium:YAG (2940-nm) laser energy is well absorbed by tissues with high water content and has a penetration depth of less than 1 μm. The laser energy is delivered via a fibre inside the aspiration port placed flush with the tip. Hoh and Fischer demonstrated that erbium laser is safe and effective for mild to moderate nuclear sclerosis [34].

Surgeons may employ a bimanual technique, separating irrigation from aspiration, or the more familiar coaxial set up. With the latter, Takayuki Akahoshi's counter prechop technique is used to effectively disassemble the lens nucleus into multiple wedge-shaped segments [2]. A horizontal chopper such as the Fine-Nagahara chopper (Rhein Medical, Tampa, FL) is inserted via the side-port, touched against the anterior lens surface and gently pushed under the distal anterior capsular flap where it falls into the golden ring. The chopper supports the nucleus while the Akahoshi Prechopper (ASICO, West-

mont, IL) is passed through the 2.5-mm corneal incision directly into the core of the nucleus. The chopper in the golden ring is held in front of the prechopper to preclude rotational movement of the nucleus. Opening the prechopper then bisects the nucleus.

The nucleus is then rotated 90° and the first hemi-nucleus is bisected in a similar fashion. The chopper supports the hemi-nucleus from the golden ring while the prechopper is inserted directly into the centre of the hemi-nucleus and opened. In this manner the nucleus may be divided into four or more segments, each of which is a suitable size for laser phacoemulsification.

Nd: YAG photolysis represents a low energy modality for cataract extraction developed by Dodick [11]. Kanellopoulos reported a mean intraocular energy use of 5.65 Joules per case [36]. This level of energy compares favourably with values previously reported for ultrasound phacoemulsification, and approximates the level of energy reported for the chop and flip phacoemulsification technique using power modulations [49]. Huetz and Eckhardt found mean total energy of 1.97 Joules for nuclear sclerosis up to grade 3, 3.37 Joules for Grade 3 and 7.7 Joules for Grade 4 [35].

Surgeons generally employ a groove and crack technique with the laser, sculpting in a bimanual fashion and cracking as soon as possible. Once superficial cortical material is aspirated, the laser tip is used to ablate and fragment the nucleus. The laser tip should only just touch the surface of the nucleus, and not be used to impale the cataract. Following central photofragmentation, the nucleus is handled much as it is with the classic divide and conquer technique. The total time that the tip is in the eye varies with the grade of nucleus, from 2.15 min for 1+ nuclear sclerosis to 9.8 min for 3+ nuclear sclerosis [36].

Using the bimanual Dodick system, a cataract may be completely extracted through two 1.5-mm incisions. Now, intraocular lens technology is becoming available to take advantage of this ultra-small incision. Wehner and Ali have reported a series of cases implanted with a dehydrated acrylic intraocular lens through a 1.5-mm incision [60].

2.5.8
Bimanual Ultrasound Phacoemulsification

The promise of bimanual, ultra-small incision cataract surgery and companion IOL technology is today becoming a reality, through both laser and new ultrasound power modulations. New instrumentation is available for bimanual surgery, including forceps for construction of the capsulorhexis, irrigating choppers and bimanual irrigation and aspiration sets. Proponents of performing phaco through two paracentesis-type incisions claim reduction of surgically induced astigmatism, improved chamber stability in every step of the procedure, better followability due to the physical separation of infusion from ultrasound and vacuum, and greater ease of irrigation and aspiration with the elimination of one, hard-to-reach subincisional region. However, the risk of thermal injury to the cornea from a vibrating bare phaco needle has posed a challenge to the development of this technique.

In the 1970s, Girard attempted to separate infusion from ultrasound and aspiration, but abandoned the procedure because of thermal injury to the tissue [30, 31]. Shearing and colleagues successfully performed ultrasound phaco through two 1.0-mm incisions using a modified anterior chamber maintainer and a phaco tip without the irrigation sleeve [50]. They reported a series of 53 cases and found that phaco time, overall surgical time, total fluid use and endothelial cell loss were comparable to those measured with their standard phaco techniques. Crozafon described the use of Teflon-coated phaco tips for bimanual high frequency pulsed phaco, and suggested that these tips would reduce friction and therefore allow surgery with a sleeveless needle [9]. Tsuneoka, Shiba and Takahashi determined the feasibility of using a 1.4-mm (19-gauge) incision and a 20-gauge sleeveless ultrasound tip to perform phaco [57]. They found that outflow around the tip through the incision provided adequate cooling, and performed this procedure in 637 cases with no incidence of wound burn [58]. Additionally, less surgically induced astigmatism developed in the eyes operated with the bimanual technique. Agarwal and colleagues developed a bimanual technique, "Phakonit," using an irrigating chopper and a bare phaco needle passed through a 0.9 clear corneal incision [1]. They achieved adequate temperature control through continuous infusion and use of "cooled balanced salt solution" poured over the phaco needle.

Soscia, Howard and Olson have shown in cadaver eye studies that phacoemulsification with the Sovereign WhiteStar system (AMO, Santa Ana, CA), using a bare 19-gauge aspiration needle, will not produce a wound burn at the highest energy settings unless all infusion and aspiration are occluded [54, 55]. WhiteStar represents a power modulation of ultrasonic phacoemulsification that virtually eliminates the production of thermal energy. Referred to as "cold phaco," WhiteStar allows reduction of the duration of energy pulses to the millisecond range.

Summary for the Clinician

- The divide and conquer technique employs ultrasonic sculpting of a deep central crater and fracturing of segments of a peripheral rim
- Phaco fracture involves ultrasonic sculpting of grooves and bimanual cracking of the nucleus into four separate quadrants
- Chip and flip means sculpting of a central bowl until a thin chip of endonucleus remains, while crack and flip is a modification of phaco fracture including hydrodelineation
- Phaco chop requires a firm hold with high vacuum and a second sharp instrument to either horizontally or vertically divide the nucleus
- Investigation of the choo choo chop and flip technique led to the conclusion that reduction of ultrasound energy is correlated with improvement of visual acuity on the first postoperative day
- Phacoemulsification with laser systems allows reduction of incision size to 1.5 mm
- Surgeons using bimanual microincision phacoemulsification have described improved chamber stability, better followability and greater ease of irrigation and aspiration

2.6
Conclusion

Since the time of Charles Kelman's inspiration in the dentist's chair (while having his teeth ultrasonically cleaned), incremental advances in phacoemulsification technology have produced ever-increasing benefits for patients with cataract. The modern procedure simply was not possible even a few years ago, and until recently prolonged hospital stays were common after cataract surgery.

The competitive business environment and the wellspring of surgeons' ingenuity continue to demonstrate synergistic activity in the improvement of surgical technique and technology. Future advances in cataract surgery will continue to benefit our patients as we develop new phacoemulsification techniques and technology.

References

1. Agarwal A, Agarwal A, Agarwal S, Narang P, Narang S (2001) Phakonit: phacoemulsification through a 0.9 mm corneal incision. J Cataract Refract Surg 27:1548–1552
2. Akahoshi T (1998) Phaco prechop: manual nucleofracture prior to phacoemulsification. Operative Techniques in Cataract and Refractive Surgery 1:69–91
3. Anis A (1991) Understanding hydrodelineation: the term and related procedures. Ocular Surg News 9:134–137
4. Arnott EJ (1981) Intraocular implants. Trans Ophth Soc UK 101:58–60
5. Brown DC, Fine IH, Gills JP et al (1992) The future of foldables. Ocular Surgery News August 15 (supplement); Panel discussion held at the 1992 annual meeting of the American Society of Cataract and Refractive Surgery
6. Ciulla TA, Starr MB, Masket S (2002) Bacterial endophthalmitis prophylaxis for cataract surgery. Ophthalmology 109:13–26
7. Colleaux KM, Hamilton WK (2000) Effect of prophylactic antibiotics and incision type on the incidence of endophthalmitis after cataract surgery. Can J Ophthalmol 35:373–8
8. Colvard DM, Kratz RP, Mazzocco TR, Davidson B (1980) Clinical evaluation of the Terry surgical keratometer. Am Intraocular Implant Soc J 6: 249–251
9. Crozafon P (1999) The use of minimal stress and the Teflon-coated tip for bimanual high frequency pulsed phacoemulsification. Presented at the 14th Meeting of the Japanese Society of Cataract and Refractive Surgery, Kyoto, Japan, July
10. Davison JA (1989) Bimodal capsular bag phacoemulsification: a serial cutting and suction ultrasonic nuclear dissection technique. J Cataract Refract Surg 15:272–282
11. Dodick JM (1991) Laser phacolysis of the human cataractous lens. Dev Ophthalmol 22:58–64
12. Faust KJ (1984) Hydrodissection of soft nuclei. Am Intraocular Implant Soc J 10:75–77
13. Fine IH (1991) Architecture and construction of a self-sealing incision for cataract surgery. J Cataract Refract Surg 17:672–676
14. Fine IH (1991) The chip and flip phacoemulsification technique. J Cataract Refract Surg 17:366–371
15. Fine IH (1992) Self-sealing corneal tunnel incision for small-incision cataract surgery. Ocular Surgery News, May 1
16. Fine IH (1992) Cortical cleaving hydrodissection. J Cataract Refract Surg 18:508–512
17. Fine IH (1993) Corneal tunnel incision with a temporal approach. In: Fine IH, Fichman RA, Grabow HB (eds) Clear-corneal cataract surgery and topical anesthesia. Slack, Thorofare, NJ, pp 5–26
18. Fine IH (1996) New blade enhances cataract surgery, techniques Spotlight. Ophthalmology Times, September 1
19. Fine IH (1997) Special report to ASCRS members: phacoemulsification incision burns. Letter to American Society of Cataract and Refractive Surgery members
20. Fine IH (1998) The choo-choo chop and flip phacoemulsification technique. Operative Tech Cataract Refract Surg 1:61–65
21. Fine IH, Fichman RA, Grabow HB (1993) Clear-corneal cataract surgery and topical anesthesia. Slack, Thorofare, NJ
22. Fine IH, Maloney WF, Dillman DM (1993) Crack and flip phacoemulsification technique. J Cataract Refract Surg 19:797
23. Fine IH, Packer M, Hoffman RS (2001) Use of power modulations in phacoemulsification. J Cataract Refract Surg 27:188–197
24. Galand A (1988) La technique de l'enveloppe. Pierre Mardaga publisher, Liege, Belgium
25. Gills JP, Gayton JL (1998) Reducing pre-existing astigmatism. In: Gills JP (ed) Cataract surgery: the state of the art. Slack, Thorofare, NJ, pp 53–66
26. Gimbel HV (1991) Divide and conquer nucleofractis phacoemulsification: development and variations. J Cataract Refract Surg 17:281–291

27. Gimbel HV (1991) Divide and conquer nucleofractis phacoemulsification. J Cataract Refract Surg 17:281

28. Gimbel HV, Neuhann T (1990) Development, advantages and methods of the continuous circular capsulorhexis technique. J Cataract Refract Surg 16:31

29. Gimbel HV, Neuhann T (1991) Letter to the editor: continuous curvilinear capsulorhexis. J Cataract Refract Surg 17:110

30. Girard LJ (1978) Ultrasonic fragmentation for cataract extraction and cataract complications. Adv Ophthalmol 37:127–135

31. Girard LJ (1984) Pars plana lensectomy by ultrasonic fragmentation 1984, part II: operative and postoperative complications, avoidance or management. Ophthalmic Surg 15:217–220

32. Girard LJ, Hoffman RF (1984) Scleral tunnel to prevent induced astigmatism. Am J Ophthalmol 97:450–456

33. Harms H, Mackensen G (1967) Intracapsular extraction with a corneal incision using the Graefe knife. In: Blodi FC (ed) Ocular surgery under the microscope. Georg Thieme, Stuttgart, pp 144–153

34. Hoh H, Fischer E (2000) Pilot study on erbium laser phacoemulsification. Ophthalmology 107: 1053–1061

35. Huetz WW, Eckhardt HB (2001) Photolysis using the Dodick-ARC laser system for cataract surgery. J Cataract Refract Surg 27:208–12

36. Kanellopoulos AJ (2001) Laser cataract surgery: a prospective clinical evaluation of 1000 consecutive laser cataract procedures using the Dodick photolysis Nd:YAG system. Ophthalmology 108: 649–654

37. Kelman CD (1967) Phacoemulsification and aspiration: a new technique of cataract removal: a preliminary report. Am J Ophth 64:23

38. Kershner RM (1997) Clear corneal cataract surgery and the correction of myopia, hyperopia, and astigmatism. Ophthalmology 104:381–389

39. Koch PS, Katzen LE (1994) Stop and chop phacoemulsification. J Cataract Refract Surg 20:566

40. Langerman DW (1994) Architectural design of a self-sealing corneal tunnel, single-hinge incision. J Cataract Refract Surg 20:84–88

41. Leaming DV (2002) Practice styles and preferences of ASCRS members-2001 survey. J Cataract Refract Surg 28:1681

42. Maloney WF, Grindle L (1988) Textbook of Phacoemulsification. Lasenda Publishers, Fallbrook, CA, pp 31–39

43. Masket S (1993) Origin of scleral tunnel methods. J Cataract Refract Surg 19:812–813 (letter to the editor)

44. McFarland MS (1990) Surgeon undertakes phaco, foldable IOL series sans sutures. Ocular Surgery News 8

45. Neuhann T (1987) Theorie und Operationstechnik der Kapsulorhexis. Klin Monatsbl Augenheilkd 190:542

46. Nichamin L (1993) Refining astigmatic keratotomy during cataract surgery. Ocular Surgery News, April 15

47. Park HJ, Kwon YH, Weitzman M, Caprioli J (1997) Temporal corneal phacoemulsification in patients with filtered glaucoma. Arch Ophthalmol 115:1375–1380

48. Paton D, Troutman R, Ryan S (1973) Present trends in incision and closure of the cataract wound. Highl Ophthalmol 14:3, 176

49. Rosen ES (1998) Clear corneal incisions: a good option for cataract patients. A roundtable discussion. Ocul Surg News, February 1

50. Shearing SP, Relyea RL, Loaiza A, Shearing RL (1985) Routine phacoemulsification through a one-millimeter non-sutured incision. Cataract 2:6–10

51. Shepherd JR (1989) Induced astigmatism in small incision cataract surgery. J Cataract Refract Surg 15:85–88

52. Shepherd JR (1990) In situ fracture. J Cataract Refract Surg 16:436

53. Shimizu K (1992) Pure corneal incision. Phaco Foldables 5:5; 6–8

54. Soscia W, Howard JG, Olson RJ (2002) Bimanual phacoemulsification through 2 stab incision. A wound-temperature study. J Cataract Refract Surg 28:1039–1043

55. Soscia W, Howard JG, Olson RJ (2002) Microphacoemulsification with WhiteStar. A wound-temperature study. J Cataract Refract Surg 28:1044–1046

56. Taher B (1997) Endophthalmitis: state of the prophylactic art. Eyeworld News (August) 42–43

57. Tsuneoka H, Shiba T, Takahashi Y (2001) Feasibility of ultrasound cataract surgery with a 1.4 mm incision. J Cataract Refract Surg 27:934–940

58. Tsuneoka H, Shiba T, Takahashi Y (2002) Ultrasonic phacoemulsification using a 1.4 mm incision: clinical results. J Cataract Refract Surg 28:81–86

59. Wasserman D, Apple D, Castaneda V et al. (1991) Anterior capsular tears and loop fixation of posterior chamber intraocular lenses. Ophthalmology 98:425

60. Wehner W, Ali I, (2002) Implantation of a 1.5 mm IOL after dodick laser photolysis cataract extraction. Symposium of the American Society of Cataract and Refractive Surgery, Philadelphia

61. Williamson CH (1993) Cataract keratotomy surgery. In: Fine IH, Fichman RA, Grabow HB (eds) Clear-corneal cataract surgery and topical anesthesia. Slack, Thorofare, NJ, pp 87–93

STEVE A. ARSHINOFF

The author of this paper has acted as a paid consultant to a number of OVD manufacturers, including all of those whose products are referred to herein.

Core Messages

- Cataract surgery is performed in a closed, fluid filled medium, and it is dependent upon fluid flow. The science of rheology, the study of the response of fluids to applied forces, is therefore key to understanding phacoemulsification (phaco) fluidics and performing better phaco surgery
- Ophthalmic viscosurgical devices (OVDs, viscoelastics) can vary in their properties from being similar to flowing air, to mimicking glass, which flows only slightly over centuries. The history of the study of OVDs has been one of working to determine which fluid properties were most important in cataract surgery and then, how to measure them
- OVDs, even those that are made with the same rheologic polymer, differ significantly depending upon the chain length of the polymer, and its concentration, such that referring to an OVD by a generically equivalent name is inaccurate and confusing
- OVDs can best be classified in a system based upon zero shear viscosity and relative degree of cohesion or dispersion, as these two factors play important roles in our surgical use of OVDs

- The soft shell technique employs a lower-viscosity dispersive OVD and a higher-viscosity cohesive OVD, sequentially to occupy adjacent spaces in the anterior chamber, and by so doing, to take maximal advantage of the desirable properties of both types of OVDs, while minimising their shortcomings. It requires meticulous ordered use of the two OVD classes to achieve optimal results
- The Ultimate Soft Shell Technique utilises a viscoadaptive OVD in conjunction with balanced salt solution, to enhance capsulorhexis, hydrodissection and OVD removal, beyond that which can be achieved using a viscoadaptive alone. Viscoadaptives provide superior space creation, stability, and clarity, when compared to use of previous OVDs, and permit us to do many things that were simply impossible before
- The science of OVD rheology is finally reaching a state of maturity, sufficient to permit the design and testing of new OVDs in the laboratory, and enabling accurate prediction of surgical performance

---

3.1
Introduction

Ophthalmic viscosurgical devices (OVDs, previously known as viscoelastics (terms which will be used interchangeably in this review) were

originally devices in search of a use. Sodium hyaluronate viscoelastic solutions were tried as vitreous substitutes as early as the 1960s, with varying success. But their eventual primary ophthalmic niche in cataract and intraocular lens (IOL) surgery did not become apparent until 1979, when Balazs, Miller and Stegmann reported success for that purpose [21]. Before the popularisation of endothelial cell protection with viscoelastics, some degree of endothelial damage had long been considered an unavoidable consequence of intraocular surgery in the anterior segment. Shortly after the introduction of OVDs, protection of the corneal endothelium and the creation and maintenance of surgical space to facilitate IOL implantation became recognised as the two chief advantages of what came to be known as viscosurgery. The evidence highlighting the enhanced safety of cataract surgery when viscosurgical devices are used is dramatic, with an extensive review demonstrating only 1/3 of the endothelial cell loss in both ECCE and phaco when viscoelastics are used compared to surgery without them [17]. The additional advantage of relatively easy and gentle viscolysis of intraocular adhesions and prevention of their reformation was soon added as a third major use. OVDs, which peculiarly exhibit some properties of both fluids and solids simultaneously, have now evolved into essential tools in ophthalmic surgery. Numerous such products are now marketed, and although each has its advocates, and some are best suited for specific surgical techniques, none has yet proven to be completely ideal, and therefore "best", for all purposes. Many surgeons' access to more than one or two specific OVDs may be limited by misguided administrative cost-containment efforts to designate one OVD as suitable in all cases or to consider two or more OVDs as therapeutically equivalent on the grounds that they are composed of a similar substance. Conversely, each OVD is most appropriately used in such a manner as to take advantage of its particular rheologic properties while coping with or limiting certain undesired effects, which every OVD has. The field of science most relevant to the comparative evaluation of OVDs and to the ultimate design of "tailored" products is rheology (the study of the deformation and flow of fluids in response to forces). Rheologists and ophthalmologists are working to ascertain the rheologic properties most and least desirable for optimal efficacy in specific ophthalmic operations and on that basis to produce OVDs tailored to specific tasks. Healon5 was the first OVD to be created rheologically, in a lab, rather than by tri-

al and error in clinical use. At the same time, efforts are underway to create new classes of OVDs that are more versatile, and therefore better approach the ideal of one OVD for every ophthalmologic surgical purpose. A major obstacle to development of the best OVD for a given purpose has been difficulty in determining which viscoelastic rheologic properties best relate to varying aspects of intraoperative performance and then devising a uniform method of measuring those properties in currently available products. Until recently, surgeons have had to rely primarily on experience and anecdotal testimony in their selection of OVDs. Moreover, as suggested above, in some practices product selection and thus comparative experience are limited by institutions intent on saving money. We now know that the OVDs currently marketed differ not only in content and properties but also in how those properties are altered by the surgical manoeuvres required in specific operations. Consequently, choosing an OVD by price alone, or a single OVD for all circumstances, may be foolhardy and even dangerous [7, 9].

3.2
History

The safety of cataract removal and lens replacement surgery was greatly improved in 1979 by the introduction of Healon, the first OVD. Healon is a sodium hyaluronate solution that maintains anterior chamber depth and protects delicate intraocular tissues, thereby facilitating IOL implantation. With far less successful results, air and autologous serum had been tried before for those purposes. Initially, there were concerns about severe postoperative intraocular pressure spikes seen when Healon was incompletely removed, a problem that would recur later, when new OVDs, such as Healon5, were developed, but removal techniques were developed to overcome these problems. Because of the tremendous advantages of corneal endothelial protection and surgical facilitation during intraocular lens implantation, Healon was rapidly adopted into the operative protocols for intracapsular cataract extraction

(ICCE) and extracapsular cataract extraction (ECCE) with IOL implantation world-wide in the early 1980s. Within a few years after the introduction of Healon, other OVDs became available. Chondroitin sulphate, Viscoat, and hydroxypropylmethylcellulose (HPMC – which was uniquely both home-made in many hospital pharmacies and commercially manufactured), appeared as competitive viscoelastic substances, and the science of rheologic study of the surgical demands and relative merits of various OVDs was born. The study of OVD efficacy was accelerated by the possibility of significant endothelial damage associated with ultrasonic phacoemulsification, which was becoming the preferred method of cataract surgery in the 1980s. Not all OVDs were found to be equal with regard to retention in the anterior chamber during the copious anterior chamber irrigation, and the consequent induced turbulence, needed to cool the phaco tip and maintain a stable deep anterior chamber during phaco. Neither were they equivalent in endothelial protection from free radicals generated by phacoemulsification, or in their ease of removal at the end of the surgical procedure. The first step in either evaluation or product design of OVDs must be to define and measure the surgically important rheologic properties of the individual OVDs now available. In the early 1980s, work to address that first step was prompted by difficulty in scientifically comparing the available products. The difficulty was partly attributable to inconsistency and non-uniformity in manufacturers' publicly reported data. Because rheology was a new and difficult field of study with varying terminology and methods, the producers of OVDs had used inconsistent methods and even varying units of measure to attain and report their data. Thus, the surgeon's preference for one product over another was necessarily based more on subjective, empirical, and anecdotal evidence than on the results of scientifically reproducible comparative study. The confusion about comparative data was addressed by the development of standardised methods to assess and compare the physical properties of OVDs using parameters that related to their use in cataract surgery [1, 2]. Recently, the International Standardization Organization (ISO) has established standards for measuring the safety and efficacy of "ophthalmic viscosurgical devices" – viscoelastic formulations intended for use in ophthalmic surgery [22]. The main goals of the ISO project was to define "requirements for minimum safety standards, and to mandate disclosure of rheologic performance characteristics in a standard fashion." Safety standards include factors relating to "accurate chemical description, required preclinical and clinical evaluation, sterilisation, product packaging, product labelling, and the information required to be supplied by the manufacturer." One of the most practically useful results of ISO standardisation is the promulgation of accepted terminology and units of measure, so that rheologic and other data about OVDs can be meaningfully and uniformly compared by surgeons who are considering using these products.

3.3
Physical Properties of OVDs

Currently available OVDs are aqueous solutions of naturally occurring long-chain polymers (sodium hyaluronate, hydroxypropylmethylcellulose [23], or chondroitin sulphate). Composed mostly of water, those products are of nearly the same density – about 1.0. The protective, retentive, cohesive, and lubricating properties of OVDs are grounded in their polymeric structure, molecular weight, electrical charge, purity, and interchain molecular interactions. The physical properties commonly recognised as differentiating the ophthalmic viscoelastics from each other include viscosity, elasticity, rigidity, pseudoplasticity, and cohesion, all of which are clinically relevant in terms of protecting tissues, maintaining space, and ease of injection and removal. Briefly stated, dynamic viscosity (the usual viscosity quoted for OVDs – the other is kinematic) is the resistance to the non-accelerated displacement of two parallel planes separated by a unit distance, the separating space being filled with the test substance. [Kinematic, or flowing, viscosity is the degree to which a fluid resists flow under an applied force (for example water flowing down a slope) and is equal to dynamic viscosity divided by specific gravity. For currently available OVDs, which consist almost entirely of water, the kinematic and dynamic viscosities are practically identical.] Elasticity is the degree to which a substance tends to reassume its original shape after having been stretched, compressed, distorted, or deformed. Rigidity is the degree of stiffness or inflexibility of a substance, and is equal to the Pythagorean sum of viscosity and elasticity ($R^2=V^2+E^2$). Plasticity is the quality of being conformable. Plastics become more conformable (exhibit decreasing viscosity) under increased applied stress, but are solid in the absence of external stress. Pseudoplastic fluids, which all of our OVDs are, exhibit decreasing viscosity as the external stress is increased, but, unlike plastics, possess a limiting viscosity as the stress is reduced, and always remain fluid. Cohesion is the tendency for similar molecules to stay together. This is a typical property of long chain entangled OVD solutions, whereas the physical opposite, dispersion is seen in solutions of small molecules, like salt in water. As we shall discuss, one challenge in evaluating the various products now available, or in assessing the potential uses of those under development, has been how to measure properties that usually change as the substance is used.

3.4
Generic or Proprietary Nomenclature

Unlike pharmacologic preparations, that we are familiar with, when considering OVDs, in which chain lengths, pH, osmolality, concentrations, other solutes present, polymeric conformations, electrical charge, molecular weight, and other factors, even within a specific polymeric molecular category of viscoelastic substances, can vary, specific trade-named products cannot be accurately designated by "generic" names. Most sodium hyaluronate products, for example, are very different even though their basic molecular structure may be identical and though they may share certain properties. For instance if one of two products of the same composition is of greater osmolality, or longer molecular chain length, than the other, it could be potentially more protective or damaging to endothelial

cells, and possess a very different pseudoplasticity profile. Nevertheless, those products within a given category do share certain qualities, so let us begin by reviewing each molecular category's similarities, before we go on to the differences within a category.

3.5
Currently Marketed Polymers

3.5.1
Sodium Hyaluronates

Hyaluronic acid, "the cement substance of tissues," is a mucopolysaccharide that is a polymer of N-acetylglucosamine and glucuronic acid. A salt of hyaluronic acid, sodium hyaluronate (NaHa) is found extensively as a gel in the intercellular matrices of vertebrate soft connective tissues, especially the skin but also in the synovial fluid and the vitreous humour of the eye. Among its purposes are wound repair, cellular growth, and lubrication and protection of musculoskeletal and eye structures. Its ophthalmic concentrations are greatest in the vitreous humour and the trabecular angle and are least in the aqueous humour and on the endothelium. Balazs, who was first to propound the use of viscoelastics in ophthalmic surgery and developed an ultrapurified sodium hyaluronate product, proposed that the corneal endothelium secretes sodium hyaluronate as a protective coat [20]. Through the use of tritiated high-molecular-weight sodium hyaluronate, Madsen et al. in Sweden have shown that human corneal endothelial cells are naturally covered in vivo by bound sodium hyaluronate, and possess specific hyaluronic acid binding sites on their surface. The cells have high affinity to binding with high-molecular-weight hyaluronate, and the greater the hyaluronate molecular weight, the greater the affinity. The sites are reported to have all the characteristics of receptors. There is no proof of a pharmacologic action of sodium hyaluronate on endothelial cells, and it is believed to play a physical protective role [24].

The sodium hyaluronate in currently available OVDs is extracted from rooster combs or streptococcal bacterial cultures and then under-

Table 3.1. Ophthalmic viscosurgical devices: content, molecular weight and zero-shear viscosity

| Higher-viscosity cohesive OVDs | | | |
OVD	Content	MW(D)	V0(mPas)
Viscoadaptives			
Healon5	2.3% NaHa	4.0M	7.0M
MicroVisc (iVisc) Phaco	2.5% NaHa	7.9M	16.0M
Super viscous-cohesive viscoelastics (V_0 > 1M):			
MicroVisc (iVisc) Plus	1.4% NaHa	7.9M	4.8M
Healon GV	1.4% NaHa	5.0M	2.0M
Viscous-cohesive viscoelastics (1M>V_0 > 100K):			
MicroVisc (iVisc)	1.4% NaHa	6.1M	1.0M
Allervisc (Viscorneal) Plus	1.4% NaHa	5.1M	500K
Provisc	1.0% NaHa	2.0M	280K
Healon	1.0% NaHa	4.0M	230K
Biolon	1.0% NaHa	3.0M	215K
Allervisc (Viscorneal)	1.0% NaHa	5.1M	200K
Amvisc	1.2% NaHa	1.0M	100K
Amvisc Plus	1.6% NaHa	1.0M	100K

| Lower-viscosity dispersive OVDs | | | |
OVD	Content	MW(D)	V0(mPas)
Medium viscosity dispersive viscoelastics (100K>V_0 > 10K):			
Viscoat	3.0% NaHa	500K	50K
	4.0% CDS	23K	
Cellugel	2.0% chemically modified HPMC	100K	40K
Vitrax	3.0% Ha	500K	25K
Very low viscosity dispersive viscoelastics (10K>V_0 > 1K):			
i-Cell	2.0% HPMC	90K	6.0K
Ocuvis	2.0% HPMC	90K	4.3K
Occucoat	2.0% HPMC	86K	4K
Hymecel	2.0% HPMC	86K	4K
Adatocel	2.0% HPMC	86K	4K
Visilon	2.0% HPMC	86K	4K

MW(D), molecular weight (Daltons); M, million; K, thousand;
V_0(mPas), zero shear viscosity (milli Pascal-seconds);
M, million; K, thousand.

NaHa, sodium hyaluronate
HPMC, hydroxypropylmethylcellulose
CDS, chondroitin sulfate.

goes a variety of purification processes. Solutions of sodium hyaluronate (like other OVDs) vary in concentration and chain length, or molecular mass, and therefore also in physical properties both in vitro and during use. Thus, not all products containing the same rheologic polymer perform alike or are necessarily useful for the same specific purpose.

Table 3.1 lists many of the hyaluronate OVDs currently marketed in western countries.

3.5.2
Chondroitin Sulphate

Chondroitin is a mucopolysaccharide found in the cornea and differing from hyaluronic acid in that it contains *N*-acetylgalactosamine in place of *N*-acetylglucosamine. The sulphate ester occurs in three forms: Chondroitin sulphate A is composed of glucuronic acid and sulphated galactosamine. In the B form, the glucuronic

constituent is replaced by L-iduronic acid. Chondroitin sulphate C differs from chondroitin sulphate B in the position of the sulphate on the galactosamine residue. All three forms of chondroitin sulphate are widespread in the connective tissues of vertebrates, particularly in cartilage. In nature, chondroitin sulphate exists as a component of a proteoglycan rather than as a free polysaccharide. For use in OVDs, chondroitin sulphate A has generally been obtained from shark-fin cartilage. As compared with sodium hyaluronate, chondroitin sulphate has an extra negative charge per repeating unit. Because the corneal endothelial cell membrane is positively charged, the greater negativity of chondroitin sulphate may increase electrostatic interaction with tissue and consequently more tenaciously bind to the cells [25]. The chain length of chondroitin sulphate is about 50 nm, and its molecular mass is about 22.5 kDa – roughly 0.5 % and 1 % of the length and mass, respectively, of sodium hyaluronate. Unlike most

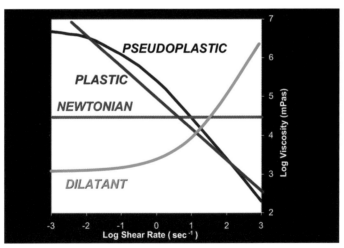

Fig. 3.1. Fluid behaviour types: rheometric patterns. The first fluids described were Newtonian. Newtonian fluids, such as air, water, and chondroitin sulfate demonstrate viscosity independent of shear rate. In other words, their viscosity is constant, independent of the degree of stress applied. Plastic fluids, however, demonstrate ever increasing viscosity with decreasing applied stress, and therefore show low viscosity at high shear rates, but infinite viscosity at infinitesimally small rates of shear. In other words, plastic fluids become solid at vanishingly small rates of shear, like

the "plastics" we use in everyday life. Pseudoplastic materials are unique in that they are similar to plastics at higher rates of shear, but have a limiting viscosity that they do not exceed, no matter how low the shear rate is reduced. In other words, they remain viscous fluids, even at very low shear rates. All currently marketed ophthalmic viscosurgical devices are pseudoplastic, as this type of behaviour is best suited to ophthalmic surgery. Dilatant fluids are unique in that their viscosity increases in response to increasing shear. Egg whites are one example of dilatant fluids

other currently available ophthalmic viscoelastics, chondroitin sulfate is a newtonian fluid (Fig. 3.1).

3.5.3
Hydroxypropylmethylcellulose (HPMC)

Another material used in the production of ophthalmic viscoelastics is ultrapurified HPMC, a cellulose ether in which about 1/3 of the hydrogen of hydroxyl groups in methylcellulose is replaced by methoxy and hydroxypropyl groups in a ratio of roughly 4:1. HPMC is more hydrophilic than methylcellulose, which although not present in mammals is a common component of plants. Methylcellulose has numerous industrial and medicinal uses and is readily available as a substrate for HPMC production. Its usual commercial source is wood pulp. Many commercially produced HPMC OVDs are on the market, but because HPMC is easily prepared (although not easily ultrapurified), some HPMC viscoelastics for use in ophthalmic surgery have been produced ad hoc in hospital pharmacies. For that reason, and because some physical properties of HPMC can depend on such factors as temperature, one batch of "home-made" HPMC will differ from another in crystalline formation and content of particulate matter. In the experimental ophthalmic application of variously formulated HPMC viscoelastics in rabbits, some older in-house formulations have been associated with severe inflammation of the vitreous [23]. Relatively inexpensive, HPMC OVDs are perhaps more commonly used in Europe and Asia than in North America. Unlike other OVDs, HPMC and modified HPMC products can undergo autoclave sterilisation and be stored for as long as 2 years at room temperature without resulting depolymerization or alteration in rheologic properties. More recent additions to the HPMC commercial offerings consist of chemically modified HPMCs, with the molecule being altered to enhance its rheological characteristics, yielding considerably increased zero shear viscosities, when compared to unmodified HPMCs. Cellugel, Ocumax and LA Gel are composed of modified HPMC.

3.6
Polymers no Longer Marketed as OVDs

3.6.1
Polyacrylamide

A synthetic polymer of acrylamide, polyacrylamide is a nonprotein, long-carbon-chain substance widely used in industrial and medical laboratories for electrophoresis and chromatography. As the principal rheologic ingredient of an OVD, Orcolon, it was marketed for human use in cataract surgery, but soon found to cause severe intractable glaucoma due to the formation of microgels that clogged the trabecular meshwork and could not be eliminated from the eye. Orcolon was rapidly removed from the market in North America and Europe, in 1991, but I have personally seen its continued sale in less affluent countries, as late as 2003 [3, 27].

3.6.2
Collagen IV

Collagen is a main supportive protein of skin, tendon, bone, cartilage, and connective tissue. Although at least theoretically the intraocular implantation of a protein could result in some adverse effects, Collagel, a viscoelastic substance prepared from type IV human placental collagen, was tried as an OVD. In comparison with other ophthalmic viscoelastics, Collagel was extremely temperature dependent, with viscosity decreasing more than a thousand-fold as temperature increased from 17° to 25°C. It behaved as a true plastic, with infinite zero-shear viscosity, and was more elastic than viscous, making its utility in intraocular surgery questionable. But the ultimate reason for its removal from the market place was the world-wide fear of possible prion contamination of human-sourced protein.

3.7
The Physical (Rheologic) Properties of OVDs and Their Measurement

As noted earlier, OVDs are peculiar in that they possess properties of both solids and fluids. In solids, internal forces are generated by a change in shape or volume. In fluids, which include liquids and gases and have no intrinsic shape, only changes in volume generate internal forces. The following are the principle parameters that have been found to be useful measures of OVD performance in cataract surgery.

3.7.1
Viscosity (Dynamic)

Some fluids, such as air, water, and chondroitin sulphate, possess constant viscosity independent of shear rate (or force applied – how fast it moves). Called Newtonian fluids, they contrast with non-Newtonian fluids, which exhibit varying viscosity at different shear rates. Plastic and pseudoplastic non-Newtonian fluids (Fig. 3.4) exhibit declining viscosity with increasing shear rate, whereas dilatant non-Newtonian fluids (e.g. egg whites) exhibit increasing viscosity with increasing shear rate. Plastic and pseudoplastic fluids differ in that pseudoplastic devices never gel: they possess a limiting viscosity at very low shear rates that does not increase further with decreasing rates of shear; thus they remain fluid even at extremely low shear rates. In the case of sodium hyaluronate solutions (typical pseudoplastic fluids), for example, the phenomenon of decreasing viscosity with increasing shear rate as the material is injected through a small-bore cannula can be explained by deformation of randomly entangled molecular coils to elongated aligned structures that flow more readily. Viscosity also varies inversely with temperature. Thus, the viscosity of non-Newtonian fluids cannot be properly measured (nor can viscosity data be relevantly interpreted) without taking into account the temperature and the shear rate at the time of measurement. Therefore, to understand and compare rheologic data about the non-Newtonian OVDs that we use in surgery, one must compare dynamic viscosities over a broad range of shear rates at a consistent temperature in a graph, and report numerically the zero-shear viscosity at that temperature. However, manufacturers, in their advertising, often report viscosities measured in various ways, at non-zero shear rates, making comparisons to other OVDs, by the reader, almost impossible.

3.7.2
Plasticity

A simple illustration of plasticity is the physical behaviour of a steel rod when a bending force is applied. After enough force has been applied to begin bending the rod, less and less force is required to continue bending it, and finally, it stays bent. The greater the plasticity of a material, the more the force required to bend it decreases as the speed of bending increases. The steel rod is a plastic solid, and not a pseudoplastic fluid, because it becomes solid at very low shear rates – that is, its zero-shear viscosity goes to infinity at low shear (it becomes solid) instead of having a limiting zero-shear viscosity and thereby remaining a viscous fluid (see Fig. 3.1).

3.7.3
Pseudoplasticity

The property of becoming less viscous with increasing shear rate, while possessing a limiting viscosity at zero shear, is called pseudoplasticity. It defines a subclass of non-Newtonian fluids. Until recently, the unit of dynamic viscosity measurement for ophthalmic viscoelastics was the centipoise (cp). [1 cp=0.01 g force per centimetre of flow per second. The current term in measurement is the milliPascal second (mPas): 1 cp=1 mPas.] It is readily apparent that surgical manoeuvres are most easily performed in a stable operative field. A corollary would be that OVDs with high zero-shear-viscosity should be better than a low-viscosity OVDs to stabilise the anterior segment and therefore also better in facilitating intraocular surgery. However, in any

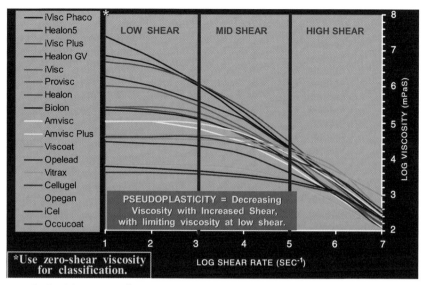

Fig. 3.2. Pseudoplasticity curves of OVDs. It is customary to plot rheologic curves of the log of viscosity vs the log of shear rate for ophthalmic viscosurgical devices. As these rheometric graphs demonstrate the pseudoplasticity of ophthalmic viscosurgical devices (OVDs), the graphs are commonly referred to as pseudoplasticity curves. They can be divided conveniently into areas of high, middle and low shear, for analysis of the behaviour of any given viscoelastic for a given surgical use. For example, it is desirable for an ophthalmic viscoelastic to possess high viscosity at low shear, thus making it better at creating and preserving intraocular surgical space, while it is also desirable for OVDs to possess low viscosity at high shear in order to facilitate injection through small bore cannulas

operation, but particularly in microsurgical procedures, any impediment to the surgeon's tactile sensitivity can complicate the procedure or even imperil the patient. A fluid that is highly viscous will require greater force for its injection into the eye than would a less viscous fluid injected through a same-sized cannula, and the greater the force required, the less able the surgeon is to judge either the required force or the sufficiency of the injection. Among the desirable characteristics of an OVD, therefore, are: (1) low viscosity during its injection (performed at very high shear rates – $1{,}000$–$10{,}000 \text{ s}^{-1}$) into the operative space, to facilitate rapid movement through a small-bore cannula while preserving the surgeon's tactile feedback sensitivity; (2) high viscosity when stationary, to create and maintain surgical spaces (shear rate 0.001–0.01 s^{-1}); and (3) intermediate viscosity at intermediate shear rates, to allow the passage of an intraocular lens or a surgical instrument as required during the operation (shear rate 0.1–10 s^{-1}). In other words, a desirable attribute

in an ophthalmic viscoelastic is a high degree of pseudoplasticity (Fig. 3.2). Pseudoplasticity is plotted as log of dynamic viscosity versus log of shear rate. Because the pseudoplasticity of an OVD is crucial in evaluating its suitability for a specific surgical operation, surgeons should be conversant with the pseudoplasticity curves of the OVDs they use, in comparison to the standards (Healon, Healon GV, Viscoat and HPMC).

3.7.4
Elasticity

Another important rheologic factor that relates to intraoperative behavior of OVDs is elasticity, which is the tendency of a substance to resume its original form after having been stretched, compressed, or deformed. By definition, viscoelastic substances have that quality, but to varying degrees. As a space occupying material becomes more viscous, it is desirable for it to also be elastic to absorb shock during surgical manipulation and increase retention in the eye in the presence of vascular pulsation. Elasticity, however, should not exceed viscosity, as that could make some surgical manoeuvres, for example. capsulorhexis, more difficult to perform. In an environment of elasticity exceeding viscosity, the capsular flap would tend to spring back to the position from which the surgeon had just moved it, when the surgeon released the flap to regrasp it. Whether an OVD is predominantly viscous or elastic at the time of measurement depends not only on molecular chain length and, concentration but also on the speed or frequency of impact as force is applied. Under low frequency impact, viscoelastics behave in a primarily viscous manner, and become ever more relatively elastic as the frequency of the applied force increases. This is due to molecular realignment under low frequency stress, and inadequate time for molecular realignment under high frequency stress.

3.7.5
Rigidity

Also referred to as complex viscosity, rigidity is the sensation of resistance, felt by the surgeon, to movement of an object through a viscoelastic substance. It is defined as the Pythagorean sum of viscosity and elasticity, i.e. $R = \sqrt{(V^2 + E^2)}$. (Mathematically, rigidity is equal to the square root of the sum of the squares of the dynamic viscosity and the elasticity.) The rigidity of a viscoelastic at any given time will depend on the shear rate and the frequency of vibration and will be nearer to the value of the dynamic viscosity or of the elasticity, whichever is the greater under the operative conditions of measurement. (Similarly, the hypotenuse of a right angle triangle is nearer in length to the longer of two unequal right angle sides of the triangle). Thus, either viscosity or elasticity will appear to predominate as the tactile "feedback" quality when the surgeon manipulates the OVD at any given shear rate, thereby yielding the surgeon's tactile sensation of the OVD's behaviour as either viscous or elastic in a given situation.

At very low shear rates, all currently available OVDs perform in a predominantly viscous

manner. For each viscoelastic product, at some specific frequency the dominant sensation of viscosity will change to elasticity – that is, on a plotted curve, the viscosity will exceed its elasticity until, at a "crossover point," the elasticity will begin to exceed the viscosity. For that reason, products with high crossover points, above $2\,s^{-1}$ will feel viscous when rubbed between the thumb and the fingers, (a manoeuvre that imposes a shear rate of about $2\,s^{-1}$), for example, Viscoat, whereas, for products with low crossover points, below $2\,s^{-1}$, the quality transmitted by rubbing will be of elasticity, for example Healon GV.

3.7.6
Cohesion and Dispersion

OVDs can be divided into two broad groups on the basis of their relative cohesion or dispersion. In reality, this behaviour really lies along a continuum; however, it is convenient, for use and study to divide viscoelastics into the above categories. To date all cohesive OVDs are of higher zero-shear viscosity, and all dispersive OVDs are of lesser zero-shear viscosity (Table 3.1). Generally, given two viscoelastic substances of the same chemical family and concentration, the greater the mean molecular weight (i.e. the greater the polymeric chain length) of a substance, the greater its cohesion and zero-shear viscosity. Cohesion correlates highly with zero shear viscosity for our current hyaluronate and HPMC viscoelastics (there are no current chondroitin sulphate containing OVDs whose primary rheologic constituent is not hyaluronic acid). However, cohesion is a different property, that is very important in surgery, and it is probably incorrect to assume that all future viscoelastics will demonstrate the same correlation. Therefore, along with zero-shear viscosity and pseudoplasticity, the relative cohesive or dispersive behaviour of an OVD is one of its most important properties, because it relates directly to how OVDs are used in surgery [26]. Cohesion is the tendency of a material's constituent molecules to adhere to one another rather than to disperse. A low concentration of high-molecular-mass polymers entangled as a

Table 3.2. Using OVDs in Phacoemulsification

Task	Shear rate	Important properties
Fill AC	1000	High pseudoplasticity
Capsulorhexis	0	High viscosity, elasticity
Emulsify nucleus	Varies with AC position	High retention
I/A cortex	Varies with AC position	High retention
Fill capsular bag	1000	High pseudoplasticity
Keep bag open	0	High viscosity, elasticity
Insert IOL	2–5	High pseudoplasticity
Removal	Varies with AC position	High cohesion, scrollability

network in solution will be cohesive, whereas a higher concentration of lower-molecular-mass polymers unentangled will be dispersive. Unlike the polymers of a predominantly cohesive viscoelastic substance, which under force will tend to move as a single mass, those of a dispersive substance (by definition) tend to separate and move apart. As we shall discuss, an understanding of the general characteristics of the two groups of products is helpful in choosing a specific formulation for use in a specific ophthalmic surgical procedure. Cohesion is actually more complicated than this, and all OVDs are really cohesive at rest, but lower molecular weight OVDs behave in a dispersive fashion under the low vacuum stress imposed by irrigation and aspiration encountered in phaco surgery. A full discussion of this is given by Arshinoff and Wong [15].

3.8
Important Viscoelastic Rheologic Properties in the Various Steps of Cataract Surgery

Intracapsular cataract extraction (ICCE) and manual extracapsular cataract extraction (ECCE) were the preferred surgical techniques for cataract removal when the first OVD, Healon, was introduced. Initially, OVDs were used primarily to maintain the depth of the anterior chamber so that an intraocular lens could be implanted without damaging the corneal endothelial cells. ICCE was soon replaced by ECCE, which in turn has now largely been dis-

placed by ultrasonic phacoemulsification in most of the world. Thus, the demands placed on surgical OVDs increased as surgical technique itself gradually became more meticulous and complex. A capsulorhexis requires much more delicate and precise manipulation than does its predecessor, the "can-opener" anterior capsulotomy. Implantation of a foldable IOL into the capsular bag is a more precise procedure than the implantation of a one-piece IOL into the ciliary sulcus. Phacoemulsification, itself, requires protection for the endothelial cells from the ultrasonic energy that was not used in earlier procedures. For those reasons, each step of modern phacoemulsification has been analysed to determine the desirable viscoelastic properties of an ideal OVD for that step (Table 3.2).

In both ECCE and phacoemulsification (followed by implantation of an IOL within the capsular bag), the first surgical step is injection of the OVD into the anterior chamber. The operative shear rate as the material is expelled through a small-bore cannula is about $1000\ s^{-1}$. At that shear rate, a desirable viscoelastic characteristic is low viscosity (therefore a highly pseudoplastic OVD is desirable) so that only a relatively gentle force of injection is required, and ocular inflation pressure can be judged and modulated by the surgeon's tactile sensitivity. If the viscosity of the OVD is excessive at high shear rates, the only feedback sensation the surgeon feels is the resistance of the cannula, and over or under inflation of the anterior chamber is a distinct possibility, often with undesirable consequences.

Having been properly injected, the OVD serves as a stable viscous and elastic mass that will resist deformation of eye structures or disruption of their anatomical relationships while the capsulorhexis is being performed. For that purpose, the operative shear rate is close to $0 s^{-1}$ as instruments are manually moved through the OVD mass that is essentially stationary as it maintains the corneal dome and anterior chamber depth, and therefore, the most desirable OVD attribute is high viscosity and elasticity at low shear.

Removal of the nucleus by ECCE entails expulsion at a shear rate of about $2-5 s^{-1}$, at which time viscoelastic pseudoplasticity is desirable to decrease the resistance that would occur if the OVD were to have high zero-shear viscosity and poor pseudoplasticity. When the nucleus is removed by phacoemulsification, however, the shear rate is irrelevant, because most of the viscoelastic substance in the area of the nucleus being emulsified, will have left the eye, irrespective of which class of OVD is used, and the anterior chamber is pressurised by the infusion pressure of the intraocular irrigant, a balanced salt solution, with viscosity very close to that of water. The cornea, however, is vulnerable to damage by ultrasonic energy and fluid turbulence. Thus, the OVD properties that are more important than viscosity during phacoemulsification are retention adjacent to the endothelium, in the concavity of the cornea, under the conditions of the procedure (to protect the endothelium), elasticity (to absorb vibration), and the ability to neutralise free radicals liberated by the phacoemulsification process.

As the nucleus is being emulsified, dispersive OVDs tend to remain within the corneal concavity of the anterior chamber better than do cohesive OVDs. However, dispersive OVDs also tend to entrap air bubbles generated by the tip of the phacoemulsification instrument and thus impede the surgeon's operative view of the lens and the posterior capsule. The problem of having to accept one liability of an OVD in order to benefit from one of its assets has been addressed in two ways. The first is the viscoelastic soft- shell technique, first presented in 1996 [10, 5, 28] and the second is the development of viscoadaptive OVDs, which despite being very viscous and cohesive exhibit high retention in the anterior chamber during phacoemulsification [15]. The first of the viscoadaptive products brought to market was Healon5, which was released at the ESCRS meeting in Nice, France, in September 1998 [8, 11, 12].

The next step, after nuclear removal, in either ECCE or phacoemulsification with IOL implantation is irrigation and aspiration of any residual lens cortex, a procedure that is identical with respect to fluidics as the demands upon the viscoelastic to phacoemulsification. The endothelial cells are still subject to the trauma of fluid turbulence, but are no longer at risk from transmitted ultrasonic energy or free radicals.

Irrigation and aspiration of the cortex is followed by injection of the OVD into the capsular bag. Because that entails the same manoeuvres and imparts the same shear rate as does filling of the anterior chamber at the beginning of the procedure, a high index of pseudoplasticity, with low viscosity at high shear rates is again desirable. Similarly, when the OVD is stable within the capsular bag and serving to maintain space, permitting easy IOL implantation, high viscosity and elasticity are preferred.

The effective shear rate during IOL insertion is about $2-5 s^{-1}$. One role of the OVD in this step is to protect the corneal epithelium from damage due to compression or drag that might occur if the lens were to approach the endothelium too closely. At low shear rates, such as when the lens is immobile, a highly viscous material between the lens and the cornea is superior in protecting the endothelium from compression by the lens. When the lens moves, however, and the shear rate increases, a cushioning material that remains highly viscous will endanger the cornea by transmitting drag forces. The most useful and versatile OVD for use in IOL insertion will therefore be highly pseudoplastic during the time of insertion – that is, it will become much less viscous where the IOL slides through it, as the shear rate increases locally. In addition, a highly viscous OVD provides excellent cushioning to the opening of foldable IOLs inside the eye.

The final step in either ECCE or phacoemulsification is removal of the viscoelastic, and here high cohesion is desirable so that removal can be accomplished expeditiously and completely. If any viscoelastic is left in the eye inadvertently, two serious specific complications can occur: severe postoperative elevation of intraocular pressure and capsulorhexis-blockade syndrome.

3.9
Choosing Viscoelastics for Specific Procedures

Most ophthalmic surgeons in clinical practice do not have a practical method to scientifically compare and evaluate the numerous OVDs now on the market. However, a useful consideration is that they can be classified generally as either higher-viscosity cohesive or lower-viscosity dispersive, according to their properties in surgical use (Table 3.1). The higher-viscosity cohesive group can be further divided into super-viscous cohesive and viscous cohesive sub groups. The attributes and disadvantages of each category and subcategory can serve as guidelines in choosing the product most suitable for a specific surgical procedure. Similarly the lower-viscosity dispersives can be sub divided into medium viscosity dispersives and very low viscosity dispersives.

Most OVDs now available are formulations of hyaluronic acid or hydroxypropyl methylcellulose (HPMC), with the hyaluronates possessing greater viscosity and more desirable rheologic attributes that the HPMCs. Any clinical differences among the hyaluronate formulations are due to differences in concentrations and lengths of the hyaluronic acid chains. Within the range of concentrations of current commercial hyaluronic acid products, those with the greatest viscosity at low shear rates are also the most elastic, rigid, and pseudoplastic.

3.9.1
Higher-Viscosity Cohesives

The property of cohesion is important for surgical removal of an OVD after it has served its purpose. Because a highly viscous product is generally desirable to increase the stability of the surgical environment, and viscosity of hyaluronates correlates highly with cohesion, these products are doubly advantageous both during surgery and at the end of the procedure and minimise postoperative spikes of intraocular pressure when removed properly by the surgeon. On the other hand, the same property of high cohesion and therefore easy removability will be less desirable when the surgeon wishes to retain some viscoelastic material within the corneal concavity throughout the phacoemulsifaction and irrigation/aspiration parts of the procedure. Viscoadaptive products were developed for precisely that reason.

OVDs within the higher-viscosity-cohesive category are particularly useful when there is a need to create space and stabilise the microsurgical environment, such as to deepen the anterior chamber, to enlarge small pupils, to dissect adhesions, to stabilise the capsular bag, or to displace the iris and vitreous temporarily during IOL implantation.

3.9.1.1
Super-Viscous Cohesives

The super-viscous cohesive OVDs are a subclass of the higher-viscosity cohesive OVDs, and exhibit extremely high zero-shear viscosity greater than 1 million mPaS (milliPascal-seconds). They are admirably suited for use in topical and intracameral anaesthesia and phacoemulsification techniques that entail confining the surgery to manoeuvres "within the capsular bag". For instance, when capsulorhexis is to be performed in a shallow-chambered hyperope under topical anaesthesia, a super-viscous cohesive OVD is especially helpful in achieving intraocular stability and creating and maintaining adequate operative space. Except when a dispersive material is specifically indicated (see Sects. 3.9.2, 3.10), the super-viscous cohesive products are often the ophthalmic surgeon's first choice in most cases.

3.9.1.2
Viscous Cohesives

The viscous cohesive OVDs (zero shear viscosity between 100,000 and 1,000,000 mPaS) consist of the original Healon and all of its copies.

They have the same utility and drawbacks as super viscous cohesive OVDs, but generally are not quite as effective [14].

3.9.2
Lower-Viscosity Dispersives

When injected as a bolus into the eye, the lower-viscosity dispersive OVDs are (by definition) more likely than viscous and cohesive products to disperse into fragments in the anterior chamber. Low viscosity and the tendency to disperse make some OVDs particularly useful when tissues must be isolated and moved selectively, as, for example, when in the presence of a zonular disinsertion the vitreous must be kept out of the operative field or when a piece of frayed iris is to be sequestered away from irrigation that would draw it toward the phaco tip. The lower-viscosity dispersives can be subdivided into the medium-viscosity dispersives and the very low-viscosity dispersives, with the medium-viscosity dispersives generally possessing better rheologic properties for cataract surgical applications, but being more expensive than the very low viscosity dispersives, which are all HPMC products. Some remnants of a lower-viscosity dispersive OVD tends to remain adjacent to the corneal endothelium, within the corneal concavity, even during phacoemulsification. However, that characteristic, which in some cases might be protective, could be detrimental if the surgeon's operative view is thereby significantly diminished. In that case, the risk of inadvertent intraocular surgical damage, for example to the posterior capsule, might be increased. Another potential drawback is that the trauma (due to drag forces from irrigation and aspiration close to the endothelial cells) required for postoperative removal of a dispersive OVD could result in more endothelial damage than was prevented by the presence of the dispersive OVD during surgery. The advantages of dispersive OVDs are maximised, and their disadvantages are minimised, by using the viscoelastic soft-shell technique for routine cases and especially for complex cases [10, 28].

3.10
The Viscoelastic Soft Shell Technique

3.10.1
Background and Rationale

Highly viscous-cohesive viscoelastics are best at creating space with their viscosity, preserving it by being elastic, and at displacing and stabilising tissues in the surgical environment. Intraocular pressure can only be induced in an unsealed eye (with a small, potentially leaking incision), with an elastic substance, consequently only the highly viscous-cohesive elastic viscoelastics are capable of neutralising positive posterior pressure, which is always present, to some extent, in cases of topical or intracameral anaesthesia (because the extraocular muscles are not paralysed), by pressurising the anterior chamber to a degree equal to the posterior pressure. I have termed this viscoelastic pressure neutralising method of cataract surgery "pressure equalised cataract surgery (PECS)", which can only be accomplished with viscous-cohesive and super viscous-cohesive OVDs (as well as viscoadaptives). A "pressure equalised anterior chamber" stabilises the lens during capsulorhexis by flattening out the anterior lens capsule, thus reducing the risk of errant tears, and facilitates foldable lens implantation, by stabilising the viscoelastic expanded capsular bag, and preventing it from developing folds in the posterior capsule as the IOL is being inserted and unfolded (Fig. 3.3). The high cohesion of viscous-cohesive and super viscous-cohesive OVDs is the factor that results in ease of removal by irrigation and aspiration at the end of the surgical procedure. But due to the same cohesive behaviour, cohesive OVDs leave the anterior chamber rapidly during phaco, except for a thin layer of hyaluronate bound to endothelial cell membrane specific binding sites [24], permitting a clear unobstructed view of the posterior capsule. But, sometimes the early disappearance of cohesive OVDs from the anterior chamber during phaco can lead to suboptimal corneal endothelial protection during the turbulence of phacoemulsification. Furthermore, cohesive OVDs are unable to partition fluid

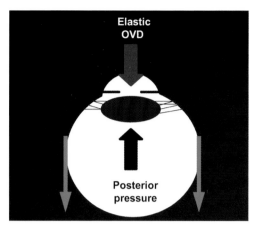

Fig. 3.3. Pressure equalised cataract surgery. When cataract surgery is performed, especially using topical or intracameral anaesthesia, once an incision is made, the eye is exposed to unbalanced forces. There is posterior vitreous pressure pushing forwards, which originates from the constant pulling of the extraocular muscles (*green arrows*), but no anterior pressure to counterbalance it, as a consequence of the incision being open, permitting aqueous escape, thus depressurising the anterior chamber. In an open eye, it is impossible to pressurise the anterior chamber with an inelastic device. Long chain hyaluronic acid OVDs are best at neutralising the posterior pressure, and permit surgery to be done in a much safer "pressure equalised" environment. This is particularly important for capsulorhexis and IOL implantation

spaces in the anterior chamber. In other words it is impossible, using a cohesive viscoelastic, to envelop a structure on one side of the anterior

chamber, and then go back in with either the I/A tip or phaco, and work on the other side of the AC, without dragging the viscoelastic mass back into the aspiration port, along with the tissue the surgeon wanted sequestered. Consequently, the higher-viscosity cohesive OVDs are best used to create space and stability where it is otherwise inadequate. This may include their use in deepening a shallow anterior chamber in a hyperope to facilitate the insertion of a phacoemulsification tip, to create a pressure-equalised environment to facilitate a difficult capsulorhexis, to enlarge small pupils, to dissect adhesions and to implant foldable intraocular lenses (Table 3.3). Surgically, the most useful properties of dispersive OVDs are their resistance to aspiration, and their ability to partition spaces. Their dispersive nature is one factor, along with negative electrical charge and the presence of hyaluronic acid (to bind to specific binding sites), that improves the retention of OVDs in the anterior chamber, adjacent to the corneal endothelium, throughout phacoemulsification and irrigation/aspiration [25]. Dispersive OVDs are also extremely useful as surgical tools in situations when it may be necessary to selectively move or isolate a single structure in the anterior chamber (e.g. holding back vitreous at an area of zonule disinsertion, or to isolate a piece of frayed iris preventing it from being constantly drawn into the phacoemulsification tip). They are capable of partitioning the anterior chamber into a viscoelastic protected space and a surgical zone in which the irrigation

Table 3.3. Best uses and disadvantages of OVD groups

Higher-viscosity cohesives	Lower-viscosity dispersives
Best uses	**Best uses**
1. Create and preserve spaces	1. Remain adjacent to corneal endothelium throughout phaco
2. Displace and stabilise tissues	2. Selectively move and isolate
3. Pressurise the AC	3. Partition spaces
4. Clear view of posterior capsule during phaco	
Disadvantages	**Disadvantages**
1. Leave AC too quickly during I/A or phaco -suboptimal endothelial protection	1. Do not maintain spaces or stabilise as well
2. Unable to partition spaces	2. Irregular fracture boundaries obscure view ofposterior capsule
3. More difficult to remove at the end of the procedure	

of phaco or I/A can be continued, without the two areas mixing. The major drawback of lower-viscosity dispersive viscoelastics is that their relatively low viscosity and elasticity do not allow them to maintain or stabilise spaces as well as higher-viscosity cohesive viscoelastics (e.g., in the performance of a capsulorhexis or implantation of a foldable intraocular lens). In other words their decreased cohesion can be used to the advantage of the surgeon, but their lower viscosity and elasticity is a definite drawback. In addition, lower-viscosity dispersive OVDs tend to be aspirated in small fragments during phaco and I/A leading to an irregular viscoelastic-aqueous interface that partially obscures the surgeon's view of the posterior capsule during phacoemulsification. The microbubbles that form during phacoemulsification, tend to become trapped in this irregular interface, further obscuring the surgeon's view of the posterior capsule, rendering surgical manoeuvres in the posterior chamber more difficult. Lower-viscosity dispersive OVDs, because of their low cohesion, are more difficult to remove at the end of the surgical procedure. Assia et al. demonstrated, in a controlled in vitro study, that lower-viscosity dispersive OVDs such as Viscoat, Occucoat and Orcolon, may take more than seven times longer to remove than higher-viscosity cohesive OVDs such as Healon and Healon GV [18]. The additional manipulation and aspiration required to completely remove dispersive viscoelastics may actually increase the likelihood of complications such as endothelial damage or puncturing of the posterior capsule. Lower viscosity-dispersive viscoelastics are most advantageous when dealing with problematic cases such as zonule disinsertions, small holes in the posterior capsule, a frayed piece of iris, and Fuch's endothelial dystrophy, the latter being a situation in which the surgeon specifically wants to isolate the corneal endothelial cells from the phaco procedure's turbulent flow (Table 3.3).

3.10.2
The Dispersive-Cohesive Viscoelastic Soft Shell Technique

The dispersive-cohesive viscoelastic soft shell technique is a method which uses both dispersive and cohesive viscoelastics sequentially, in order to derive the benefits of both viscoelastic types and eliminate the drawbacks of each (see discussion above). The viscoelastics should not mix in the eye, but should occupy adjacent spaces within the anterior chamber, if optimal results are to be achieved. The technique relies upon three principles:

1. A pressurising elastic device (e.g., a higher-viscosity cohesive OVD) in a confined space, will transmit pressure through adjacent fluids, within the confined space, to pressurise the entire space.
2. A dispersive viscoelastic will maintain it's dispersive characteristics when subjected to moderate pressure from an adjacent cohesive fluid.
3. Two rheologically dissimilar, but both transparent, OVDs can be placed in adjacent spaces within the anterior chamber, without mixing, and without blurring the surgeon's view, in order to take maximum advantage of the unique properties of each viscoelastic, in the exact location where it is most needed.

3.10.3
Method

At the commencement of the surgical cataract procedure (Fig. 3.4), a lower-viscosity dispersive OVD is injected into the anterior chamber first, and a mound is formed centrally on the anterior surface of the lens. A higher-viscosity cohesive OVD is then injected into the posterior centre of the lower-viscosity dispersive OVD mound, such that the incoming higher viscosity cohesive OVD fills the centre of the eye, and pushes the lower-viscosity dispersive OVD upwards and outwards, eventually forming a smooth, even, pressurised layer adjacent to the corneal endothelium . The higher-viscosity cohesive OVD permits creation of space and pres-

surisation of the anterior chamber, to deepen
and stabilise it and facilitate capsulorhexis, in a
manner that could never be achieved with a
lower-viscosity dispersive alone, while the lower-viscosity dispersive is fashioned into a
smooth, even protective layer adjacent to the
corneal endothelial cells, where it will remain
throughout the turbulence of the surgical procedure. A continuous curvilinear capsulorhexis
is then performed followed by hydrodissection.
As the phaco is begun, the higher-viscosity cohesive OVD is aspirated out, leaving a smooth,
ironed out layer of lower-viscosity dispersive
OVD adjacent to the corneal endothelial cells,
without irregular fracture boundaries, allowing
for clearer visualisation of the posterior capsule, while simultaneously protecting the delicate endothelial cells against fluid turbulence.
After the lens has been emulsified and irriga-
tion/aspiration of the cortical remnants completed, but before implantation of the IOL, the
OVDs are injected in reverse order: the higher-
viscosity cohesive OVD is injected first, followed by the lower-viscosity dispersive into its
centre. The higher-viscosity cohesive OVD pres-
surises the anterior chamber and expands the

Fig. 3.4 a–f. The viscoelastic soft shell technique.
a The lower-viscosity dispersive OVD (*violet*) is injected first to form a mound on the surface of the centre of the cataractous lens. **b** The higher-viscosity cohesive OVD (*green*) is injected into the posterior
centre of the lower-viscosity dispersive OVD, such
that continued injection pushes the lower-viscosity
dispersive OVD upward and outward, finally pressurising it into a smooth layer against the corneal endothelial cells. **c** After performance of the capsulorhexis, when the phaco is begun, the higher-viscosity cohesive OVD (*green*) rapidly leaves the eye, leaving behind the smooth layer of lower-viscosity dispersive OVD (*violet*) ironed out against the corneal
endothelial cells, which remains largely intact
throughout the phaco and I/A procedures. **d** After
completion of removal of the nucleus and cortex the
OVDs are injected in reverse order. The higher-viscosity cohesive OVD (*green*) is injected first to stabilise the iris, capsule and anterior chamber. The lower-viscosity dispersive OVD (*violet*) is then injected
into its centre, placing the cannula tip approximately
in the geographic centre of the capsulorhexis. Figure
3.4 e,f see next page

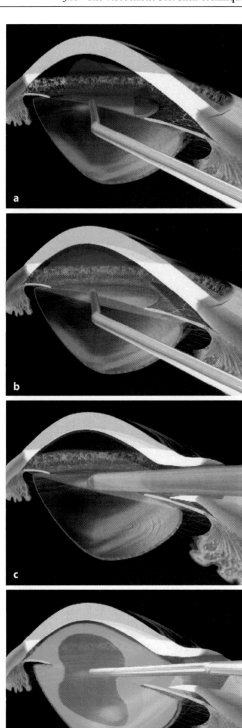

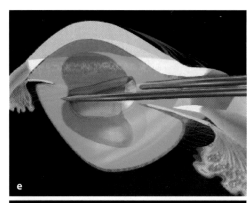

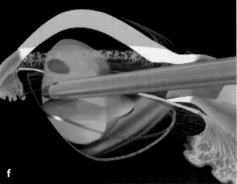

Fig. 3.4. e The presence of the lower-viscosity dispersive OVD (*violet*) in the centre of the higher-viscosity cohesive OVD mass (*green*) allows freer movement of the incoming IOL with better stabilisation of the surrounding iris and capsular bag. **f** Because the lower-viscosity dispersive OVD (*violet*) is enveloped within the higher-viscosity cohesive OVD (*green*), both are easily aspirated out of the eye together at the end of the procedure, as if only a higher-viscosity cohesive OVD had been present.

capsular bag to prevent wrinkles in the posterior capsule and facilitate foldable lens implantation. It's presence in the periphery of the anterior chamber stabilises the iris and lens capsule so that they do not move when the IOL is introduced. It also protects the delicate structures of the eye against the sometimes rapid unfolding of silicone IOLs. The lower-viscosity dispersive OVD, occupying the centre of the anterior

chamber and capsular bag, permits easier movement of instruments and the IOL through the OVD mass. Because of the concentric partitioning of the anterior chamber into two different OVD filled spaces, the unfolding of the IOL in the central lower-viscosity dispersive filled space transmits less force into the surrounding higher-viscosity cohesive OVD filled space, than would occur with either type of viscoelastic alone. As a consequence IOL implantation is achieved through a much better stabilised anterior chamber, and the tendency for a haptic to catch on the iris or posterior capsular folds, or to be reluctant to drop into the capsular bag, is greatly reduced. Furthermore, the anterior chamber, iris and capsular bag are all more stable during IOL implantation. The incision is enlarged, if necessary, to the appropriate size to allow implantation of the selected IOL after both OVDs have been injected. Once the lens has been implanted, the OVDs are aspirated from the eye. Because the lower-viscosity dispersive OVD is enveloped by the higher-viscosity cohesive, removal of both OVDs is quick and easy, similar to the experience of removing a higher-viscosity cohesive viscoelastic alone.

3.10.4
Using the Soft Shell Technique

I have been using this soft shell technique to manage difficult phacoemulsification cases, and complications, for about 15 years, using Healon or Healon GV in combination with Viscoat. The cost of using two syringes of viscoelastic for each case precluded the use of soft shell for every case. It is a bit tedious, because of the extra step involved with the extra viscoelastic syringe, but advantageous, especially in difficult cases. The more recent advent of DuoVisc (Alcon Laboratories, Fort Worth, TX), consisting of one syringe each of Provisc and Viscoat, also manufactured by Alcon, has somewhat overcome this logistical issue.

3.10.5
Application of the Soft Shell Technique to specific problems

3.10.5.1
Fuchs' Endothelial Dystrophy

In cases of Fuchs' endothelial dystrophy, the soft shell technique is performed in the usual fashion, except that no attempt is made to remove the Viscoat layer residing adjacent to the endothelium at the end of the case. Instead the patient is treated with intraocular pressure reducing agents (preferably a cholinergic) to prevent an unacceptable postoperative intraocular pressure spike [17].

3.10.5.2
Broken Zonules

The management of cases of broken zonules, whether in traumatic or congenital subluxation cases, is an example of slight modification of the soft shell technique in order to accommodate a specific area of the anterior chamber in need of protection from the turbulence of the irrigation of the phaco or I/A. In this case the lower-viscosity dispersive OVD is injected to cover the area of disinserted zonules, whereas in the routine soft shell technique the target for protection is the endothelium. As the higher-viscosity cohesive viscoelastic is injected behind the lower-viscosity dispersive, the AC is pressurised, and any protruding vitreous is pushed backwards, along with some of the lower-viscosity dispersive OVD, away from the area of the planned phacoemulsification procedure. A capsular tension ring is inserted into the capsular bag to preserve the relationships just created with the OVDs, and further enhance the safety of the procedure. As the phaco is begun, the higher-viscosity cohesive OVD is aspirated out, but the lower-viscosity dispersive remains behind to isolate and protect the vitreous surface in the area of the broken zonules.

3.10.5.3
A Small Hole in the Posterior Capsule

Sometimes, during phaco, a small round hole is punched in the posterior capsule. In this case, the following is done. First the surgeon must examine the hole and be sure that there it has a smooth round border. If not, a posterior capsulorhexis should be completed under viscoelastic, using the soft shell technique, by first covering the area with lower-viscosity dispersive OVD, and then filling the AC with a higher-viscosity cohesive OVD without pressure (pressure could extend the tear). Then the posterior capsulorhexis is done with forceps. Once the boundary of the hole is determined to be intact and continuous, more higher-viscosity cohesive viscoelastic is gently injected to slightly pressurise the AC, as this serves to push any protruding vitreous back through the hole, along with some of the lower-viscosity dispersive OVD. Subsequently, now that the AC and capsular bag have been stabilised, the phaco and I/A can be completed under low flow conditions.

3.10.5.4
Frayed Iris Strands

The problem of how to deal with a piece of unintentionally frayed iris, or any other semi-attached fragment in the anterior chamber is not dissimilar to the problem of disinserted zonules. The area of frayed iris is covered with the lower-viscosity dispersive viscoelastic, and the higher-viscosity cohesive viscoelastic is injected behind it to pressurise the AC and move the tail of frayed iris out of the way. When the phaco is recommenced, the higher-viscosity cohesive OVD comes out with the fluid flow, but the lower-viscosity dispersive remains behind to isolate and protect the area of frayed iris strands.

3.10.5.5
Other Problems

With a bit of thought, given the above examples, the surgeon can apply the principles of the viscoelastic soft shell technique to deal better with other problems that may arise during surgery. The surgeon must simply keep in mind that the lower-viscosity dispersive OVD is used to isolate and protect an area of concern, whereas the higher viscosity cohesive is used to create and preserve spaces, and to pressurise. The cohesive will rapidly be aspirated out, once phaco is recommenced, while the dispersive will largely remain where it was placed.

3.11
Viscoadaptives – Healon5

3.11.1
Development

The viscoelastic soft shell technique was introduced to avoid the detriments of both classes of OVDs by using one viscoelastic, from each of the two major classes, sequentially, in a logical system that takes advantage of the best properties of each type of OVD, while avoiding the problems associated with each, when used alone. The disadvantage of the soft shell technique is that it requires the use of two separate syringes of OVDs which must be used sequentially, with correct sequence and precise positioning, instead of a single OVD syringe, thus increasing cost and inconvenience. There is the risk that the wrong one may be injected first, a problem that can require additional steps to correct, and may negate some of the advantages of the soft shell technique. Healon5, "the world's first viscoadaptive", was the first OVD to be designed rheologically. The desired rheologic parameters were determined based upon what was thought to be optimal for modern phacoemulsification surgery at the turn of the Millenium, and rheologic knowledge of hyaluronic acid solutions was used to engineer about 20 "candidate formulations," which were then extensively tested in masked trials of simulated phacoemulsification, before the final version

was chosen. The goal of the exercise was to create a highly viscous OVD that possessed the best properties of Healon GV (generally considered to be the best of the super viscous cohesive OVDs), but was also highly retentive in the anterior chamber throughout all the steps of phacoemulsification (higher-viscosity cohesive viscoelastics generally have poorer retention than dispersive viscoelastics), at least as well as the best of the lower-viscosity dispersive OVDs, thus conforming to our current concept of an "ideal" viscoelastic. The world-wide launch of Healon5 was at the European Society of Cataract and Refractive Surgery meeting, Nice, France, on September 7, 1998. Other competitive viscoadaptives have appeared since then (IVisc Phaco, MicroVisc Phaco and BD MultiVisc, all manufactured by Bohus Biotech). It can be seen from Table 3.1 that viscoadaptives have the highest zero shear viscosities of any OVDs yet marketed. Like Healon GV and Healon, Healon5 and other viscoadaptives are very pseudoplastic (see Fig. 3.2), making injection into the anterior chamber through a small bore cannula similar, with respect to required force and feedback sensation, to Healon GV. The molecular weight of viscoadaptives has not been increased, but their concentrations have. It is the increased concentration of hyaluronic acid at this high molecular weight, that allows viscoadaptives to display their unique characteristics. Not only does increasing concentration affect zero shear viscosity, but, in addition, given constant molecular mass, ophthalmic OVDs will appear to the surgeon to be more dispersive as concentration is increased, and will exhibit increased retention during surgery. I will discuss design issues of viscoadaptives, using Healon5 as the example, as it was first. The problem in the design of Healon5 was the fact that all preceding higher-viscosity cohesive ophthalmic viscoelastics were very good at space creation and maintenance, but sometimes, in a long or complicated surgical case, tended to come out of the eye, in a bolus, too early in the procedure. The essence of Healon5 is it's rheological idiosyncrasy that makes it unique in being both very highly viscous cohesive and retentive. Figure 3.5 illustrates the outstanding characteristic of Healon5. The attribute of the surgical environ-

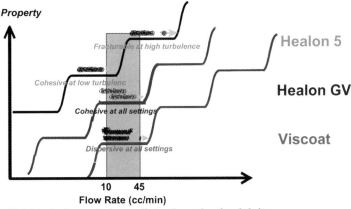

Property

Fracturable at high turbulence

Cohesive at low turbulence

Cohesive at all settings

Dispersive at all settings

Healon 5

Healon GV

Viscoat

10   45

Flow Rate (cc/min)

Fluid turbulence in immediate viscoelastic vicinity

Fig. 3.5. The response of Healon5 to turbulence. Healon GV and Viscoat retain their respective cohesive and dispersive natures over the normal range of fluid turbulence to which they are exposed in cataract surgery, with fluid flow rates rarely going below 10 cc/min and rarely exceeding 45 cc/min. Healon5 is uniquely viscoadaptive in that it becomes fracturable (like a solid), as a consequence of its extremely high viscosity and cohesion, at flow rates around 25 cc/min (in the middle of the surgical range), thus allowing surgeons to merely turn up the flow rate to make it behave in a fracturable, pseudo-dispersive fashion. Similarly, compartmentalisation of the anterior chamber (for example by working in the capsular bag, beneath an intact capsulorhexis, will yield differential flow rates above and below the capsulorhexis, and cause fracturing of Healon5 at the pupil plane. This is the "viscoadaptive" behaviour of Healon5

ment that causes stress to be placed upon OVDs is fluid turbulence. Because the ultrasonic phaco energy itself is felt only for a very short distance from the phaco tip, the OVD present remote from the immediate vicinity of the phaco tip remains unaffected by the power used. Fluid turbulence, however, as well as being an important factor in potential endothelial damage, is roughly constant throughout the anterior chamber during phaco, except when the phaco or I/A tip is kept within the capsular bag behind an intact capsulorhexis. Lower-viscosity dispersive OVDs behave as dispersives over the entire range of fluid turbulence normally encountered in the AC during cataract surgery. Similarly higher-viscosity cohesive viscoelastics behave as viscous devices over the entire range of turbulence normally encountered. Both of these classes are therefore appropriately named, because their behaviour is consistent, under the conditions that we expose them to. Healon5 is referred to as viscoadaptive because under conditions of low turbulence it behaves just like a super viscous cohesive device, whereas when the turbulence is increased Healon5 fractures into smaller pieces and therefore somewhat mimics the behaviour of dispersive viscoelastics, but in a different way, referred to as pseudo-dispersion [15]. What actually happens as OVDs are made ever more viscous and cohesive from, for example, Ocucoat to Viscoat to Healon to Healon GV to Healon5, is that they begin to approach the properties of solids somewhat, and start to become brittle or fracturable. This is somewhat analogous to what happens to viscous chocolate pudding when it is placed in the refrigerator for varying periods of time. If tested after different periods of cooling, the pudding will be found to have become more and more viscous, until it reaches a point when it appears to be almost solid, but a spoon inserted into it can very easily fracture out a piece, which can be extracted with a relatively solid mound of pudding sitting on the spoon. The unique fracturable quality of Healon5 is what makes it viscoadaptive. What it means at the molecular level, is that the inter-chain hydrogen bonding secondary to the intertwining of the chains, is stronger than the intrachain carbon–carbon bonds, preventing the deformation seen when less viscous OVDs are exposed to stress. This fracturability, exhibiting different characteristics post-fracture than before, is what allows Healon5 to be used throughout surgery as a highly viscous-cohesive OVD, somewhat like Healon GV, except that it can be fractured to improve retention during phaco, or for removal. Healon5 can be broken at the iris plane and the cataract procedure can be carried out in the capsular bag, while the anterior chamber, exposed to lower flow and protected from turbulence by an intact capsular bag, can remain full of Healon5, yielding superlative protection of the endothelial cells. On the other hand, when removal from the anterior chamber is desired, we need only turn up the flow rate to fracture the viscoelastic matrix, rotate the I/A tip so that an infusion port is directed up into the OVD mass, and use high vacuum to aspirate the viscous pieces. It is the fracturable characteristic of Healon5 which allows it to be used in cases of Fuchs' endothelial dystrophy, congenital or traumatic subluxated cataracts, frayed iris, small holes in the posterior capsule, and other circumstances when tissue isolation and protection is desired. Healon5 can therefore compete with the viscoelastic soft shell technique in that it can be adapted to almost any intraocular surgical circumstance, as long as the concept of fracturability is understood and utilised properly by the operating surgeon. It should however be remembered, that during injection, Healon5 remains a large cohesive mass, and cases without an intact posterior capsule, at the time of OVD injection, will still benefit from the concomitant use of a dispersive OVD, like Viscoat, to surround and protect delicate unstable structures, before Healon5 is injected to pressurise. The author acted as a consultant to Pharmacia and Upjohn for the development of Healon5. During the process of development, we wanted to see if this type of viscoadaptive device was really superior to conventional higher viscosity cohesive and lower viscosity dispersive viscoelastics during all phases of routine cataract surgery. World leading cataract surgeons were therefore asked to take part in masked handling tests on eye bank eyes in sim-

ulated phaco surgery, using the Miyake type preparation of eye bank eyes. The cumulative results of these tests were that although Healon5 was not judged as absolutely the best at every stage of phacoemulsification, it was judged either best, or insignificantly different from the best at each and every stage of phaco surgery, whereas cohesive and dispersive viscoelastic groups both had decidedly weak performance in some aspects of phaco surgery. In fact, Healon5 is unique in having been judged as excellent for every surgical task.

3.11.1
Viscoadaptive Use in Complications

As explained above, viscoadaptives possess the unique property of being fracturable when exposed to high turbulence, giving them a desirable dual personality. Strategies of viscoelastic fracturing, instead of layering two OVDs can be used in the examples above (see Sect. 3.10) of desired partitioning of the anterior chamber into a viscoelastic filled space and an operative zone to deal with complications such as broken zonules, Fuchs' endothelial dystrophy, a piece of frayed iris, a small hole in the posterior capsule etc.

3.11.2
The Ultimate Soft Shell Technique

3.11.2.1
Why a Soft Shell Technique for Viscoadaptives?

Initial experience with viscoadaptives demonstrated, that like with any other new device, some aspects of use would present problems for some surgeons. Three areas were found to present difficulty to significant numbers of surgeons:

1. Capsulorhexis – The surgical environment of an AC full of viscoadaptive was found by many to be too viscous to work in. Many found the increased stability of the AC to be an advantage, and increasing AC pressure by increasing the amount of viscoadaptive in-

jected, allowed easy customisation of the diameter of the capsulorhexis performed. However, some found that the capsulorhexis flap gets tangled too easily in such a viscous environment

2. Hydrodissection – Filling the AC with viscoadaptive blockades the incision. When BSS is injected to perform hydrodissection, the intraocular pressure can be severely elevated before the viscoadaptive is expelled. If the OVD does not expel easily, hydrodissection becomes difficult because of the increased intraocular pressure caused by the attempted BSS injection. If the lens is unstable, as in cases of pseudoexfoliation, this increased injection pressure could be dangerous

3. Viscoadaptive removal – Viscoadaptives were designed to be fracturable. So, one of the logical places for them to fracture is on the edges of the new sharp edged IOLs, resulting in failure to remove all the OVD behind the IOL and possible undesirable severe postoperative IOP spikes. Tetz et al. had introduced the two compartment technique, suggesting that viscoadaptive can be removed behind the IOL by simply placing the I/A tip behind the lens, but not all surgeons are comfortable with that procedure, despite it having been shown to be safe, and fairly easy [29].

3.11.2.2
The Ultimate Soft Shell Technique (USST)

The first, or pre-capsulorhexis step of the USST (Fig. 3.6) is a method to blockade the cataract wound with viscoadaptive, while filling the area just above the lens surface with BSS, thus creating a situation where the eye is pressurised as if a viscoadaptive alone was used, but the resistance to surgical manoeuvres on the lenticular surface (capsulorhexis) is that of BSS. This overcomes concern (1) above with viscoadaptives, and is well described in the reference at the end of this section. To perform hydrodissection, in a low resistance environment, which is desired, the surgeon merely wiggles the hydrodissection cannula, while simultaneously slowly injecting BSS, as it enters the AC, to break out the small piece of viscoadaptive that is blockading the

wound, thus establishing free BSS irrigation and exit from the eye below the viscoadaptive mass filling the corneal concavity, and resolving the second concern above. The second step of the USST, the pre-IOL implantation step, merely involves injecting the viscoadaptive into the AC, across rather than into the capsular bag, after completion of the I/A, until the viscoadaptive begins to enter the capsular bag. At this point the wound and the capsulorhexis have been blockaded by OVD, and the OVD syringe is exchanged for the BSS syringe. BSS is injected into the capsular bag by placing the end of the cannula underneath the capsulorhexis edge, in a manner similar to what is done for hydrodissection, and continued until the bag is seen to fill, and the eye becomes fairly firm. As the IOL is inserted into the eye, the leading haptic will fall into the BSS filled capsular bag and begin to open, whereas the trailing haptic remains folded in the OVD. When the I/A is reinserted into the AC to remove the OVD, the IOL is seen to fall backwards into the BSS filled capsular bag when irrigation is engaged and the trailing haptic opens. The viscoadaptive is now entirely anterior to the IOL, in the AC, and is easily removed in about 5–10 seconds, with gentle "Rock 'n' Roll" [4, 6]. I have been using the USST for four years, and it is the easiest and safest technique of phacoemulsification that I have yet found [13].

3.11.3
Removal of Viscoadaptives

As in all innovation, the work with viscoadaptives has taught us an important lesson. Like all OVDs, Healon5, and other viscoadaptives, must be removed as completely as possible from the eye at the end of the surgical procedure to avoid unacceptable postoperative elevations of intraocular pressure. Historically, a number of studies in a Miyake lab ascertained optimal removal techniques for OVDs. "Rock 'n' Roll" had been confirmed by a comparative study of different removal techniques by Auffarth et al. in 1994 to be the most effective technique to date [19]. To remove Healon5 using the "Rock 'n' Roll" technique settings causing sufficient turbulence to achieve easy fracturing of the

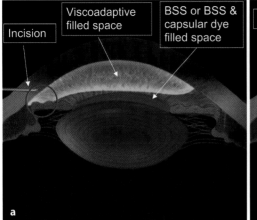

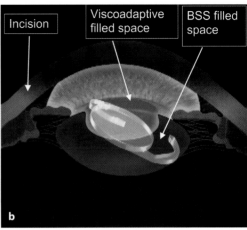

Fig. 3.6 a, b. Ultimate soft shell technique. **a** In the pre-capsulorhexis step of the USST the AC is first filled about 70% with viscoadaptive through the main incision, being sure to blockade the incision by injecting OVD as the cannula is withdrawn. Balanced salt solution is then injected through the same incision, with the tip of the cannula remote from the incision and slightly indenting the anterior lens capsule, until the eye begins to become firm. The capsulorhexis is performed with the resistance of water, but the AC is pressurised as if only viscoadaptive was being used. After completion of the capsulorhexis, the BSS cannula is again introduced, but this time wiggled as the eye is entered, slowly injecting BSS all the time, which breaks out the small piece of OVD in the *red circle*, permitting free circulation of BSS under the viscoadaptive protective dome. When it is desired to use capsular dyes, the dye is gently painted over the capsular surface, before the BSS injection step. Very little trypan blue is required, about one drop, and the subsequent injection of the BSS visually clears the field, making capsulorhexis easy in these otherwise difficult cases. **b** In the pre-IOL implantation step of the USST, after completion of the phaco and I/A, viscoadaptive is injected into the eye, across the capsulorhexis, not into it. When the AC begins to fill, OVD is seen to begin to enter the capsular bag. At that point injection stops, and the BSS cannula is retrieved. BSS is injected into the capsular bag, by placing the tip of the cannula under the capsulorhexis edge, in the same manner as is done with hydrodissection. As BSS fills the capsular bag, the bag is seen to distend, and the OVD moves upwards out of the bag toward the incision. As the eye begins to become firm, injection stops. The IOL may be implanted with forceps or an injector, but I use a little more OVD, and less BSS, when implanting the IOL with forceps. When an injector is used, the leading IOL haptic is observed to open as it enters the BSS filled capsular bag. The trailing haptic, however, remains folded, as it remains in viscoadaptive. When the I/A is reinserted to begin OVD removal, the trailing haptic is observed to fall into the bag and open as soon as irrigation is begun, thus pressurising the eye. All of the viscoadaptive is now in front of the IOL and can be removed in less than 10 s with gentle "Rock 'n' Roll"

Healon5 matrix, are necessary. This technique takes less than 30 seconds with Healon5, but as with all viscoelastics, the end point is complete removal, and not any time period: the time estimate being only a general guide. The two compartment technique (TCT) of Tetz [29], and the ultimate soft shell technique (USST) [13] have proved to be more effective and popular viscoadaptive removal techniques than simple "Rock 'n' Roll". When Healon5 first appeared, severe postoperative IOP spikes were reported when it was incompletely removed, but it has since been shown that postop IOP spikes are a function of incomplete removal, and patient susceptibility, and are not significantly different with different OVDs [16].

3.12
Conclusion

The purpose of this chapter is to inspire interest in how an understanding of physical mechanics of OVDs, in the practice of ophthalmic surgery, can enable the development of newer, better OVDs and viscosurgical techniques, enhance the surgeon's skills, the likelihood of operative success, and the patient's safety. Phacoemulsification surgery is really just a sequence of rheologic manoeuvres, because everything is done with fluid flow, and the better we understand rheology, the better our surgery will be.

Attempts to comparatively evaluate the many available OVDs have been complicated by the varying methods, units of measurement, and technologic terminology cited in technical data. Now, however, the confusion imposed by such variation is giving way to consensus and understanding as the International Standardization Organization (ISO) establishes guidelines for uniformity and precision in assuring chemical safety and presenting to the surgeon data derived from research on OVDs that is understandable and comparative, while being expressed in a manner directly comparable to methods of surgical use. That standardisation in turn assists not only in the surgeon's choice of products but also in the researchers' development of products with the rheologic and biologic properties most likely to enhance the efficacy and safety of ophthalmic surgery. Another benefit of standardisation, I hope, will be the recognition that OVDs do differ in rheologic properties that are directly relevant to clinical practice. For example, higher-viscosity cohesive OVDs and lower-viscosity dispersives are essentially different and each is especially suitable for specific operative situations. Whether or not viscoadaptives will fulfil their goal of being the ideal viscosurgical device for all surgical procedures awaits broader world-wide experience. Undoubtedly, the future will not end, and newer better OVDs await development. For now, to minimise complications and thereby to enhance surgical quality and improve outcomes, a reasonable range of a few OVD products from the different categories should be made available to ophthalmologic surgeons at all times. Healon5 was the first OVD to be designed at the rheological bench, rather than by trial and error in animal and human surgery. Surely there will be more to come.

References

1. Arshinoff S (1989) Comparative physical properties of ophthalmic viscoelastic materials. Ophthalmic Pract 7:16–37
2. Arshinoff S (1991) The physical properties of ophthalmic viscoelastics in cataract surgery. Ophthalmic Pract 9:2–7
3. Arshinoff S (1994) The safety and performance of ophthalmic viscoelastics in cataract surgery and its complications. In: Proceedings of the National Ophthalmic Speakers Program, 1993. Montreal, PQ, Medicopea
4. Arshinoff SA (1996) Rock 'n' Roll removal of Healon GV (video). In: American Society of Cataract and Refractive Surgery Film Festival, Seattle, Washington
5. Arshinoff SA (1996) Soft shell' technique uses 2 types of viscoelastics to achieve good results. In: Reported by Harvey Black. Ocul Surg News
6. Arshinoff SA (1997) Rock 'n' Roll removal of Healon GV. In: Proceedings of the 7th annual National Ophthalmic Speakers Program, Ottawa, Canada, June 1996. Medicopea, Montreal, Canada
7. Arshinoff S (1998) Dispersive and cohesive viscoelastic materials in phacoemulsification revisited 1998. Ophthalmic Pract 16:24–32
8. Arshinoff SA (1998) Healon5 entering selected countries in Europe. Ocul Surg News 9:11–12
9. Arshinoff SA (1998) Myths and facts about viscoelastics. Ophthalmol Manage Nov, pp 48–52
10. Arshinoff SA (1999) Dispersive-cohesive viscoelastic soft shell technique. J Cataract Refract Surg 25:167–173
11. Arshinoff SA (1998) Healon5. In: Buratto L, Giardini P, Bellucci R (eds) Viscoelastics in ophthalmic surgery. Slack, Thorofare, NJ, pp 24–32
12. Arshinoff S (1999) The unusual rheology of viscoadaptives, and why it matters. Video. In: American Society of Cataract and Refractive Surgery Film Festival, Seattle, Washington., April 10–14
13. Arshinoff SA (2002) Using BSS with viscoadaptives in the ultimate soft-shell technique. J Cataract Refract Surg 28:1509–1514
14. Arshinoff SA, Hofman I (1998) Prospective, randomized trial comparing Micro-Visc Plus and Healon GV in routine phacoemulsification. J Cataract Refract Surg 24:814–820
15. Arshinoff SA, Wong E (2003) Understanding, retaining, and removing dispersive and pseudo-dispersive ophthalmic viscosurgical devices. J Cataract Refract Surg 29:2318–2323
16. Arshinoff SA, Albiani DA, Taylor-Laporte J (2002) Intraocular pressure after bilateral cataract surgery using Healon, Healon5, and Healon GV. J Cataract Refract Surg 28:617–625

17. Arshinoff SA, Calogero DX, Bilotta R, Eydelman M, Haber S, Hadi H, Senft S (1999) Post operative IOP, endothelial cell counts, and pachymetry after viscoelastic use in cataract surg (in press). Presented in parts by S. Senft at the Amer Soc Cataract Refract Surgery annual meetings San Diego, April 1998, and Seattle, April 1999

18. Assia EI, Apple DJ, Lim ES, Morgan RC, Tsai JC (1992) Removal of viscoelastic materials after experimental cataract surgery in vitro. J Cataract Refract Surg 18:3–6

19. Auffarth GU WT, Solomon K et al (1994) Evaluation of different removal techniques of a high-viscosity viscoelastic. J Cataract Refract Surg. In: ASCRS Symposium on Cataract, IOL, and Refractive Surgery, Boston

20. Balazs E (1986) Viscosurgery: features of a true viscosurgical tool and its role in ophthalmic surgery. Montreal, PQ, Medicopea, pp 121–128

21. Balazs EA MD, Stegmann R (1979) Viscosurgery and the use of ultrapure Na-hyaluronate in intraocular lens implantation. In: Paper presented at the International Congress and First Film Festival on Intraocular Lens Implantation, Cannes, France

22. International Standards Organization ISO 15798 (2001) Ophthalmic implants – Ophthalmic viscosurgical devices

23. Koster R, Stilma JS (1986) Comparison of vitreous replacement with Healon and with HPMC in rabbits' eyes. Doc Ophthalmol 61:247–253

24. Madsen K SU, Apple DJ, Harfstand A (1989) Histochemical and receptor binding studies of hyaluronic acid binding sites on corneal endothelium. Ophthalmic Pract 7:92–97

25. Poyer JF, Chan KY, Arshinoff SA (1998) New method to measure the retention of viscoelastic agents on a rabbit corneal endothelial cell line after irrigation and aspiration. J Cataract Refract Surg 24:84–90

26. Poyer JF, Chan KY, Arshinoff SA (1998) Quantitative method to determine the cohesion of viscoelastic agents by dynamic aspiration. J Cataract Refract Surg 24:1130–1135

27. Siegel MJ, Spiro HJ, Miller JA, Siegel LI (1991) Secondary glaucoma and uveitis associated with Orcolon. Arch Ophthalmol 109:1496–1498

28. Arshinoff Steve A (1996) The dispersive/cohesive viscoelastic soft shell technique for compromised corneas and anterior chamber compartmentalization. In: American Society of Cataract and Refractive Surgery Film Festival, June 1–5, Seattle, Washington

29. Tetz MR, Holzer MP (2000) Two-compartment technique to remove ophthalmic viscosurgical devices. J Cataract Refract Surg 26:641–643

Foldable Intraocular Lenses

Liliana Werner, Nick Mamalis

Core Messages

- Foldable intraocular lenses are manufactured from silicone or acrylic (hydrophobic or hydrophilic) biomaterials, in three-piece or single-piece designs. Single-piece lenses can be found in plate configurations, or with two or more haptic components
- The most important isolated IOL design feature for prevention of posterior capsule opacification is the square, truncated optic edge. This feature has been incorporated to foldable IOLs manufactured from silicone, hydrophobic acrylic and hydrophilic acrylic biomaterials
- Foldable silicone and acrylic lenses are also available in designs providing special features. These include multifocality and toric corrections, lenses with a modified prolate profile to compensate for the corneal spherical aberration, yellow lenses to protect the retina against blue light rays, accommodative lenses, lenses that can be inserted through sub 1.5-mm incisions, and light adjustable power lenses

4.1
Introduction and Brief Overview of Biomaterials Used for the Manufacture of Foldable Intraocular Lenses

Although sporadic early attempts to implant foldable intraocular lenses (IOLs) probably occurred in the 1970s, in general the development of small incision lenses occurred in the past two decades [3]. More recently, the majority of effort and funding appears to be spent on the development of complex foldable IOLs that not only restore the refractive power of the eye after cataract extraction through small incisions, but also provide some special features. These include multifocality, toric corrections, pseudoaccommodation, and postoperative adjustment of the IOL refractive power, among others [46].

In this text we present an overview of foldable IOL designs, focusing on modern lenses that are currently available or under investigation. Our intention is to provide a general scan of the subject, which is therefore not intended to be an exhaustive list. For some of these lenses, formal peer-reviewed publications are not yet available. The information provided is sometimes based on non peer-reviewed publications, advertising material, or preliminary results from experimental studies performed in our laboratory. Some of the designs discussed in this chapter are not yet approved by the United States Food and Drug Administration (FDA).

Biomaterials (polymers) currently used for the manufacture of IOL optics can be divided into two major groups, namely acrylic and silicone [13, 25, 40, 41]. Acrylic lenses can be further divided as follows:

– Rigid, e.g. manufactured from poly(methyl methacrylate) (PMMA)
– Foldable, manufactured from hydrophobic acrylic materials, or from hydrophilic acrylics also known as hydrogels

Polymerization is the process by which the repeating units of monomers linked by covalent stable bonds form a polymer. Three-dimensional, flexible acrylic polymers can be created by a process known as cross-linking. When different monomers are polymerized together, the process is called copolymerization. Each currently available foldable acrylic lens design is manufactured from a different copolymer acrylic, with a different refractive index, glass transition temperature (above this temperature the polymer exhibits flexible properties and below it remains rigid), water content, and mechanical properties, etc.

Silicones are known chemically as polysiloxanes based on their silicon-oxygen molecular backbone, which confers mechanical flexibility to the materials. Pendant to the silicone backbone are organic groups, which determine mechanical and optical properties. The first silicone material used in the manufacture of IOLs was poly(dimethyl siloxane), which has a refractive index of 1.41. Poly(dimethyl diphenyl siloxane) is a later generation silicone IOL material that has a higher refractive index than poly(dimethyl siloxane) (1.46). While foldable acrylics display glass transition temperatures at around room temperature, the glass transition temperature of silicones can be significantly below room temperature. Acrylic lenses in general unfold in a more controlled manner, while silicone lenses have the tendency to rapidly spring open. Another differentiating property between foldable acrylics and silicones is the refractive index, which is higher in the first group (1.47 or greater) so acrylic lenses are thinner than silicone lenses for the same refractive power.

Other important elements of the IOL optic component are represented by the ultraviolet-absorbing compounds (chromophores). These are incorporated into the IOL optic in order to protect the retina from ultraviolet radiation in the 300–400 nm range, a protection normally provided by the crystalline lens. In general, two classes of ultraviolet-absorbing chromophores are used for the manufacture of pseudophakic IOLs: benzotriazole and benzophenone. Four materials are currently being used for the manufacture of the haptic component (loops) of three-piece foldable lenses: PMMA, polypropylene (Prolene), polyimide (Elastimide) and poly(vinylidene) fluoride (PVDF). Polypropylene is less rigid than PMMA, polyimide and PVDF. We have recently performed a laboratory study comparing the shape recovery ratios after compression of three-piece silicone lenses with haptics manufactured from these four materials. The three later materials exhibited similar loop memories, which were found to be higher than that of polypropylene [19].

Summary for the Clinician

• Currently available intraocular lenses are manufactured from silicone and acrylic (hydrophobic or hydrophilic) biomaterials
• Acrylic lenses in general unfold in a more controlled manner, and have higher refractive indexes than silicone lenses

4.2
Silicone Intraocular Lenses

4.2.1
Plate Intraocular Lenses

Development of single-piece soft IOL designs, including plate lenses, began in the 1970s and early 1980s. By the late 1980s, the design and manufacture had markedly improved and modern foldable silicone plate lenses, first characterized by the presence of small positioning holes on either side of the optic (0.3 mm in diameter), emerged (Fig. 4.1a) [3]. These became very popular, because they were relatively easy to insert using an injector through a small incision. The designs with small holes are now considered obsolete and have been replaced by silicone lenses with larger fenestrations (1.15 mm in diameter).

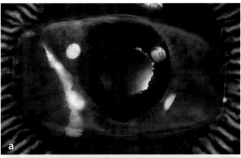

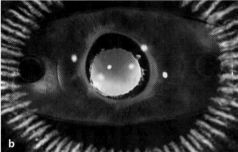

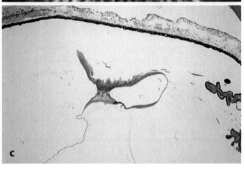

Fig. 4.1 a–c. Silicone plate lenses. **a, b** Gross photographs from a posterior or Miyake-Apple view of human eyes obtained postmortem implanted with a silicone plate small hole lens (**a**), and a silicone plate large hole lens (**b**). **c** Photomicrograph illustrating the growth of fibrocellular tissue through the large fenestrations of a silicone plate large hole lens, which should ensure better lens fixation (Masson's trichrome stain; X40)

These latter have been incorporated to enhance postoperative lens fixation, as fibrous adhesions occur between the anterior and posterior capsules through the holes to lock the lens to the equator of the capsular bag, assuring optic centration and long-term stability (Fig. 4.1b,c) [22, 50].

Silicone plate lenses available in the US are basically manufactured by Staar Surgical (Elastic Lens, Monrovia, CA), and Bausch & Lomb Surgical (Rochester, NY). Staar also uses the platform of the silicone plate lens with large holes for the manufacture of toric lenses (see Sect. 4.4.2). A similar design is used for lenses manufactured from the Collamer material (see Sect. 4.3.2). The biconvex optic of silicone plate lenses is 5.5 or 6.0 mm in diameter, and lenses with an overall length of 10.5, 10.8 or 11.2 mm are available.

4.2.2
Three-Piece Intraocular Lenses

The optic component of currently available three-piece silicone lenses is, in general, manufactured from silicone materials with a refractive index higher than those of silicone plate lenses. Thus three-piece lenses are thinner for the same refractive power. There is a manufacturer tendency to use haptic materials that are relatively rigid, with good material memory, such as PMMA, polyimide or PVDF (Fig. 4.2). Studies have demonstrated that anterior capsule opacification/fibrosis is more significant with silicone lenses, especially the plate designs, due to the larger area of contact between the biomaterial and the inner surface of the anterior capsule [43, 44]. In the case of the three-piece designs, haptics with appropriate rigidity provide better resistance to postoperative contraction forces within the capsular bag, preventing lens decentration in cases of asymmetric capsule fibrosis/contraction.

Another recent manufacturing tendency is the incorporation of square optic edges to silicone lenses. This is probably the most important isolated design feature for posterior capsule opacification (PCO) prevention, regardless of the biomaterial used for the lens [6, 24, 35]. Examples of square-edged silicone lenses are the CeeOn Edge IOL, model 911 (Pfizer Global Pharmaceuticals, Peapack, NJ), and the ClariFlex with OptiEdge (Advanced Medical Optics, Santa Ana, CA). The first is a three-piece silicone optic-PVDF haptic lens, in a cap C haptic design with a 90° exit and an angulation of 6°. The sec-

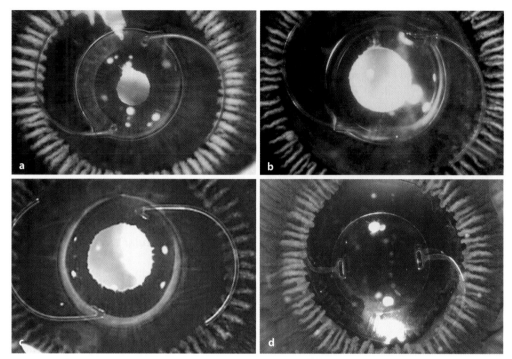

Fig. 4.2. a–d. Gross photographs from a posterior or Miyake-Apple view of human eyes obtained postmortem implanted with three-piece silicone lenses. **a** SI30 (AMO), with Prolene haptics. **b** SI40 (AMO), with PMMA haptics. **c** AQ2003 V (Staar), with Elastimide haptics. **d** CeeOn Edge (Pfizer), with PVDF haptics

ond is a three-piece silicone optic-PMMA haptic lens, in a modified-C haptic design with an angulation of 10°. The OptiEdge technology incorporated to the ClariFlex lens is described in details in Sect. 4.3.1.

Summary for the Clinician

• Anterior capsule opacification is more significant with silicone lenses, especially the plate designs
• Silicone lenses with square, truncated posterior optic edges for the prevention of posterior capsule opacification are also available

4.3
Acrylic Intraocular Lenses

4.3.1
Hydrophobic Acrylic Intraocular Lenses

The first hydrophobic acrylic lens introduced on the market (December 1994) was the three-piece AcrySof (Alcon Laboratories, Fort Worth, TX). Some of the characteristics of the currently available three-piece AcrySof designs are provided in Table 4.1. The optic component of the lenses is manufactured from a material with a contact angle in water of 73°, made of a copolymer of phenylethyl acrylate and phenylethyl methacrylate, crosslinked with butanediol diacrylate. The material has the highest refractive index available (1.55). The haptics of the lenses are made of blue-coloured PMMA in a modified-C design. The lenses can be implanted with

Table 4.1. Characteristics of the currently available AcrySof intraocular lenses

Model	Optic diameter	Overall length	Haptic angle	A-constant	Power range
MA30AC	5.5 mm	12.5 mm	5°	118.4	+10 to +30
MA60AC	6.0 mm	13 mm	10°	118.4	+6 to +30
MA50BM	6.5 mm	13 mm	10°	118.9	+6 to +30
MA60MA	6.0 mm	13.0 mm	5°	118.9	–5 to +5
SA60AT	6.0 mm	13.0 mm	–	118.4	+6 to +40
SA30AT	5.5 mm	13.0 mm	–	118.4	+10 to +30
SA30AL	5.5 mm	12.5	–	118.4	+10 to +30

MA, three-piece models; SA, single-piece models

forceps, or injected with the Monarch II IOL delivery system.

The AcrySof lens was also the first lens manufactured with square optic edges, a design feature that was proved to be associated with lower rates of PCO (Fig. 4.3 a, b). The square edge creates a barrier where it maintains contact with the posterior capsule, preventing migration of cells from the equatorial region of the capsular bag onto the central posterior capsule. In a study on pseudophakic human eyes obtained postmortem, the three-piece AcrySof IOL with square optic edges was associated with the lower Nd:YAG posterior capsulotomy rates [4]. In other studies on cadaver eyes, this lens was also associated with the lower rates of anterior capsule opacification (ACO) [44, 43]. Some studies suggest that the adhesive nature of the AcrySof material also plays a role in the maintenance of the clarity of the capsular bag. The "sandwich" theory states that IOLs having a bioadhesive surface would allow only a monolayer of lens epithelial cells to attach to the capsule and the IOL, preventing further cell proliferation and capsular bag opacification [26]. Recent studies performed in our laboratory revealed that this bioadhesion, in the case of AcrySof lenses is mostly mediated by fibronectin [27, 28].

The occurrence of glistenings has been described in association with the AcrySof material. In vitro studies have suggested that it may be related to variations in the temperature (Δt), with formation of vacuoles within the submersed acrylic polymer when there is a transient increase in temperature above the glass transition temperature, approximately 18.5 °C for AcrySof. Clinical studies on this lens have demonstrated that contrast sensitivity has been decreased to a small degree in some patients, but clinically significant decrease on visual acuity has been rare [16].

The one-piece AcrySof lens (Alcon Laboratories, Fort Worth, TX), model SA30AL was approved by the FDA in 1999, but was semi-officially launched at the 2000 ASCRS Symposium on Cataract, IOL and Refractive Surgery, in Boston [11, 15]. Three models are currently available (Table 4.1). The single-piece AcrySof has square, truncated optic and haptic edges, which present a "velvet" finishing (Consistent Edge Technology); it is claimed to reduce the glare phenomenon that has been described in association with IOLs having square optic edges and a high refractive index. This lens has the modified "L" shape of Alcon's previous one-piece "slimplant" PMMA IOLs, rather than the Sinskey-style appearance of three-piece foldable IOLs to which we have become accustomed. It has solid extended haptics that are made of the same acrylic copolymer as the optic. The haptics are more flexible than the traditional three-piece acrylic foldable design, and are purported to retain the same good memory. The haptics of three-piece lenses often create striae by applying pressure to the edges of the capsular bag. In addition to the undesired optical effects, striae can create a pathway for the migration of lens epithelial cells and increase the risk for PCO formation. The haptics of the single-piece AcrySof have increased the IOL

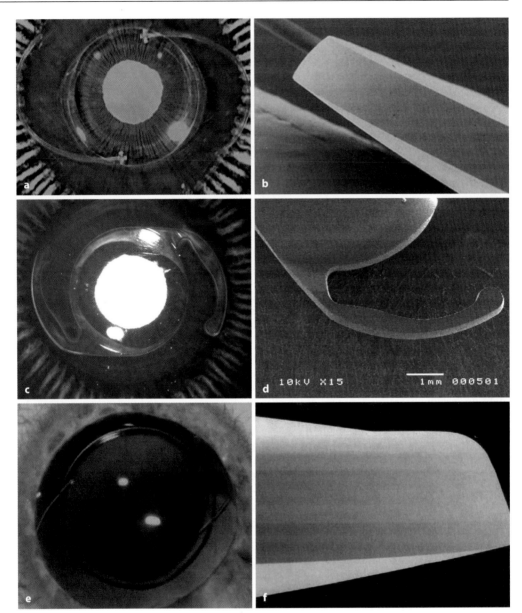

Fig. 4.3. a–f. Hydrophobic acrylic lenses. **a** Three-piece AcrySof lens in a human eye obtained postmortem (posterior or Miyake-Apple view). **b** Scanning electron microscopy showing the square optic edge of the same design as in (**a**). **c** Single-piece AcrySof lens in a human eye obtained postmortem (posterior or Miyake-Apple view). **d** Scanning electron microscopy showing the square optic and haptic edges of the same design as in (**c**). **e** Clinical photograph of a patient implanted with the Sensar lens (courtesy of AMO). **f** Scanning electron microscopy showing the characteristics of the OptiEdge design

surface contact area, resulting in fewer posterior capsule wrinkles and excellent centration (Fig. 4.3 c,d).

Because of the memory and flexibility of the AcrySof material, the haptics can literally be bent back on themselves, twisted and contorted to a much greater degree than PMMA haptics. They conform to the equatorial region of the capsular bag instead of pushing into it like the PMMA haptic design. The single-piece design is strong enough not to break or permanently deform when folded or squeezed through an injector or a tight incision. In this respect it has an advantage over the three-piece IOLs, which occasionally suffer permanent haptic deformation under the stress of implantation. This IOL was solely designed for capsular implantation. It should be used only with both an intact capsulorhexis and intact bag, because of the very flexible nature of the haptics, which unfold slowly like the IOL. The optic-haptic angulation is planar. The optic is biconvex; the convexity of the posterior surface is fixed and that of the anterior surface varies according to the IOL power. The single-piece can be implanted either with forceps or the Alcon Monarch II injector.

We recently accessioned the first 14 pseudophakic human eyes obtained postmortem implanted with this IOL design [20]. From a posterior or Miyake-Apple view, all the lenses showed excellent centration. According to our scoring methods, central and peripheral PCO, Soemmering's ring formation and ACO were only minimal. Also, histopathological analyses of these specimens demonstrated the barrier effect of the square edge, and the presence of "sandwich" structures, composed of the anterior or posterior capsules, a monolayer of lens epithelial cells and the IOL.

The single-piece AcrySof platform is being used for the manufacture of three different lenses with special features (see Sect. 4.4). The ReSTOR is a multifocal diffractive lens; model SA60TT was designed to provide toric corrections, and the AcrySof Natural (SN60AT) contains a covalently bonded, blue light-filtering chromophore, which more closely mimics the light transmission spectrum of the pre-cataractous adult human crystalline lens.

The other currently available hydrophobic acrylic lens is the Sensar lens with the OptiEdge Technology (Advanced Medical Optics, Santa Ana, CA), approved by the FDA and introduced on the US market in February 2000. The optic component of the lens is manufactured from a material with a contact angle in water of 88°, made of a copolymer of ethyl acrylate and ethyl methacrylate. The material has a refractive index of 1.47. The haptics of the lens are made of blue-coloured PMMA in a modified-C design, with an optic-haptic angulation of 5°. The optical diameter of the lens is 6.0 mm and the overall diameter is 13.0 mm. Implantation with the Unfolder Sapphire Series implantation system is recommended.

The hydrophobic acrylic copolymer used for the manufacture of this lens is stated to be "vacuoles free." An in vitro study comparing glistening formation induced by temperature among hydrophobic acrylic lenses available in the US has recently been published [18]. The authors confirmed that glistening quantity varied among hydrophobic acrylic lenses and was temperature dependent. Glistening quantity observed with the Sensar lens in the same study was more stable than with the other IOL types upon cooling.

The Sensar lens with the OptiEdge technology is the successor model of the Sensar IOL, which had smooth, slightly rounded edges to scatter internal reflections and eliminate glare. The new OptiEdge design (also incorporated to the ClariFlex design; see Sect. 4.2.2) combines three elements: a rounded anterior edge, a sloping side edge and a sharp, vertical posterior edge (Fig. 4.3 e, f). The rounded anterior edge was designed to minimize glare. It spreads out rays that pass through its surface and disperses light rays reflected from the edge. The sloping side edge is designed to reduce the area of the surface that can cause internal reflections and to scatter internal reflections away from the retina. The squared posterior optic rim design has proven to be effective in the prevention of PCO. Thus, the new Sensar lens with OptiEdge was designed to reduce the occurrence of PCO, without introducing unwanted internal glare symptoms (dysphotopsia).

A clinical study by Buehl et al. [10] confirmed that incorporation of the OptiEdge with a sharp posterior edge design led to significantly less PCO 1 year postoperatively in comparison to the previous rounded-edge Sensar. Also, implantation of currently available single-piece and three-piece hydrophobic acrylic lenses in rabbit eyes showed no statistically significant difference among the groups of lenses, with regard to PCO formation [47].

4.3.2
Hydrophilic Acrylic (Hydrogel) Intraocular Lenses

Foldable hydrophilic acrylic (hydrogel) IOLs have been marketed by several firms for several years in international markets [46]. Many surgeons have adopted the use of hydrophilic acrylic IOLs because of their easier-handling properties and biocompatibility, with low inflammatory cytological response. Most of the currently available hydrophilic acrylic lenses are manufactured from different copolymer acrylics with water content ranging from 18% to 38%, and an incorporated UV absorber. They are packaged in a vial containing distilled water or a balanced salt solution, thus being already implanted in the hydrated state and in their final dimensions. Hydration renders these lenses flexible, enabling the surgeons to fold and insert/inject them through small incisions. In the past 2 years, we have been witnessing an increasing introduction of hydrophilic acrylic posterior chamber lenses in international markets. Different companies, mostly European, are manufacturing lenses from hydrophilic acrylic materials in a great variety of designs. They are, in general, single-piece plate lenses, some of which have clearly defined three or four fixation points to the capsular bag.

One of the US manufactured hydrophilic acrylic designs is the Hydroview lens, manufactured by Bausch and Lomb (Rochester, NY). The optic material of the lens is composed of a cross-linked copolymer of 2-hydroxyethyl methacrylate and 6-hydroxyhexyl methacrylate, with a bonded benzotriazole-type UV absorber. The water content of this material is 18%

and the refractive index is 1.474. The haptics are modified-C loops made of blue-coloured PMMA, polymerically cross-linked with the optics by means of an interpenetrating polymer network, which provides a one-piece design with a true optic zone of 6.0 mm (Fig. 4.4a) [46]. Its launch in the US was postponed because of reports of calcium precipitation on its surfaces, clustered in some centres [42]. An in vitro model, according to the manufacturer, revealed a migration of silicone from a gasket in the lens packaging (SureFold system) onto the surface of the IOL. The experimental model also showed that, in addition to silicone, fatty acids had to be present to attract calcium ions to the lens surface. A compromised blood–retinal barrier seemed to be associated with the appearance of calcified deposits. Changes in the packaging of the lens were performed and no cases of calcification were reported 2 years after implantation of the lenses in the modified packaging.

The MemoryLens manufactured by Ciba Vision (Duluth, GA) is the only pre-folded acrylic IOL available on the market. It can be implanted directly from the container without any requirement of folding instruments, thus reducing the surgical time. The container with the lens is kept at a temperature of 8 °C. Following intraocular insertion and under the influence of body temperature, the lens unfolds slowly (approximately 15 min) providing an atraumatic and controlled implantation (Fig. 4.4b, c). The polymer used for the manufacture of the optic of this lens contains 59% of 2-hydroxyethyl methacrylate, 16% of methyl methacrylate, 4% of 4-methacryloxy 2-hydroxy benzophenone UV absorber and 1% of ethylene glycol dimethacrylate. The haptics are made of Prolene. The optic material has a water content of 20% and a refractive index of 1.473. The optic diameter of the MemoryLens is 6.0 mm, the overall length is 13.4 mm and the optic-haptic angulation is 10°. Reports on traces of a polishing compound on the MemoryLens causing postoperative inflammatory reactions in approximately 0.1% of the lenses implanted led Ciba Vision to voluntarily withdraw the lens from the market [21]. After identifying and correcting the problem, the manufacturer received

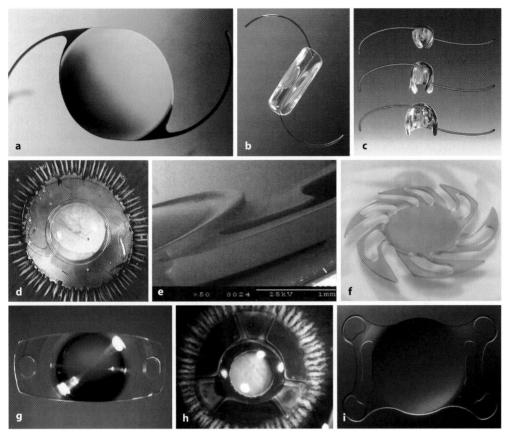

Fig. 4.4. a–i. Examples of hydrophilic acrylic lenses. **a** Gross photograph showing the Hydroview design (Bausch & Lomb). **b, c** Gross photographs showing the unfolding of the MemoryLens (Ciba Vision). **d** Experimental implantation of the CenterFlex model 570C (Rayner) in a human eye obtained postmortem, prepared according to the Miyake-Apple technique. **e** Scanning electron microscopy showing the enhanced square edge of the model 570C, at the level of the optic-haptic junction. **f** Gross photograph showing the Concept 360 (Corneal). (Courtesy of Dr. Philippe Sourdille, Nantes, France.) **g** Gross photograph showing the Acqua (Mediphacos) lens in a dry state. **h** Gross photograph of a human eye obtained postmortem implanted with the Stabibag lens, manufactured by Ioltech (La Rochelle, France). Note the fibrotic tissue formed through the holes of the haptic component, which certainly helps in the fixation of the lens (case from Dr. G. Ravalico, Trieste, Italy). **i** Gross photograph showing the Quattro lens, which was manufactured by Corneal (Pringy, France)

approval from both the US FDA and the European regulatory authorities to return the lens to the market in September 2000. Cases of surface lens calcification were also reported in association with specific lots of MemoryLens IOLs manufactured in 1999 by using a special polishing process. This has been discontinued, and no similar cases have been reported with this lens design to date.

Staar Surgical (Monrovia, CA) manufactures single-piece and three-piece foldable lenses from "Collamer," Staar's proprietary material, which is said to be highly biocompatible [8, 9]. This material is composed of a proprietary hydrophilic collagen polymer (copolymer of 63% hydroxy-ethyl-methyl-acrylate, 0.2% porcine collagen and 3.4% of a benzofenone for UV absorption), with a water content of 34%, a light transmission of 99%, and a refractive index of 1.45 at 35°C. Model CC4204BF is a plate haptic design (see Sect. 4.2.1). The overall length of the IOL is 10.8 mm with an optic diameter of 5.5 mm. The haptic component has two 0.9 mm fenestrations to help stabilize the IOL and reduce the risk of decentration. This IOL has the wound size benefits of injectable silicone foldable lenses but with intraocular unfolding characteristics closer to acrylic IOLs. Model CQ2003 V is a three-piece design, with modified-C Elastimide haptics. The overall length of the lens is 13.0 mm with an optic diameter of 6.0 mm, and no optic-haptic angulation. The high water content properties require the Collamer IOLs to be wet packed. They have a distinct, almost shiny patina that is easily seen under the slit lamp. This material is also used for the manufacture of the Staar Implantable Contact Lens (ICL).

The CenterFlex lens (model 570H; Rayner Intraocular Lenses Ltd., Brighton-Hove, East Sussex, UK) is a newly developed one-piece, hydrophilic acrylic IOL. It is not a traditional plate haptic design, but has extended loops or haptics that resemble three-piece modified-C loop IOL designs. The optic size of this lens is 5.75 mm, with an overall diameter of 12.0 mm. The CenterFlex is made of a copolymer of hydrophilic and hydrophobic methacrylates with a water content of 26%, namely 2-hydroxyethyl methacrylate and methyl methacrylate, which is the main component of PMMA. The lens material (Rayacryl) also comprises ethylene glycol dimethacrylate and a benzophenone ultraviolet absorbing agent. This lens design has been developed to provide maximum stability and centration while incorporating a square edge to the optic and the haptics. The haptics have been designed to resist an excessive or asymmetrical capsular contraction, which provides the benefit of increasing support for the lens as the capsule contracts. This also prevents dislocation due to buckling or twisting the haptics. The CenterFlex is a non-angulated lens style that can be inserted either by forceps or by the Rayner Injection System.

We recently performed a study in our laboratory on the evaluation of PCO formation after implantation of the CenterFlex lens. The results were comparable to those of the single-piece AcrySof [37]. In a second study, we compared minus power (−7 D) to regular power (+21 D) CenterFlex lenses [38]. The minus power lenses had a thicker square optic edge as well as a ridged posterior-peripheral aspect of the posterior concave optic surface that appeared to increase the barrier effect. Indeed, the minus power lenses were significantly associated with less PCO formation. The manufacturer has developed a new design of the CenterFlex lens (model 570C) incorporating the ridged posterior-peripheral aspect of the low power lenses to all dioptric powers (Fig. 4.4d,e). This created an enhanced square edge for 360 degrees around the IOL optic. This later design performed better than the standard 570H model, with regard to PCO formation in a rabbit model [48].

The Concept 360 (Corneal Laboratoire, Pringy, France) is a single-piece IOL manufactured from a foldable hydrophilic acrylic material with water content of 26%. The lens has an optical diameter of 6.0 mm, an overall diameter of 11.5 mm, and square optic and haptic edges. It can be injected through a 3.0-mm incision. The overall design is that of a disc-shaped lens, with six haptic components having a 10° posterior optic-haptic angulation. Once implanted, the periphery of the lens stays in contact with the equatorial region of the capsular bag for 360°, having the effect of a complete capsular tension ring (Fig. 4.4f). This design is also aimed at keeping the anterior capsule away from the anterior IOL optic surface in order to prevent capsular opacification and shrinkage. The square edges of the lens, in association with the maintenance of the overall geometry of the capsular bag by the capsular tension ring effect are expected to help in the prevention of PCO.

The Acqua (Mediphacos, Belo Horizonte, MG, Brazil), IOL is a single-piece plate design manufactured from a proprietary copolymer hydrophilic acrylic (Acryfil CQ) with high water content (73.5%) and an incorporated UV absorber. The refractive index of this material is 1.409. In a dry state, this IOL is 7.1 mm long and 3.2 mm wide (Fig. 4.4g). This allows its direct intraocular insertion through a small incision without folding. Once in the capsular bag the IOL material becomes hydrated. After 2–3 min the degree of expansion obtained allows for general centration of the lens inside the capsular bag. The IOL reaches its final and permanent dimensions after 20 min (10.8 mm long and 5.1 mm wide), but a complete hydration of the optic component is observed 8–24 h after implantation. The fixation holes measure 1.00 × 0.65 mm, when the lens is fully expanded. This is the only "expandable" IOL currently available on the international market. It was determined in experimental studies that this lens may absorb minimal residual amounts of trypan blue, presenting postoperative blue discoloration. Thus, it should not be implanted in cases where this capsular dye has been used for staining the anterior capsule while performing capsulorhexis [45].

Examples of other European hydrophilic acrylic designs, with three and four points of fixation are shown in Fig. 4.4 h, i.

Summary for the Clinician

- Two hydrophobic acrylic lenses are available on the market: the Alcon AcrySof (one or three-piece), and the AMO Sensar with OptiEdge (three-piece)
- Hydrophilic acrylic lenses are available in a great variety of designs, including three-piece designs, or single-piece designs in a plate configuration or with multiple haptic components

4.4
Specialized Foldable Intraocular Lenses

4.4.1
Multifocal Intraocular Lenses

Before choosing multifocal IOLs, astigmatism control and precise biometry are required, as well as careful patient selection. This is especially true because of concerns related to the possibility of higher incidence of decreased contrast sensitivity and glare with these lenses.

The Array lens (Advanced Medical Optics, AMO, Santa Ana, CA) is a three-piece multifocal IOL manufactured from a silicone material having a refractive index of 1.46. It has angulated "C" haptics made of extruded PMMA [17, 39]. It

is the first multifocal IOL approved by the FDA. The optical design of this lens is a zonal-progressive multifocal optic with five concentric zones (Fig. 4.5 a). This lens design is a distance-dominant, zonal progressive optic. The center of the lens is primarily for distance but has some near effect. All of the other zones have distance and near in different proportions – 50 % of the available light is devoted to distance vision, 13 % to intermediate vision and 37 % to near vision. No available light is lost in the lens because the optic is refractive and not diffractive. The addition for near is +3.5 dioptres.

The ReSTOR (Alcon Laboratories, Fort Worth, TX) is a diffractive multifocal IOL under investigation, manufactured by using the platform of the single-piece AcrySof design. The lens is designed so that the diffractive grating is present only in the central 3.6 mm of the optic. The largest diffractive step is at the lens centre and sends the greatest portion of energy to the near focus. As the steps move away from the centre, they gradually decrease in size, blending into the periphery, and sending a decreasing proportion of energy to the near focus (Fig. 4.5 b). As a result of this design, when the pupil is small, such as during reading tasks, the lens provides appropriate near and distance vision. However, in large pupil situations, such as during the night, the ReSTOR lens becomes a distant-dominant lens, providing appropriate distance vision while reducing unwanted visual phenomena, as the defocused near image has less energy and is smaller.

The MF4 manufactured by Ioltech Laboratoires (La Rochelle, France) is a single-piece, biconvex hydrophilic acrylic design with three points of fixation (tripod design). The optic diameter of the lens is 6.0 mm and the overall diameter is 10.5 mm. It has four refractive zones, alternating near and distance vision (Fig. 4.5 c). The manufacturer states that the surface of the different optic zones has been calculated to provide optimal near and distance vision, according to the natural diameter of the pupil. The refractive addition obtained with this lens for near vision is +4 dioptres [46].

Acri.Tec GmbH (Berlin, Germany) developed three-piece silicone-optic, PMMA-haptic multifocal lenses, the Acri.Twin. The two models

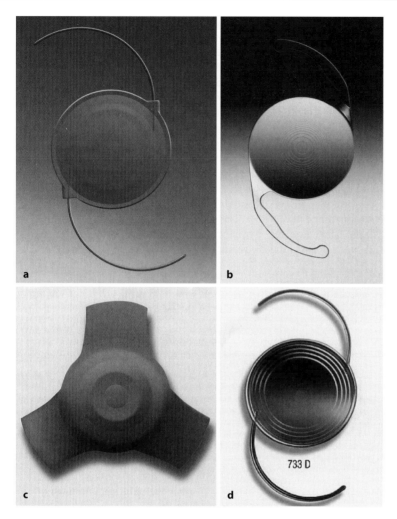

Fig. 4.5 a–d. Gross photographs of multifocal intraocular lenses. **a** Array lens (AMO). **b** ReSTOR lens (Alcon). **c** MF4 (Ioltech). **d** Acri.Twin (Acri.Tec)

(737 D and 733 D) have the same design, but an asymmetric optic configuration for near and far vision (Fig. 4.5 d). The overall diameter of the lenses is 12.5 mm, and the diameter of the diffractive optic is 6.0 mm. The addition obtained with these lenses for near vision is +4 dioptres. They are aspheric, biconvex, and equiconvex. According to the manufacturer, better results are obtained with implantation in the dominant eye of the model 737 D, with 70 % of the light intensity used for far vision, while the other eye is implanted with the model 733 D, with 30 % of the light intensity used for near vision [46].

4.4.2
Toric Intraocular Lenses

For the manufacture of lenses to reduce pre-existing astigmatism in cataract patients, it is very important to use a design that provides appropriate centration, fixation, and stability, without rotational movements.

Staar Surgical (Monrovia, CA) manufactures silicone posterior chamber IOLs with toric optics (models AA4203TF and AA4203TL) [12, 36]. These toric IOLs are single-piece, plate haptic, injectable lenses with biconvex optics designed to be implanted within the capsular bag (Fig. 4.6 a). They incorporate a cylindrical cor-

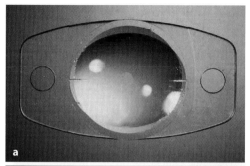

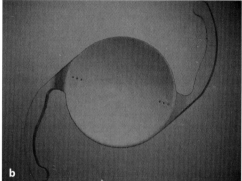

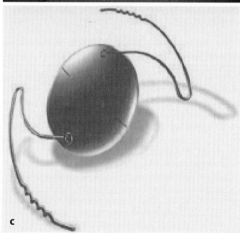

Fig. 4.6 a–c. Gross photographs of toric intraocular lenses. **a** AA4203TF (Staar). **b** AcrySof SA60TT (Alcon). **c** MicroSil (HumanOptics)

tre increments. The cylindrical powers of the IOLs are of 2 dioptres and 3.5 dioptres in the long axis of the lens. The cylindrical power of the toric IOLs at the corneal plane for a 2-dioptre lens is about 1.4 dioptres, and about 2.3 dioptres for the 3.5-dioptre IOL.

Another toric lens, now under investigation, is the model SA60TT, manufactured by using the platform of the single-piece AcrySof IOL (Alcon Laboratories, Fort Worth, TX). The SA60TT is available in three models for the ongoing study that offer 1.50 dioptres (SA60T3), 2.25 dioptres (SA60T4), or 3 dioptres (SA60T5) of power at the IOL plane. The IOLs feature three alignment marks on each side of the lens to assist with axis orientation. Implantation is also performed by injection with the Monarch II system (Fig. 4.6 b).

The MicroSil toric IOL (HumanOptics, Erlangen, Germany) is a three-piece silicone-optic, PMMA-haptic lens. It has sharp edges, a spherical front surface and a toric back surface. The overall diameter of the lens is 11.6 mm, with an optical diameter of 6.0 mm. The haptics have a special "Z"-shaped design, which is said to increase the rotational stability of the lens within the capsular bag, and to balance any mechanical forces during postoperative capsular bag shrinkage (Fig. 4.6 c). The lens has no optic-haptic angulation, and it is available in dioptric powers between –3.0 to +31.0 dioptres, and cylindrical powers between 2.0 and 12.0 dioptres. It can be inserted with a forceps through a 3.2- to 3.4-mm incision.

4.4.3
Aspheric Intraocular Lenses

The Z-Sharp Optic Technology developed at Pfizer (Pfizer Global Pharmaceuticals, Peapack, NJ) is being implemented on the CeeOn Edge IOL, model 911 platform (Tecnis Z 9000 IOL) [7, 23, 31, 33]. The principle of this technology, which has FDA approval, is based on the fact that spherical aberrations of the human eye vary with age [5]. The cornea has positive spherical aberration, which means peripheral rays are focused in front of the retina. This positive spherical aberration of the cornea remains

rection to a spherical optic to create a toric lens. The toric IOL has an overall diameter of 10.8 mm in the TF version and of 11.2 mm in the TL version to fit in the capsular bag of eyes of different sizes. These IOLs are available in powers from +4 dioptres to +35 dioptres, in 0.5 diop-

throughout life. In young people, the crystalline lens corrects this defect, as it is dominated by negative spherical aberration. The crystalline lens undergoes changes with age, which cause a shift of spherical aberration towards positive. This adds to the positive spherical aberration of the cornea, with possible increased sensitivity to glare and also reduced appreciation of contrast. The Tecnis lens has an aspheric surface, more specifically a modified prolate profile. This means that the lens has less refractive power at the periphery (contrary to spherical lenses, which have more refractive power at the periphery), therefore all the rays are coming to the same point, leading to a higher contrast sensitivity. The Z-Sharp Optic Technology could actually be applied to any lens biomaterial, as it is based on the modified prolate profile of the lens optic.

4.4.4
Intraocular Lenses with Special Blockers (Blue Blocker)

The AcrySof Natural (SN60AT) is the first IOL that provides incremental light protection above and beyond traditional ultraviolet protection [46]. This lens is manufactured by using the platform of the single-piece AcrySof. It contains a proprietary, integrated polymer dye (blue light-filtering chromophore – ImprUV) designed to filter both invisible ultraviolet rays and visible blue rays of light. The addition of a covalently bonded yellow dye results in an IOL ultraviolet/visible light transmittance curve that mimics the protection provided by the natural, pre-cataractous adult human crystalline lens. While the traditional ultraviolet-absorbing lenses provide light filtration from 200–400 nm, the AcrySof Natural lens would provide filtration properties from 200–550 nm. Prolonged exposure to visible blue light rays are widely considered to be a causative factor for damage to the retina and macula, and are believed to be a primary contributor to age-related macular degeneration. Studies performed at various intervals after cataract surgery and IOL implantation showed no significant differences between the AcrySof Natural and the standard SA30AL with regard to visual acuity, contrast sensitivity, or colour perception.

4.4.5
Accommodative Intraocular Lenses

In general, IOLs proposed to restore accommodation have been designed to do so by enabling a forward movement of the optic component during the efforts for accommodation. However, it is still not known whether the ability of these new IOL designs to move their optic forward will not be impaired by long-term postoperative fibrosis/opacification within the capsular bag. This involves not only PCO, but also ACO, which has been only considered a significant complication in cases such as capsulorhexis phimosis.

The C&C Vision (Aliso Viejo, CA) CrystaLens (model AT-45) is a modified plate haptic lens manufactured from a high-refractive index (1.430), third generation silicone material (Biosil), which contains an ultraviolet filter [14]. The lens is hinged adjacent to the optic and has small looped polyimide haptics, which have been shown to fixate firmly in the capsular bag. The grooves across the plates adjacent to the optic make the junction of the optic with the plate haptic the most flexible part of the optic-haptic design. The overall length of the lens is 11.5 mm (loop tip to loop tip measurement), while the overall length, as measured from the ends of the plate haptics, is 10.5 mm. The optic is biconvex and is 4.5 mm in diameter; the recommended A-constant is 119.24, and the lens is designed for placement in the capsular bag (Fig. 4.7 a). The theoretical mechanism of efficacy of this lens is based on the concept that with accommodative effort, redistribution of the ciliary body mass will result in increased vitreous pressure which will move the optic forward anteriorly within the visual axis, creating a more plus powered lens. One drop of atropine administered at the time of surgery and one drop on the first day after surgery would allow the lens to remain in the maximal posterior position within the capsular bag and not move forward during the period of fibrosis around the lens haptics. This would result in a greater potential for forward movement

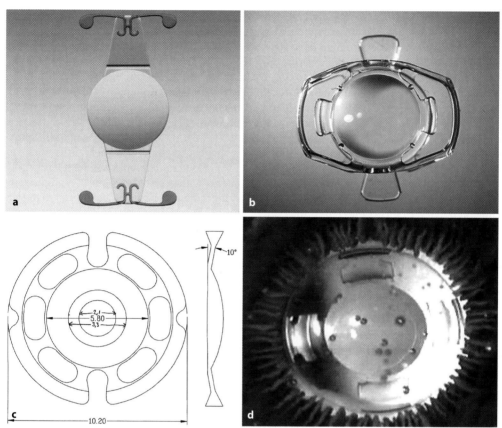

Fig. 4.7 a–d. Accommodative intraocular lenses. **a** Gross photograph of the CrystaLens (C&C Vision). **b** Gross photographs of the Synchrony IOL (Visiogen). **c** Schematic drawing showing the BioComFold model 43E (Morcher). **d** Experimental implantation of the Akkommodative 1CU in a human eye obtained postmortem, prepared according to the Miyake-Apple technique. (Courtesy of Dr. Gerd U. Auffarth, Heidelberg, Germany)

of the lens upon ciliary body constriction. The hinge was incorporated to facilitate the forward movement of the optic by minimizing the resistance to the possible pressure exerted on the lens by the forward movement of the vitreous body by contraction of the ciliary muscle. The lens has recently been approved by the FDA.

The Synchrony IOL (Visiogen Inc. Irvine, CA) is a one-piece lens manufactured from silicone [30, 49]. The lens, which is under investigation, has two major components (anterior and posterior), each having the general design of a plate-haptic silicone lens connected by a bridge through the haptics, with spring function. The posterior aspect of the device is designed with a significantly larger surface area than the anterior, in order to maintain stability within the capsular bag during the accommodation/un-accommodation process. The anterior optic has two expansions oriented parallel to the haptic component that lift the capsulorhexis edge up, thus preventing complete contact of the anterior capsule with the anterior surface of the lens (Fig. 4.7b). In this dual optic lens system the anterior lens has a high plus power beyond that required to produce emmetropia, while the posterior lens has a minus power to return the eye to emmetropia. The lens is designed to work in concert with the capsular bag, according to the traditional Helmholtz theory of accommodation. The distance between the two optics is stated to be minimum in the un-accommodated state and maximum in the accommodated state, with anterior displacement of the anterior optic.

The BioComFold, manufactured by Morcher GmbH (Stuttgart, Germany) is composed of a hydrophilic copolymer of PMMA and poly(2-hydroxyethyl methacrylate) with a water content of 28% and a refractive index of 1.46 [46]. The first available model had an overall length of 10.0 mm with a 5.8 mm diameter. BioComFold has square edges for PCO prevention. A peripheral bulging ring is connected to the optic via an intermediate, forward-angled (10°) perforated ring section. With accommodation efforts for near vision, the centripetal force of the elastic hollow ring of the equator narrows the peripheral ring, thereby steepening the intermediate ring section of the lens, which pushes the optical part forward. For distance vision, the elastic properties of the bulging ring and of the intermediate ring section of the lens return the optic to its primary position. The current version, the 43E, has an overall length of 10.2 mm, and an optic diameter of 5.8 mm (Fig. 4.7 c). The diameter of the perforations in the perforated ring section is also larger. Model 43S also has a refractive zone of +2 dioptres.

The Akkommodative 1CU, manufactured by HumanOptics (Erlangen, Germany), is also manufactured from a hydrophilic acrylic material [32]. The optical diameter of this lens is 5.5 mm with an overall diameter of 9.8 mm (Fig. 4.7 d). The refractive index of the lens material is 1.46. As with the other above-mentioned lenses, the special design and mechanical properties of this IOL are also stated to enable the lens to change power by a forward movement of the optic during the contraction of the ciliary muscle.

4.4.6
Intraocular Lenses for Very Small Incisions

The advent of microincision surgical techniques rendered cataract removal through clear corneal incisions as small as 1.6 mm possible. The natural consequence of this advance is the development of IOLs that can be inserted through such small incisions [2].

One of the recently developed lenses that can be inserted through a sub 2.0-mm incision (1.45 mm) is the UltraChoice 1.0 Rollable Thin-Lens (ThinOptX, Abingdon, VA) lens [34]. It is manufactured from a hydrophilic acrylic material with 18% water content. The refractive index of the material is 1.47. As of April 2003, the dioptric power of this lens ranges from +15 to +25 dioptres. The optical thickness is 300–400 μm, with a biconvex optical configuration having a meniscus shape. The overall diameter of the lens is 11.2 mm, and the optical diameter is 5.5 mm. After implantation, the natural temperature of the eye causes the lens to open gradually within the capsular bag, approximately 20 s. The teardrop shaped holes in the haptic component should point in a clockwise direction.

The ultrathin properties of the lens are attributable to its optical design. The optic features three to five concentric optical zones with steps of 50 μm (Fig. 4.8 a,b). Each Fresnel-like ring or segment of the lens has a small change in the radius to correct for spherical aberration. The difference in radius is stated to ensure that each ring of the lens focuses light at nearly the same point as the prime meridian. According to the manufacturer, by making the lens thinner, other aberrations such as coma, as well as the potential for distortion and glare, are reduced. The four tips of the haptic component have a thickness of 50 μm. They can roll once in the capsular bag, absorbing capsular contraction forces. The edge of the lens is also 50 μm thick, which is stated to reduce the potential for halos and glare. It has been hypothesized that the thin nature of this design provides increased amplitude of pseudoaccommodation, which will be further investigated. One explanation could be that the thin lens is associated with increased depth of field. Another possibility is that the lens would move with the capsular bag during efforts for accommodation, as it is thin and light, and exerts little force against the equator.

Another recently developed lens for insertion through very small incisions is the Acri.Smart lens (model H44-IC-1, Acri.Tec GmbH, Berlin, Germany) [1]. This is a one-piece

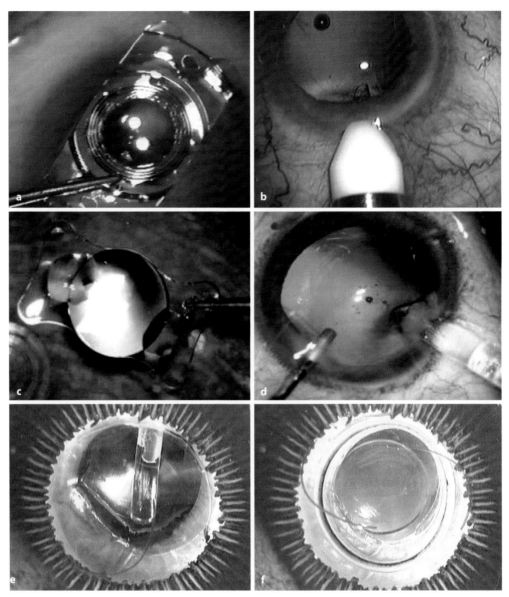

Fig. 4.8 a–f. Intraocular lenses for very small incisions. **a** Gross photograph showing the UltraChoice lens and its optic steps. (Courtesy of ThinOptX.) **b** Clinical picture obtained under an operating microscope, showing injection of the UltraChoice lens through a 1.45-mm incision, using a newly developed roller/injector system. (Courtesy of ThinOptX.) **c** Gross photograph showing the Acri.Smart lens model 48 S. **d** Implantation of the Acri.Smart lens through a 1.5-mm incision using a specially designed injector. (Courtesy of Dr. Sunita Agarwal, Banglore, India, and Dr. Suresh K. Pandey, Salt Lake City, UT) **e, f** Gross photographs of a human eye obtained postmortem (Miyake-Apple posterior view) implanted with a prototype of the three-piece SmartIOL. The rod gradually transformed into a three-piece lens, after instillation of balanced salt solution at body temperature

hydrophilic acrylic lens that has an optical diameter of 6.0 mm and a total length of 12.3 mm. The lens is pre-folded as follows: after dehydration up to 27%, the optic of the lens is rolled onto itself to create a pre-folded lens that is shorter in diameter. A folded +19-dioptre lens has a width of about 1.2 to 1.3 mm. Over the next minutes following implantation in the capsular bag, the Acri.Smart unfolds gradually, being completely unfolded after 23–30 min. Other models of the Acri.Smart lens (model 48 S with a 5.5-mm optic, and model 46S with a 6.0-mm optic) have been developed for implantation with a specially designed injector through a 1.5-mm incision. These are hydrophilic acrylic (25% water content) lenses with a hydrophobic coating. The overall design is that of plate haptic lenses with square edges, which are loaded into the injector already in a hydrated state, thus the unfolding is faster (Fig. 4.8 c,d). Model 36A, with a special aspherical design, has also been developed to compensate for the positive spherical aberration of the cornea, in a mechanism similar to that of the Tecnis lens.

A new concept of very-small-incision IOLs is being developed at Medennium Inc. (Irvine, CA), called the SmartIOL. This lens uses a thermodynamic hydrophobic acrylic material that is packaged as a solid rod approximately 30.0 mm long and 2.0 mm wide. The refractive index of the material is 1.47, and the glass transition temperature is 20–30° C. When implanted through a small incision, body temperature transforms the solid into a soft gel-like material, which has the shape of a full-sized biconvex lens that completely fills the capsule. The entire transformation takes less than 30 s and results in a lens about 9.5 mm wide and from 2.0 to 4.0 mm thick (but averaging about 3.5 mm) at the centre, depending on dioptric power. The lens is highly flexible, more closely resembling a gel, and it recovers its full shape when not compressed. Before it forms into a rod, the precise dioptric power and dimensions that the transformed material will take upon thermal activation in each eye can potentially be imprinted.

Besides being implanted through a very small incision, another potential advantage is to restore accommodation. By combining a full-sized optic with a very flexible material, Medennium scientists hope to be able to mimic the accommodative action of the young, natural lens and achieve a larger potential accommodation than other optical-mechanical designs, according to the classical Helmholtz theory. Also, complete filling of the capsular bag eliminates space for cell growth. The hydrophobic acrylic material of this lens exhibits high tackiness, which might promote its attachment to the capsular bag, further enhancing PCO prevention. A new design of this lens is being developed, which is a three-piece lens, having PVDF haptics (Fig. 4.8 e,f). This will probably eliminate potential problems related to the different diameters of the capsular bags in different eyes.

4.4.7
Adjustable Power Intraocular Lenses

Calhoun Vision (Pasadena, CA) is developing a three-piece silicone optic-PMMA haptic lens with photosensitive silicone subunits, which move within the lens upon fine tuning with a low intensity beam of near-ultraviolet light (light adjustable lens – LAL). The refractive power of the lens can thus be adjusted non-invasively after implantation to give the patient a definitive refraction (Fig. 4.9) [46].

When the eye is healed at 2–4 weeks after implantation, the refraction is measured and a low intensity beam of light is used to correct any residual error. The mechanism for dioptric change is akin to holography and is pictorially displayed in Fig. 4.9. The application of the appropriate wavelength of light onto the central optical portion of the LAL polymerizes the macromer in the exposed region, thereby producing a difference in the chemical potential between the irradiated and non-irradiated regions. To reestablish thermodynamic equilibrium, unreacted macromer and photoinitiator diffuses into the irradiated region. As a consequence of the diffusion process and the material properties of the host silicone matrix, the LAL will swell producing a concomitant decrease in the radius of curvature of the lens. This process may be repeated if further refractive change in the LAL is desired, or an irradiation of the entire lens may be applied consuming the remaining,

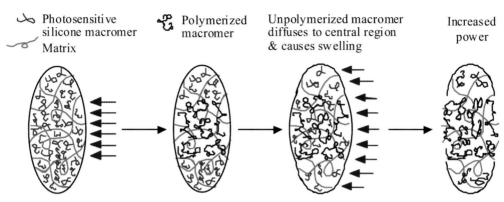

| ꙮ Photosensitive silicone macromer | ꙮ Polymerized macromer | Unpolymerized macromer diffuses to central region & causes swelling | Increased power |

Fig. 4.9. Proposed mechanism of swelling. Selective irradiation of the central zone of the IOL polymerizes macromer creating a chemical potential between the irradiated and non-irradiated regions. To reestablish equilibrium, excess macromer diffuses into the irradiated region causing swelling. Irradiation of the entire IOL "locks" the macromer and the shape change. (Courtesy of Calhoun Vision)

undiffused, unreacted macromer and photoinitiator. This action has the effect of "locking" in the refractive power of the LAL.

It should be noted that it is possible to induce a myopic change by irradiating the peripheral portion of the LAL to effectively drive macromer and photoinitiator out of the central region of the lens, thereby increasing the radius of curvature of the lens and decreasing its power. A new digital delivery system for light application has recently been developed in conjunction with Carl Zeiss Meditec (Jena, Germany). Correction of higher order aberrations such as the tetrafoil pattern, besides hyperopic, myopic, and astigmatic corrections, is now possible. Preliminary in vitro and in vivo studies with the rabbit model have demonstrated appropriate accuracy and reproducibility of the corrections obtained with the new digital system.

Summary for the Clinician

- Careful patient selection is important in multifocal IOL implantation, because of concerns of decreased contrast sensitivity and glare
- Designs used for the manufacture of toric IOLs should provide appropriate centration, fixation, and stability without rotational movements
- An IOL with an aspheric surface compensates for the positive spherical aberration of the cornea, improving the contrast sensitivity
- An IOL with an incorporated blue light blocker mimics the protection provided by the natural crystalline lens to the retina
- Accommodative IOLs currently available or in development are designed to enable a forward movement of the optic during efforts for accommodation
- IOLs that can be inserted through sub 1.5-mm incisions are already available
- Development of the light adjustable lens will allow non-invasive postoperative adjustment of the refractive power and full customization of the lens

4.5 Summary

Foldable lenses have been implanted over the past two decades with increasing success as better manufacture and surgical techniques become available. A recent survey of the complications associated with these lenses revealed that some of the common causes for explantation of foldable IOLs are not specifically related to them, e.g. incorrect lens power [29]. New technology available, such as the LAL, will allow non-invasive postoperative adjustment of these errors in power calculation. Also, we expect in the near future an increase in the popularity of other specialized foldable lenses, including multifocal and accommodative lenses, with increasing performance of procedures such as refractive lens exchange.

Acknowledgements. Supported in part by a grant from Research to Prevent Blindness, Inc., New York, N.Y., to the Department of Ophthalmology and Visual Sciences, University of Utah.

The authors would also like to point out that they have no financial or proprietary interest in any product mentioned in this text.

References

1. Agarwal A, Agarwal S, Agarwal A (2003) Phakonit with an AcriTec IOL. J Cataract Refract Surg 29:854–855
2. Alio JL, Rodriguez-Prats JL, Galal A (2003) Micro incision cataract surgery (MICS). In: Buratto L, Werner L, Zanini M, Apple DJ (eds) Phacoemulsification: principles and techniques, 2nd edn. Slack, Thorofare, NJ, pp 259–263
3. Apple DJ, Auffarth GU, Peng Q, Visessook N (2000) Foldable intraocular lenses: evolution, clinicopathologic correlations, and complications. Slack, Thorofare, NJ
4. Apple DJ, Peng Q, Visessook N, Werner L, Pandey SK, Escobar-Gomez M, Ram J, Auffarth GU (2001) Eradication of posterior capsule opacification: documentation of a marked decrease in Nd:YAG laser posterior capsulotomy rates noted in an analysis of 5416 pseudophakic human eyes obtained postmortem. Ophthalmology 108:505–518
5. Artal P, Berrio E, Guirao A, Piers P (2002) Contribution of the cornea and internal surfaces to the change of ocular aberrations with age. J Opt Soc Am A Opt Image Sci Vis 19:137–143
6. Auffarth GU, Golescu A, Becker KA, Völcker HE (2003) Quantification of posterior capsule opacification with round and sharp edge intraocular lenses. Ophthalmology 110:772–780
7. Bellucci R (2003) Optical aberrations and intraocular lens design. In: Buratto L, Werner L, Zanini M, Apple DJ (eds) Phacoemulsification: principles and techniques, 2nd edn. Slack, Thorofare, NJ, pp 454–455
8. Brown DC, Ziémba SL (2001) Collamer intraocular lens: clinical results from the US FDA core study. J Cataract Refract Surg 27:833–840
9. Brown DC, Grabow HB, Martin RG, Rowen SL, Shepherd JR, Williamson CH, Ziémba SL (1998) Staar Collamer intraocular lens: clinical results from the phase I FDA core study. J Cataract Refract Surg 24:1032–1038
10. Buehl W, Findl O, Menapace R, Rainer G, Sacu S, Kiss B, Petternel V, Georgopoulos M (2002) Effect of an acrylic intraocular lens with a sharp posterior optic edge on posterior capsule opacification. J Cataract Refract Surg 28:1105–1111
11. Caporossi A, Casprini F, Tosi GM, Baiocchi S (2002) Preliminary results of cataract extraction with implantation of a single-piece AcrySof intraocular lens. J Cataract Refract Surg 28:652–655
12. Chang DF (2003) Early rotational stability of the longer Staar toric intraocular lens: fifty consecutive cases. J Cataract Refract Surg 29:935–940
13. Christ FR, Buchen SY, Deacon J et al (1995) Biomaterials used for intraocular lenses. In: Wise DL, Trantolo DJ, Altobelli DE et al (eds) Encyclopedic handbook of biomaterials and bioengineering. Part B: applications, vol 2. Marcel Dekker, New York, pp 1261–1313
14. Cumming JS, Slade SG, Chayet A (2001) Clinical evaluation of the model AT-45 silicone accommodating intraocular lens: results of feasibility and the initial phase of a Food and Drug Administration clinical trial. Ophthalmology 108:2005-9; discussion 2010
15. Davison JA (2002) Clinical performance of Alcon SA30AL and SA60AT single-piece acrylic intraocular lenses. J Cataract Refract Surg 28:1112–1123
16. Dhaliwal DK, Mamalis N, Olson RJ, Crandall AS, Zimmerman P, Alldredge OC, Durcan FJ, Omar O (1996) Visual significance of glistenings seen in the AcrySof intraocular lens. J Cataract Refract Surg 22:452–457
17. Fine IH, Hoffman RS (2000) The AMO array foldable silicone multifocal intraocular lens. Int Ophthalmol Clin 40:245–252
18. Gregori NZ, Spencer TS, Mamalis N, Olson RJ (2002) In vitro comparison of glistening formation among hydrophobic acrylic intraocular lenses(1). J Cataract Refract Surg 28:1262–1268
19. Izak AM, Werner L, Apple DJ, Macky TA, Trivedi RH, Pandey SK (2002) Loop memory of haptic materials in posterior chamber intraocular lenses. J Cataract Refract Surg 28:1229–1235
20. Izak AM, Werner L, Pandey SK, Apple DJ (2004) Pathological evaluation of human eyes obtained postmortem implanted with a new single-piece hydrophobic acrylic lens. J Cataract Refract Surg (in press)

21. Jehan FS, Mamalis N, Spencer TS et al (2000) Postoperative sterile endophthalmitis (TASS) associated with the MemoryLens. J Cataract Refract Surg 26:1773–1777
22. Kent DG, Peng Q, Isaacs RT et al (1997) Security of capsular fixation: small- versus large-hole plate-haptic lenses. J Cataract Refract Surg 23:1371–1375
23. Kershner RM (2003) Retinal image contrast and functional visual performance with aspheric, silicone, and acrylic intraocular lenses. Prospective evaluation. J Cataract Refract Surg 29:1684–1694
24. Kruger AJ, Schauersberger J, Abela C, Schild G, Amon M (2000) Two year results: sharp versus rounded optic edges on silicone lenses. J Cataract Refract Surg 26:566–570
25. Legeais JM, Werner L, Werner LP, Renard G (2001) Les matériaux pour implants intraoculaires. Partie III: les implants intraoculaires acryliques souples. J Fr Ophthalmol 24:309–318
26. Linnola RJ (1997) Sandwich theory: bioactive-based explanation for posterior capsule opacification. J Cataract Refract Surg 23:527–535
27. Linnola RJ, Werner L, Pandey SK et al (2000) Adhesion of fibronectin, vitronectin, laminin and collagen type IV to intraocular lens materials in human autopsy eyes. Part I: histological sections. J Cataract Refract Surg 26:1792–1806
28. Linnola RJ, Werner L, Pandey SK et al (2000) Adhesion of fibronectin, vitronectin, laminin and collagen type IV to intraocular lens materials in human autopsy eyes. Part II: explanted IOLs. J Cataract Refract Surg 26:1807–1818
29. Mamalis N (2002) Complications of foldable intraocular lenses requiring explantation or secondary intervention-2001 survey update. J Cataract Refract Surg 28:2193–2201
30. McLeod SD, Portney V, Ting A (2003) A dual optic accommodating foldable intraocular lens. Br J Ophthalmol 87:1083–1085
31. Mester U, Dillinger P, Anterist N (2003) Impact of a modified optic design on visual function: clinical comparative study. J Cataract Refract Surg 29:652–660
32. Nguyen NX, Langenbucher A, Huber S, Seitz B, Kuchle M (2002) Short-term blood–aqueous barrier breakdown after implantation of the 1CU accommodative posterior chamber intraocular lens. J Cataract Refract Surg 28:1189–1194
33. Packer M, Fine IH, Hoffman RS, Piers PA (2002) Prospective randomized trial of an anterior surface modified prolate intraocular lens. J Refract Surg 18:692–696
34. Pandey SK, Werner L, Agarwal A et al (2002) Phakonit: cataract removal through a sub-1.0 mm incision and implantation of the ThinOptX rollable intraocular lens. J Cataract Refract Surg 28:1710–1713
35. Schauersberger J, Amon M, Kruger A, Abela C, Schild G, Kolodjaschna J (2001) Comparison of the biocompatibility of 2 foldable intraocular lenses with sharp optic edges. J Cataract Refract Surg 27:1579–1585
36. Till JS, Yoder PR, Wilcox TK, Spielman JL (2002) Toric intraocular lens implantation: 100 consecutive cases. J Cataract Refract Surg 28:295–301
37. Vargas LG, Peng Q, Apple DJ, Escobar-Gomez M, Pandey SK, Arthur SN, Hoddinott DS, Schmidbauer JM (2002) Evaluation of 3 modern single-piece foldable intraocular lenses: clinicopathological study of posterior capsule opacification in a rabbit model. J Cataract Refract Surg 28:1241–1250
38. Vargas LG, Izak AM, Apple DJ, Werner L, Pandey SK, Trivedi RH (2003) Implantation of a single-piece, hydrophilic, acrylic, minus-power foldable posterior chamber intraocular lens in a rabbit model: clinicopathological study of posterior capsule opacification. J Cataract Refract Surg 29:1613–1620
39. Weghaupt H, Pieh S, Skorpik C (1996) Visual properties of the foldable Array multifocal intraocular lens. J Cataract Refract Surg 22(Suppl 2):1313–1317
40. Werner L, Legeais JM (1998) Les matériaux pour implants intraoculaires. Partie I: les implants intraoculaires en polyméthylméthacrylate et modifications de surface. J Fr Ophthalmol 21:515–524
41. Werner L, Legeais JM (1999) Les matériaux pour implants intraoculaires. Partie II: les implants intraoculaires souples, en silicone. J Fr Ophthalmol 22:492–501
42. Werner L, Apple DJ, Escobar-Gomez M, Ohrström A, Crayford BB, Bianchi R, Pandey SK (2000) Postoperative deposition of calcium on the surfaces of a hydrogel intraocular lens. Ophthalmology 107:2179–2185
43. Werner L, Pandey SK, Escobar-Gomez M, Visessook N, Peng Q, Apple DJ (2000) Anterior capsule opacification: a histopathological study comparing different IOL styles. Ophthalmology 107:463–471
44. Werner L, Pandey SK, Apple DJ, Escobar-Gomez M, McLendon L, Macky TA (2001) Anterior capsule opacification: correlation of pathologic findings with clinical sequelae. Ophthalmology 108:1675–1681
45. Werner L, Apple DJ, Crema AS, Izak AM, Pandey SK, Trivedi RH, Ma L (2002) Permanent blue discoloration of a hydrogel intraocular lens by intraoperative trypan blue. J Cataract Refract Surg 28:1279–1286

46. Werner L, Apple DJ, Schmidbauer JM (2003) Ideal IOL (PMMA and foldable) for year 2002. In: Buratto L, Werner L, Zanini M, Apple DJ Phacoemulsification: principles and techniques, 2nd edn. Slack, Thorofare, NJ pp 435–451

47. Werner L, Mamalis N, Izak AM et al (2004) Posterior capsule opacification in rabbit eyes implanted with single-piece and three-piece hydrophobic acrylic intraocular lenses. J Cataract Refract Surg (in press)

48. Werner L, Mamalis N, Pandey SK et al (2004) Posterior capsule opacification in rabbit eyes implanted with hydrophilic acrylic intraocular lenses with enhanced square edge. J Cataract Refract Surg (in press)

49. Werner L, Pandey SK, Izak AM et al (2004) Capsular bag opacification after experimental implantation of a new accommodating intraocular lens in rabbit eyes. J Cataract Refract Surg 30: 1114–1123

50. Whiteside SB, Apple DJ, Peng Q et al (1998) Fixation elements on plate IOLs. 3. Large positioning holes to improve security of capsular fixation. Ophthalmology 105:837–842

"Accommodative" IOLs

Oliver Findl

Core Messages

- Current designs of "accommodative" IOLs are supposed to work by the focus-shift principle to allow true pseudophakic accommodation
- Studies that biometrically assessed "accommodative" IOL optic shift found no or only low amplitudes of forward movement
- The amount of forward movement, if present, is highly variable between patients
- To date, most studies present psychophysical data for the proof of concept which seems insufficient
- Capsule bag performance and posterior capsule opacification with "accommodative" IOLs seems worse than that with standard IOLs

5.1
Introduction

5.1.1
Background

Accommodation is the change of overall refractive power of the eye to produce a sharp image of near objects on the retina. The age-dependent loss of the ability to accommodate, named presbyopia, is primarily attributed to a decrease in lens elasticity [18]. Other possible causal factors for presbyopia include the increase in equatorial diameter of the lens, loss of elasticity of Bruch's membrane and reduced mobility of the ciliary muscle [6].

One of the most challenging tasks of modern cataract surgery is restoration of the accommodative ability in pseudophakic patients. Various attempts to solve the problem of presbyopia correction after cataract surgery have been made to enable satisfying distance and near vision without spectacles. One example are multifocal intraocular lenses (IOL) that provide improved uncorrected near vision at the expense of reduced contrast sensitivity and disturbing optical phenomena [40]. Since the optics of current IOLs do not change in shape during ciliary muscle contraction, it is the general understanding that pseudophakic patients cannot accommodate.

5.1.2
Apparent Accommodation or Depth of Field

As a result of several factors such as small pupil size [43], myopic astigmatism [29], corneal aberrations [47], corneal multifocality [17] and good visual perception [25], pseudophakic patients may have an adequate depth of field to reach satisfying far and near visual acuity without any correction. This clinical phenomenon is referred to as apparent accommodation or pseudoaccommodation. It is also found in aphakic patients, proving that this phenomenon does not rely on the presence of an IOL.

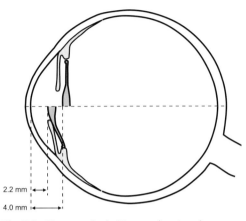

2.2 mm

4.0 mm

Fig. 5.1. The pseudophakic eye showing the extent of IOL movement necessary to achieve 3 dioptres of true pseudophakic accommodation

5.1.3
Focus Shift Principle

Provided that the ciliary muscle maintains its potential for contraction with increasing age [56], a forward shift, or movement, of the IOL optic under ciliary muscle contraction and the concomitant shift of the focal plane would result in true pseudophakic accommodation. For an eye of the usual dimensions, an IOL forward movement of about 0.60 mm would cause 1 D of accommodation in the spectacle plane [27]. The mechanism of such an IOL movement could be based either on the Helmholtz theory of accommodation [57], hypothesising force transmission from the ciliary muscle to the lens via the zonular apparatus, or the "hydraulic suspension theory" by Coleman [3], that assumes changes in vitreous pressure to be responsible for lens shape changes. "Accommodative" IOLs are designed to transform such forces of the ciliary muscle into a forward movement of the IOL optic (optic-shift concept) by anterior flexing of the optic in relation to the haptics. However, in order to attain an accommodative amplitude of 3 D to enable reading at the usual reading distance of 33 cm, an IOL movement of 1.8 mm is needed for an eye of normal dimensions. The distance from the posterior corneal surface to the IOL, or anterior chamber depth, obviously depends on the IOL design and size of the anterior segment of the eye, but will be about 4 mm on average. Therefore, to attain an IOL induced accommodative amplitude of 3 D, the resulting anterior chamber depth under ciliary muscle contraction would need to be rather shallow with about 2.2 mm (Fig. 5.1). Such a change of IOL position seems unrealistic considering the anatomical setting. An IOL movement of such magnitude could be potentially harmful to the eye by, for example, causing pigment dispersion because of contact between the IOL and the iris.

However, an accommodative effect of an IOL by movement of the optic would be supported by the apparent accommodation which is always present. The amplitude of apparent accommodation is in the order of 1–2 D [10, 25, 44], depending on which method of assessment was used. Therefore, if an "accommodative" IOL would cause at least 1 D of true pseudophakic accommodation, then most patients should be able to read without near addition. Consequently, the minimum induced IOL movement would need to be in the order of at least 0.6 mm for an accommodative IOL to be of clinical use.

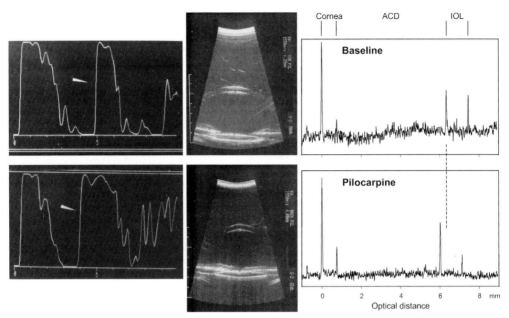

Fig. 5.2. Biometric measurement methods for evaluation of IOL movement: a-scan ultrasound [39] (*left*), ultrasound biomicroscopy [2] (*middle*), laser interferometry (*right*). Scans under disaccommodation (*upper*) and pilocarpine induced ciliary muscle contraction (*lower*)

5.1.4
Clinical Assessment

5.1.4.1
Psychophysical Assessment

For rating the accommodative effect of "accommodative" IOLs, most clinical studies use psychophysical methods such as near visual acuity with distance spectacle correction. However, such visual acuity data is strongly influenced by depth of field, or apparent accommodation, which in turn is influenced by many factors as mentioned above. Obviously, patient compliance and observer bias are also confounding factors in such subjective testing. Additionally, there are differences in optotype size between different reading charts. This is even the case for reading charts of the same type but from different manufacturers, for example the Rosenbaum chart [28]. Therefore, psychophysical assessment is not appropriate for a proof of principle of "accommodative" IOLs.

5.1.4.2
Refraction Measurement

A large number of techniques for measurement of refraction and it's dynamic changes are available [53]. Unfortunately, these methods do not work well for eyes with small pupils, and for pseudophakic eyes because of the bright Purkinje images.

5.1.4.3
Biometric Measurement

Measurement of IOL movement with ciliary muscle contraction is the direct way of proving that an IOL has an "accommodative" potential. Different methods of measurement have been used (Fig. 5.2).

Ultrasound

Ultrasound has been used for quantification of IOL movement during accommodation in the human eye [2, 38, 39]. Both a-scan ultrasound and b-scan mode with ultrasound biomicroscopy have been used (Fig. 5.2). The ultrasound approach is mainly limited by the reproducibility of the technique which is in the order of 0.15 mm for the anterior eye segment [42]. One problem is that the eye that is measured cannot fixate since the ultrasound probe is in front of the eye. Therefore, the contra-lateral eye must be used for fixation. This results in a change in direction of gaze due to convergence that varies with extent of accommodation. The axis of the ACD measurement is therefore not constant which leads to a low reproducibility of measurement. Additional problems are echo artefacts caused by the iris or the IOL optic material, that can make identification of the actual IOL peak impossible. Better reproducibility data was reported for dedicated laboratory ultrasound equipment [45].

Optical and Photographic Techniques

Haag-Streit slitlamp pachymetry has been used to assess anterior chamber depth in pseudophakic eyes with a reproducibility of 0.1 mm under cyclopentolate cycloplegia and mydriasis [24]. However, the reproducibility of this technique was not reported for pseudophakic eyes under small pupil conditions, as seen during pilocarpine induced accommodation.

Photographic techniques, such as Scheimpflug photography or automated slit-lamp photography, as found in the Orbscan (Bausch & Lomb, Rochester, NY) or IOL-Master (Carl Zeiss Meditec, Jena, Germany), have been shown to suffer from poor accuracy mainly because of artefactual measurements of anterior chamber depth to the posterior IOL surface or the iris instead of the anterior IOL surface, especially under miosis [2, 32].

Laser Interferometry

Dual beam partial coherence interferometry, or laser interferometry, is a new optical technique which has been developed for high precision biometry [11]. This technique was used to perform accurate biometry in phakic and pseudophakic eyes [8, 9, 13]. Since the eye being measured is used for fixation and scans can only be attained when measuring along the optical axis, the reproducibility of this method is about 4 μm for measurements of the anterior segment, more than ten times better than that of conventional ultrasound. Sample scans are shown in Fig. 5.2, illustrating the slim peaks of the laser interferometric a-scans. Currently, laser interferometry seems to be the most promising technology for assessing lens movement in pseudophakic eyes.

5.1.4.4
Accommodative Stimulus

When attempting to measure change of IOL position in pseudophakic eyes, ciliary muscle contraction must be stimulated. In monkey eyes this has been done effectively by direct stimulation of the Edinger Westphal nucleus which results in a maximal contraction of the ciliary muscle [5]. For clinical studies in humans, near-point stimulation and pharmacological means of inducing ciliary muscle contraction have been used.

Near-Point Stimulus

In the clinical setting with patients there are two options for stimulating the ciliary muscle: voluntary near-point stimulation and pharmacological stimulation. Clearly, a near-point stimulus is more physiological. However, the stimulus, usually an optotype used as the target, should be presented to the eye being measured for reasons mentioned previously. This is technically not possible in most of the above-mentioned apparatus set-ups. Also, when using a near-point stimulus, the examiner relies on patient compliance during the measurement procedure. Prolonged fixation of a near target can be difficult and tiring, especially for elderly pseudophakic patients.

Table 5.1. Main properties of "accommodative" IOLs

IOL	Haptic angulation	Overall size (mm)	Optic size (mm)	Material
BioComfold, 43 A, Morcher	−10°	9.8	5.8	Hydrophilic acrylic
1CU, Humanoptics	0°	9.8	5.5	Hydrophilic acrylic
Crystalens AT-45, C&C Vision	0°	10.5 (11.5 between loop tips)	4.5	Silicone

Pharmacological Stimulus

Advantages of using pharmacological means of stimulating ciliary muscle contraction are that it allows more time for measuring the biometric changes within the eye and is probably more reproducible, especially, in a pseudophakic population. Combining these measurements with IOL position under cycloplegia, performed with cyclopentolate in most studies, results in the difference between maximal stimulation and relaxation of the ciliary muscle. This maximal amplitude of IOL movement is an indicator of the accommodative potential of a new IOL design. Possible drawbacks of pharmacological stimulation are that it may act "unphysiologically" by inducing a pattern of muscle contraction that cannot be reproduced by patients in daily life, and therefore over- or possibly under-estimating the real accommodative effect of an IOL. Also, the concomitant miosis of the pupil can hinder measurement with some of the mentioned techniques.

Pilocarpine is the most commonly used drug for this purpose, usually in a concentration of 1% or 2%, in some studies even as high as 6%. The maximum effect was reached after 33 min in phakic eyes [59] and 60 min in pseudophakic eyes [33]. It was shown that application of pilocarpine was effective in inducing changes in lens thickness [12], anterior chamber depth and lens curvature [1, 50] that were similar to those found during near-point fixation in young phakic subjects. In presbyopic phakic subjects, near-point stimulation did not induce any biometric changes, as expected; however, pilocarpine induced a forward shift of the lens of about 0.15 mm [31]. Therefore, it seems as if pilocarpine acts as an "unphysiological superstimulus" in the elderly presbyopic eye and may also do so in the pseudophakic eye.

5.1.4.5
Capsule Bag Performance

Current "accommodative" IOLs are made of well known materials, but have an altered haptic design compared to conventional open loop or plate haptics to allow optic movement during ciliary muscle contraction. Such design alterations also carry the risk of a compromised capsule bag performance by deviating from the well-tested conventional IOL designs. Therefore, meticulous evaluation of the safety of such new IOLs is of great clinical importance. The main variables concerning capsule bag performance are lens centration and tilt, fibrotic changes of the capsule and posterior capsule opacification (PCO).

5.1.5
Accommodative IOLs

The so-called accommodative intraocular lenses are made of flexible silicone or acrylate, and have in common a thin and flexible "hinge" at the haptic–optic junction which should allow forward movement of the optic with haptic compression (Table 5.1).

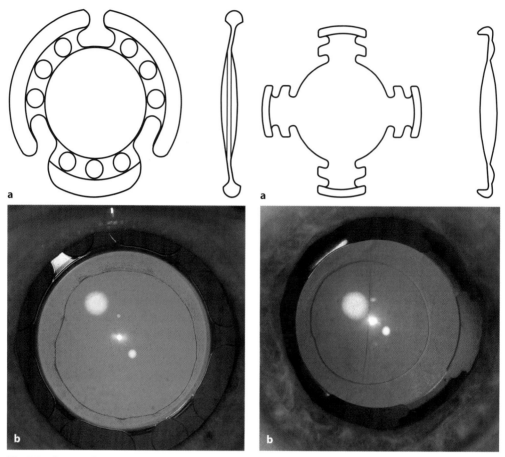

Fig. 5.3 a, b. Ring-haptic IOL: type 43 A (**a**) and retroillumination photograph of type 43 E (**b**)

Fig. 5.4 a, b. 1CU IOL: drawing (**a**) and retroillumination photograph (**b**)

5.1.5.1
Ring-Haptic IOL

The first "accommodative" IOL that was available on the market was the ring-haptic IOL designed by H. Payer and produced by Morcher GmbH in Stuttgart, Germany [48]. Two designs were marketed in the 1990s, under the names Biocomfold 43 A and 43 E, the latter with a few minor modifications in design. This foldable, single-piece, disc-like IOL is made of hydrophilic acrylate and has a peripheral bulging discontinuous ring (Fig. 5.3). The ring is connected to the optic by an intermediate forward angled perforated ring section. The IOL optic is positioned in front of the haptic plane to ensure that centripetal compression of the haptic by the ciliary muscle will result in a forward shift of the optic and not in the reverse direction.

5.1.5.2
1 CU IOL

The second "accommodative" IOL that became available in 2001 is based on a concept by K.D. Hanna and is produced under the name "1CU" by HumanOptics AG, Erlangen, Germany [34]. This foldable, single-piece IOL is made of hydrophilic acrylate and has four flexible haptics that have transmission elements at their attachment to the optic (Fig 5.4). A centripetal pressure of the ciliary body on these haptic elements should result in a forward shift of the optic. The haptic ends are formed in such a way as to simulate the equator of the crystalline lens, probably to allow for a ciliary body – zonula – capsule relationship similar to that seen in the phakic eye. A finite element model was used to develop this design.

5.1.5.3
Crystalens IOL

The third "accommodative" IOL that became available in Europe in 2002 and has been FDA approved since 2003, was designed by S. Cumming and is produced under the name Crystalens AT-45 by C&C Vision (Aliso Viejo, CA) [7]. The Crystalens is a modified three-piece plate haptic silicone IOL with small t-shaped polyimide haptics at the end of the plate (Fig. 5.5). The optic has an unusually small diameter of 4.5 mm with hinges at the optic–haptic junction to allow shift of the optic relative to the haptic plane. Forward movement of this lens under accommodation is supposedly mediated by an increase in vitreous pressure pushing the lens forward as a result of a mass redistribution under ciliary muscle contraction as postulated by Coleman [3, 4].

5.1.5.4
Future Concepts

IOL with Two Optics

As early as 1990, T. Hara introduced the concept of an IOL with two optics which he named spring IOL [21, 22]. The IOL is positioned inside the capsule bag, with one optic positioned at the posterior capsule and connected to the other optic, which rests behind the anterior capsule, through spring-like loops. With this IOL the entire capsule bag space is occupied. With deformation of the capsule bag during ciliary muscle contraction, the optics should move apart and vice versa under disaccommodation. A prototype of an IOL with a similar concept which is also foldable has recently been presented by F.M. Sarfarazi [52]. However, no clinical data in humans is yet available.

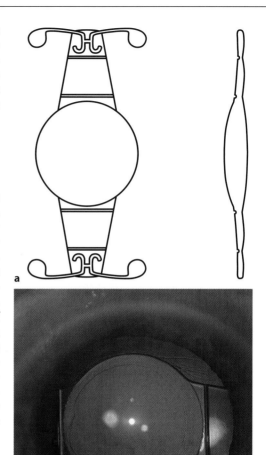

Fig. 5.5 a, b. Crystalens IOL: drawing (**a**) and retroillumination photograph (**b**)

IOL with Magnets

Recently, the concept of shifting the entire capsule bag-IOL complex instead of the IOL within the capsule bag was introduced by P.R. Preussner [51]. Tiny permanent magnets are introduced into a special capsular tension ring and opposing magnets are positioned under the rectus muscles on the sclera. With ciliary muscle contraction and zonular relaxation the entire capsule bag should shift forward resulting in a concomitant shift of the optic. No clinical data in humans is yet available.

5.1.6
Lens Refilling

One approach, albeit still experimental, is to preserve accommodation by lens refilling. Thereby, a special phacoemulsification technique is used to remove the lens through a small capsular opening. The capsule bag is filled with a refilling material. Such a material must be transparent, non-toxic and elastic.

At present, in animal experiments, lens refilling still faces great difficulties [20, 23, 26, 46]. Especially due to the refilling procedure and material, postoperative refraction is still unpredictable, and the long-term problem of secondary cataract, has not been solved. No clinical data in humans is yet available.

5.2
Clinical Experience with Available IOLs

5.2.1
Conventional IOLs

5.2.1.1
IOL Movement Data

Measurement of IOL movement under pharmacologically and near-point stimulated ciliary muscle contraction was reported for pseudophakic eyes with conventional IOLs in five studies (see Table 5.2). Hardman Lea et al. observed a slight backward shift of rigid PMMA IOL reaching a maximum of 0.25 mm in single cases and no shift with a foldable IOL, as assessed with optical pachymetry under pilocarpine stimulation [24]. Gonzalez et al. observed essentially no shift for PMMA IOLs and a forward shift of 0.42 mm for hydrogel IOLs [19]. In a study by Niessen et al., an average forward shift of 0.08 mm was found for a disc IOL with near-point stimulation in 15 eyes using a dedicated ultrasound set-up [45]. Lesiewska-Junk et al. reported on adolescent pseudophakic patients and found a forward shift of 0.42 mm under near-point stimulation as measured with ultra-

Table 5.2. Clinical data on IOL movement with conventional IOL designs

Study	Measurement method	IOL style	Eyes (n)	Average IOL movement (mm)[a]	Remarks
[24]	Optical pachymetry	PMMA	21	0.25	
		Hydrogel	8	0	
[19]	Ultrasound	PM	8	0.08	
		Hydrogel	12	−0.42	
[45]	Ultrasound	Disc	15	−0.08	
[39]	Ultrasound	PC IOL	45	−0.42	Adolescents, no reproducibility data
[15]	Laser interferometry	Plate	10	−0.16	
		PMMA c-loop	10	−0.06	
		Acrylic c-loop	8	0.04	
		Acrylic j-loop	12	0.16	

[a] Negative values indicate forward movement.

sound [39]. Unfortunately, no reproducibility data for the measurement method was reported in that study. A sample a-scan is shown in Fig. 5.2.

In a study on 40 eyes that used laser interferometry as the measurement technique, Findl et al. assessed a plate haptic IOL and three different open-loop three-piece IOLs that differed in haptic angulation and rigidity [15]. The conventional plate haptic IOL showed a slight, but statistically significant, forward shift of 0.162 mm, with a large variability ranging from no shift to a forward shift of 0.5 mm. With the three-piece IOLs, the c-loop lenses did not show any change, irrespective of haptic angulation. However, the j-loop lens with a haptic angulation of 10°, showed a slight backward shift of 0.156 mm. The shifts detected were too small to provide relevant refractive changes.

Psychophysical Data

There is an extensive literature on apparent accommodation of patients with conventional IOLs. The amount of apparent accommodation in most studies was about 2 D, ranging from 0.7 to 5.1 D [10, 17, 25, 44, 47, 60], depending on the method of assessment.

5.2.2
Accommodative IOLs

5.2.2.1
Ring-Haptic IOL

Functional Performance

All three studies that assessed IOL shift found a slight forward movement with this IOL under pilocarpine induced ciliary muscle contraction. Payer found a mean forward shift of 0.29 mm with a large variability (0.2–1.0 mm) [48]. In another study using ultrasound, a forward shift of 0.72 mm was found also with a large variability, ranging from a backward shift of 0.40 mm to a forward shift of 1.53 mm [38]. However, the shift data did not correlate with the accommodative amplitudes measured. In the largest sample of 22 eyes, assessed with laser interferometry, the mean forward shift was 0.17 mm, varying from no shift up to 0.75 mm in a single case (Fig. 5.6) [15].

Fig. 5.6. IOL movement with "accommodative" IOLs as measured with laser interferometry. The *box* indicates the interquartile range, the *line* the median, the *whiskers* the minimum and maximum, the *stars* the outliers

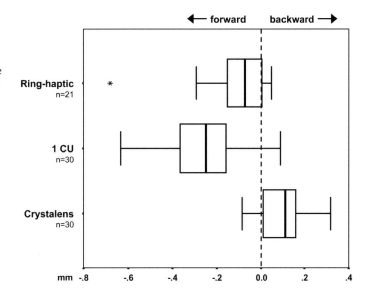

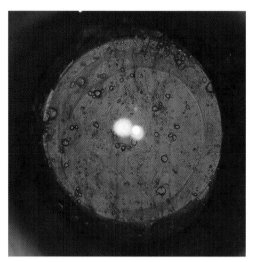

Fig. 5.7. Ring-haptic IOL with regeneratory PCO 1 year after surgery

Capsule Bag Performance

Since the optic plane is in front of the haptic plane in this lens style, there is frequently a gap between the posterior capsule and the IOL optic surface. This retrolental space and the insufficient barrier function of the IOL optic edge resulted in increased PCO rates (Fig. 5.7).

5.2.2.2
1CU IOL

Functional Performance

In a study that assessed accommodation with several techniques, the authors found the 1CU to have better near acuity with distance correction (0.32 versus 0.14) and better results in video refractometry, retinoscopy and defocusing with minus glasses compared to a conventional IOL [37]. However, one weakness of that study was that the control group was not randomised. In another study, the pilocarpine induced IOL forward shift was measured to be 0.63 mm with the 1CU using a photographic technique [36]. However, this technique has been shown to be of poor accuracy in pseudophakic eyes [2, 32] and is explicitly stated not to be used in pseudophakic eyes for measurement of anterior chamber depth in the operating manual.

A study using only psychophysical measures to evaluate the 1CU IOL, found a large difference in accommodative amplitude between the 1CU (1.90 D) and the control group (0.00 D) using a near-point procedure, 6 months after surgery [41]. It is surprising that in the control group of that study, during the entire follow-up which included four examinations, the mean distance corrected near acuity and it's standard deviation remained unchanged to the second decimal figure. Also, a mean accommodative amplitude of 0 D is unlikely for the pseudophakic control group.

Using laser interferometry, pilocarpine induced ciliary muscle contraction caused a forward movement of the 1CU IOL of 0.314 mm compared to a randomised control group which showed no IOL movement [16]. The estimated accommodative effect, as calculated from the IOL movement data with ray-tracing, was less than 0.5 D in a little more than half of the eyes examined. Extensive anterior capsule polishing, an attempt to optimise IOL performance by reducing capsule fibrosis and preserving capsule bag elasticity, did not influence the "accommodative" performance of the 1CU IOL. The amount of IOL movement with the 1CU showed a large inter-patient variability as was seen from the found standard deviation of more than 300 μm (see Fig. 5.6). There was even a slight backward movement in one case. On the other hand, there was one eye that showed an IOL movement of 0.7 mm which resulted in a pseudophakic accommodative amplitude of more than 1 D. The amount of IOL movement observed in the randomised trial using laser interferometry was comparable to that found in a series of seven eyes using ultrasound biomicroscopy [2].

Two recently presented studies using defocus curves to assess the accommodative ability of the 1CU IOL, showed slightly better results when comparing it to a randomised control group [49, 54]. However, the amount of additional accommodative performance was only about 0.5 D, which is in good agreement with the laser interferometric data described above.

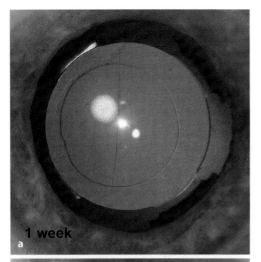

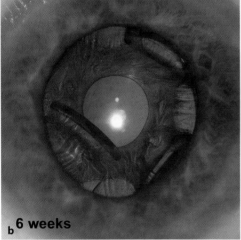

Fig. 5.8 a,b. 1CU IOL with "infolding" of haptics 6 weeks after uneventful surgery, causing a hyperopic shift of more than 2 D. Explantation of the IOL followed

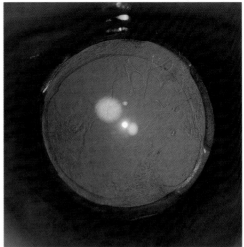

Fig. 5.9. 1CU IOL with thin regeneratory PCO 3 months after surgery

there are currently eight photodocumented cases of such haptic subluxation with 1CU IOLs, of these several IOLs had to be explanted because of the hyperopic shift, or astigmatism induced by the tilt. In these cases, surgery had been uneventful and it is not clear what the risk factors may be to developing such a complication.

Concerning PCO, the 1CU IOL seems to perform worse compared to current sharp edge open-loop IOLs. This may be a consequence of the absence of an effective sharp optic edge in the junction zone of the four haptics with an inferior barrier effect, or the hydrophilic material, or both (Fig. 5.9). However, long-term follow-up is necessary to assess the PCO performance of this IOL.

5.2.2.3
Crystalens IOL

Functional Performance

This lens was reported to result in excellent uncorrected distance and near visual acuity (VA) [7]. However, as discussed in a commentary by T. Werblin in the same issue of the journal [58], this study was not randomised and had no internal control group. This is the major weakness, especially when using psychophysical as-

Capsule Bag Performance

Although the 1CU IOL has been reported to be safe [35, 36], there have been a number of reported cases of "infolding" of 1CU haptics in front of the optic underneath the capsulorhexis. An example is shown in Fig. 5.8, where the patient reported blurred vision 6 weeks after uneventful cataract surgery. The refraction had changed from +0.25 D 1 week after surgery to +2.5 D 5 weeks later. To the author's knowledge,

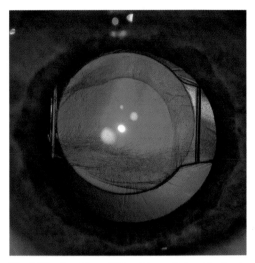

Fig. 5.10. Crystalens IOL with partial optic-rhexis buttonholing in lower half 6 months after surgery due to fibrosis and the small optic diameter

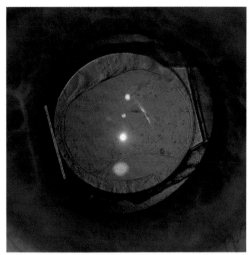

Fig. 5.11. Crystalens IOL with regeneratory PCO invading along the haptic–optic junction 2 years after surgery

sessment for proof of the accommodative ability of the Crystalens. As mentioned earlier, visual acuity data is primarily dependent on apparent accommodation. Comparing visual acuity data from this study to that of historic controls of other studies which used different near acuity cards probably under different lighting conditions and in different study populations is problematic.

Using laser interferometry with the identical measurement protocol as for the ring-haptic and 1CU IOLs, pilocarpine caused a small backward movement of the Crystalens [14] (see Fig. 5.6). Such a backward movement should result in a slight disaccommodation and, therefore, be counterproductive for an "accommodative" IOL. Obviously, if an eye has good apparent accommodation, the patient will still be able to read small print with distance corrected spectacles; however, the IOL is not the enabling factor.

Capsule Bag Performance

Surprisingly, the small optic diameter of 4.5 mm has not been reported to cause dysphotopsias. Concerning fibrotic after-cataract, buttonholing of the optic, due to the small optic size, is seen more commonly with this IOL than with conventional 6-mm optic diameter IOLs (Fig. 5.10). However, we have not seen any decentrations due to these buttonholings. Even though the Crystalens has a sharp optic edge, as with all plate haptic designs, there is a junction phenomenon with PCO ingrowth behind the IOL optic along the haptic plates (see Fig. 5.11). Therefore, the incidence of PCO is predicted to be higher than that of current conventional open-loop IOLs. However, to date there is no published data on the PCO incidence with this lens.

5.3
Current Clinical Practice and Recommendations

Assessment of "accommodative" IOLs remains a problem. Obviously, biometric methods that directly measure the IOL optic movement and therefore can prove the "accommodative" capability of such an IOL are preferable over indirect psychophysical measures that are influenced by many different factors. When using biometric methods, a physiological stimulus would be preferable; however, this is still difficult in many of the procedures currently used.

Fig. 5.12. The change in ciliary body configuration from the relaxed state (*grey*) to pilocarpine contraction (*red*) in a presbyopic eye. Contour lines extracted from 3-D ultrasound data by Stachs and coworkers [30, 55]. For this example, the axial and radial components of the vector of the anterior apex of the ciliary body were calculated. The possible change in IOL haptic position are illustrated

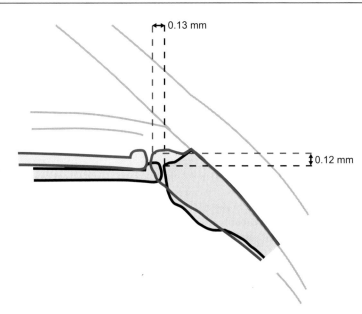

The question arises whether the presented focus-shift concept can be applied to the human eye. As can be seen from Fig. 5.1, to attain a sufficient amplitude of true pseudophakic accommodation, the IOL needs to shift far forward and would need to displace the iris anteriorly. Just from inspecting the geometrical and anatomical changes needed, such a concept seems unlikely if a full 3 D were the goal. However, with the addition of apparent accommodation to the focus shift effect, a movement of the IOL optic of about 1 mm would probably suffice to allow functional near vision with distance correction.

Analysing the pilocarpine induced movement data as assessed with laser interferometry of the conventional and "accommodative" IOLs, it becomes clear that there are large inter-patient differences in all the IOL groups. However, there are distinct differences between some IOL types. Most open-loop IOLs showed no significant movement upon ciliary muscle contraction. The only exception was the Acyrsof three-piece IOL that has a modified j-loop haptic design and a pronounced haptic angulation of 10°, in contrast to the c-loop haptic designs and the lower amounts of angulation of the other open-loop IOLs examined. Therefore, one could

hypothesise that a radial compression of the haptics by the ciliary muscle induces a backward vaulting in the Acrysof, however, less or no significant vaulting in the c-loop designs. The reason could be that the latter tend to absorb such radial compressive forces within the haptic, whereas the j-loop design conveys this compression directly to the optic with the result of an increase in posterior vault. This hypothesis would speak in favour of radial haptic compression occurring. This is in accordance with the changes seen in 3D ultrasound imaging of presbyopic subjects after pilocarpine application. For illustration purposes, a ciliary body contour has been extracted from a publication by Stachs and coworkers [30, 55]. This contour was overlaid onto an ultrasound biomicroscopic image of a pseudophakic eye (see Fig. 5.12). The resulting radial and axial vectors were calculated. For the most anterior point of the contour of the example displayed, these are 0.13 and 0.12 mm, respectively. Therefore, the amount of anterior displacement of the ciliary body-zonule-capsule plane is similar to the radial compressive vector. For an IOL that is posteriorly vaulted when the ciliary muscle is relaxed, the radial vector of the contracting ciliary muscle will cause an increase in vault pushing the optic backwards. This may be compensated, at least in part, by the forward displacement of the entire ciliary body-capsule-IOL plane. This could explain the differences found between the open-loop IOL designs. Interestingly, the conventional plate haptic design showed forward movement under ciliary muscle contraction. In these cases, the radial action may not induce a backward vault, but instead the IOL is just pulled forward by the axial displacement movement.

With the "accommodative" IOLs, the relatively far posterior positioned Crystalens, which accordingly also has the highest IOL constant for power calculation, probably is slightly backward vaulted during the resting state, with the optic plane behind the haptic plane. With muscle contraction, the IOL vault increases causing the slight backward movement. This movement does not speak in favour of the vitreous pressure theory by Coleman. Another argument that speaks against the Coleman theory, especially in the pseudophakic eye, is that a forward push of the optic by increased vitreous pressure should be lost or only of short duration in the case of a liquified vitreous, as found in most cataract patients, since the aqueous fluid from the posterior eye segment would pass the zonules to flow into the posterior chamber. This would result in initially good reading acuity which diminishes within seconds to minutes. There have not been any reports on patients experiencing such fluctuations with time.

The 1CU was the IOL style that showed the most forward movement, even though too little to allow useful near vision in most patients examined. With this IOL, and also with the ring-haptic to a lesser degree, the radial compression may actually result in a forward shift of the optic and this is enhanced by the axial forward displacement of the ciliary body-capsule-IOL plane. However, there was a high degree of variability between patients. This may be a result of differences in residual ciliary muscle mobility, or the positioning of the IOL haptics relative to the ciliary body. If the haptic ends are too far from the ciliary body apex, then the radial compression may not be used effectively.

Summary for the Clinician

- There is a trade-off between questionable accommodation and worse PCO and capsule bag performance with "accommodative" IOLs
- More studies are needed that measure IOL shift to prove the functioning of an accommodative IOL, instead of using near visual acuity data, which is determined by many factors that are not IOL related

References

1. Abramson DH, Coleman DJ, Forbes M, Franzen LA (1972) Pilocarpine. Effect on the anterior chamber and lens thickness. Arch Ophthalmol 87:615–620
2. Auffarth GU, Martin M, Fuchs HA, Rabsilber TM, Becker KA, Schmack I (2002) Validity of anterior chamber depth measurements for the evaluation of accommodation after implantation of an accommodative Humanoptics 1CU intraocular lens. Ophthalmologe 99:815–819
3. Coleman DJ (1986) On the hydraulic suspension theory of accommodation. Trans Am Ophthalmol Soc 84:846–868
4. Coleman DJ, Fish SK (2001) Presbyopia, accommodation, and the mature catenary. Ophthalmology 108:1544–1551
5. Crawford K, Terasawa E, Kaufman PL (1989) Reproducible stimulation of ciliary muscle contraction in the cynomolgus monkey via a permanent indwelling midbrain electrode. Brain Res 503: 265–272
6. Croft MA, Glasser A, Kaufman PL (2001) Accommodation and presbyopia. Int Ophthalmol Clin 41:33–46
7. Cumming JS, Slade SG, Chayet A (2001) Clinical evaluation of the model AT-45 silicone accommodating intraocular lens: results of feasibility and the initial phase of a Food and Drug Administration clinical trial. Ophthalmology 108:2005–2009
8. Drexler W, Baumgartner A, Findl O, Hitzenberger CK, Fercher AF (1997) Biometric investigation of changes in the anterior eye segment during accommodation. Vision Res 37:2789–2800
9. Drexler W, Baumgartner A, Findl O, Hitzenberger CK, Sattmann H, Fercher AF (1997) Submicrometer precision biometry of the anterior segment of the human eye. Invest Ophthalmol Vis Sci 38: 1304–1313

10. Elder MJ, Murphy C, Sanderson GF (1996) Apparent accommodation and depth of field in pseudophakia. J Cataract Refract Surg 22:615–619

11. Fercher AF, Roth E (1986) Ophthalmic laser interferometer. Proc SPIE 658:48–51

12. Findl O (2001) IOL movement induced by ciliary muscle contraction. In: Guthoff R, Ludwig K (eds) Current aspects of human accommodation. Kaden, Heidelberg, pp 119–133

13. Findl O, Drexler W, Menapace R, Hitzenberger CK, Fercher AF (1998) High precision biometry of pseudophakic eyes using partial coherence interferometry. J Cataract Refract Surg 24:1087–1093

14. Findl O, Kriechbaum K, Koeppl C, Menapace R, Drexler W (2003) Laserinterferometric measurement of IOL movement with "accommodative" IOLs. In: Symposium on Cataract, IOL, and Refractive Surgery. San Francisco

15. Findl O, Kiss B, Petternel V, Menapace R, Georgopoulos M, Rainer G, Drexler W (2003) Intraocular lens movement caused by ciliary muscle contraction. J Cataract Refract Surg 29:669–676

16. Findl O, Kriechbaum K, Koeppl C, Sacu S, Wirtitsch M, Buehl W, Drexler W (2003) Laserinterferometric measurement of the movement of an "accommodative" intraocular lens. In: Guthoff R, Ludwig K (eds) Current aspects of human accommodation II. Kaden, Heidelberg, pp 211–221

17. Fukuyama M, Oshika T, Amano S, Yoshitomi F (1999) Relationship between apparent accommodation and corneal multifocality in pseudophakic eyes. Ophthalmology 106:1178–1181

18. Glasser A, Campbell MC (1999) Biometric, optical and physical changes in the isolated human crystalline lens with age in relation to presbyopia. Vision Res 39:1991–2015

19. Gonzalez F, Capeans C, Santos L, Suarez J, Cadarso L (1992) Anteroposterior shift in rigid and soft implants supported by the intraocular capsular bag. Graefes Arch Clin Exp Ophthalmol 230:237–239

20. Haefliger E, Parel JM, Fantes F, Norton EW, Anderson DR, Forster RK, Hernandez E, Feuer WJ (1987) Accommodation of an endocapsular silicone lens (Phaco-Ersatz) in the nonhuman primate. Ophthalmology 94:471–477

21. Hara T, Yasuda A, Yamada Y (1990) Accommodative intraocular lens with spring action. Part 1. Design and placement in an excised animal eye. Ophthalmic Surg 21:128–133

22. Hara T, Yasuda A, Mizumoto Y, Yamada Y (1992) Accommodative intraocular lens with spring action–Part 2. Fixation in the living rabbit. Ophthalmic Surg 23:632–635

23. Hara T, Sakka Y, Sakanishi K, Yamada Y, Nakamae K, Hayashi F (1994) Complications associated with endocapsular balloon implantation in rabbit eyes. J Cataract Refract Surg 20:507–512

24. Hardman Lea SJ, Rubinstein MP, Snead MP, Haworth SM (1990) Pseudophakic accommodation? A study of the stability of capsular bag supported, one piece, rigid tripod, or soft flexible implants. Br J Ophthalmol 74:22–25

25. Hayashi K, Hayashi H, Nakao F, Hayashi F (2003) Aging changes in apparent accommodation in eyes with a monofocal intraocular lens. Am J Ophthalmol 135:432–436

26. Hettlich HJ, Lucke K, Asiyo-Vogel MN, Schulte M, Vogel A (1994) Lens refilling and endocapsular polymerization of an injectable intraocular lens: in vitro and in vivo study of potential risks and benefits. J Cataract Refract Surg 20:115–123

27. Holladay JT (1993) Refractive power calculations for intraocular lenses in the phakic eye. Am J Ophthalmol 116:63–66

28. Horton JC, Jones MR (1997) Warning on inaccurate Rosenbaum cards for testing near vision. Surv Ophthalmol 42:169–174

29. Huber C (1981) Myopic astigmatism a substitute for accommodation in pseudophakia. Doc Ophthalmol 52:123–178

30. Kirchhoff A, Stachs O, Guthoff R (2001) Three-dimensional ultrasound findings of the posterior iris region. Graefes Arch Clin Exp Ophthalmol 239:968–971

31. Koeppl C, Findl O, Kriechbaum K, Drexler W (2003) Comparison of pilocarpine-induced and stimulus-driven accommodation in phakic eyes. In: XXI Congress of the European Society of Cataract and Refractive Surgery, Munich, p 71

32. Kriechbaum K, Findl O, Kiss B, Sacu S, Petternel V, Drexler W (2003) Comparison of anterior chamber depth measurement methods in phakic and pseudophakic eyes. J Cataract Refract Surg 29:89–94

33. Kriechbaum K, Findl O, Koeppl C, Wirtitsch M, Sacu S, Menapace R, Drexler W (2003) Comparison of stimulus-driven and pilocarpine-induced accommodation in pseudophakic eyes. In: XXI Congress of the European Society of Cataract and Refractive Surgery, Munich, p 203

34. Kuchle M, Langenbucher A, Gusek-Schneider GC, Seitz B, Hanna KD (2001) First results of implantation of a new, potentially accommodative posterior chamber intraocular lens. Klin Monatsbl Augenheilkd 218:603–608

35. Kuchle M, Nguyen NX, Langenbucher A, Gusek-Schneider GC, Seitz B (2002) Two years experience with the new accommodative 1 CU intraocular lens. Ophthalmologe 99:820–824.

36. Kuchle M, Nguyen NX, Langenbucher A, Gusek-Schneider GC, Seitz B, Hanna KD (2002) Implantation of a new accommodative posterior chamber intraocular lens. J Refract Surg 18:208–216

37. Langenbucher A, Huber S, Nguyen NX, Seitz B, Gusek-Schneider GC, Kuchle M (2003) Measurement of accommodation after implantation of an accommodating posterior chamber intraocular lens. J Cataract Refract Surg 29:677–685

38. Legeais JM, Werner L, Abenhaim A, Renard G (1999) Pseudoaccommodation: BioComFold versus a foldable silicone intraocular lens. J Cataract Refract Surg 25:262–267.

39. Lesiewska-Junk H, Kaluzny J (2000) Intraocular lens movement and accommodation in eyes of young patients. J Cataract Refract Surg 26:562–565

40. Leyland M, Zinicola E (2003) Multifocal versus monofocal intraocular lenses in cataract surgery: a systematic review. Ophthalmology 110:1789–1798

41. Mastropasqua L, Toto L, Nubile M, Falconio G, Ballone E (2003) Clinical study of the 1CU accommodating intraocular lens. J Cataract Refract Surg 29:1307–1312

42. Mutti DO, Zadnik K, Egashira S, Kish L, Twelker JD, Adams AJ (1994) The effect of cycloplegia on measurement of the ocular components. Invest Ophthalmol Vis Sci 35:515–527

43. Nakazawa M, Ohtsuki K (1983) Apparent accommodation in pseudophakic eyes after implantation of posterior chamber intraocular lenses. Am J Ophthalmol 96:435–438

44. Nakazawa M, Ohtsuki K (1984) Apparent accommodation in pseudophakic eyes after implantation of posterior chamber intraocular lenses: optical analysis. Invest Ophthalmol Vis Sci 25:1458–1460

45. Niessen AGJE, de Jong LB, van der Heijde GL (1992) Pseudo-accommodation in pseudophakia. Eur J Implant Ref Surg 4:91–94

46. Nishi O, Hara T, Hayashi F, Sakka Y, Iwata S (1989) Further development of experimental techniques for refilling the lens of animal eyes with a balloon. J Cataract Refract Surg 15:584–588

47. Oshika T, Mimura T, Tanaka S, Amano S, Fukuyama M, Yoshitomi F, Maeda N, Fujikado T, Hirohara Y, Mihashi T (2002) Apparent accommodation and corneal wavefront aberration in pseudophakic eyes. Invest Ophthalmol Vis Sci 43:2882–2886

48. Payer H (1997) Ringwulstlinse mit Zoomwirkung zur Verstärkung einer Pseudoakkommodation und deren Erklärung aus erweiterter Akkommodationstheorie. Spektr Augenheilkd 11: 81–89

49. Pieh S, Schmiedinger G, Italon C, Simader C, Kriechbaum K, Menapace R, Skorpik C (2003) Comparing visual acuities at different distances of an accommodative IOL and a monofocal IOL. In: XXI Congress of the European Society of Cataract and Refractive Surgery, Munich, p 104

50. Poinoosawmy D, Nagasubramanian S, Brown NA (1976) Effect of pilocarpine on visual acuity and on the dimensions of the cornea and anterior chamber. Br J Ophthalmol 60:679–679

51. Preussner PR, Wahl J, Gerl R, Kreiner C, Serester A (2001) Accommodative lens implant. Ophthalmologe 98:97–102

52. Sarfarazi FM (2003) Long-term results of the Sarfrazi elliptical accommodating IOL in monkeys. In: Symposium on Cataract, IOL and Refractive Surgery, San Francisco

53. Schaeffel F (2003) Optical techniques to measure the dynamics of accommodation. In: Guthoff R, Ludwig K (eds) Current aspects of human accommodation II. Kaden, Heidelberg, pp 71–94

54. Spalton D, Heatley C (2003) Depth of focus with an accommodating IOL vs monofocal IOLs. In: XXI Congress of the European Society of Cataract and Refractive Surgery, Munich, p 122

55. Stachs O, Martin H, Kirchhoff A, Stave J, Terwee T, Guthoff R (2002) Monitoring accommodative ciliary muscle function using three-dimensional ultrasound. Graefes Arch Clin Exp Ophthalmol 240:906–912

56. Strenk SA, Semmlow JL, Strenk LM, Munoz P, Gronlund-Jacob J, DeMarco JK (1999) Age-related changes in human ciliary muscle and lens: a magnetic resonance imaging study. Invest Ophthalmol Vis Sci 40:1162–1169

57. von Helmholtz H (1855) Über die Akkommodation des Auges. Graefe's Arch. Klin Exp Ophthalmol 1:1–74

58. Werblin TP (2001) Discussion of article "Clinical evaluation of the model AT-45 silicone accommodating intraocular lens: results of feasibility and the initial phase of a Food and Drug Administration clinical trial". Ophthalmology 108:2010

59. Wold JE, Hu A, Chen S, Glasser A (2003) Subjective and objective measurement of human accommodative amplitude. J Cataract Refract Surg 29:1878–1888

60. Yamamoto S, Adachi-Usami E (1992) Apparent accommodation in pseudophakic eyes as measured with visually evoked potentials. Invest Ophthalmol Vis Sci 33:443–446

Rupert M. Menapace

Core Messages

- Pearl formation and capsular fibrosis represent the two types of after-cataract that derive from two different subpopulations of the lens epithelial cells (LECs)
- Thorough surgical clean-up and the use of a sharp-edge optic implant are readily available methods that effectively reduce posterior capsule opacification
- Circumferential overlap of the optic by the rhexis leaf is crucial for the formation of a mechanical barrier along the optic rim which is mediated by the capsular bend and mechanical pressure created at the posterior optic edge
- Slim haptics designed to conform to the capsular bag support circumferential barrier formation, while preserving the integrity of the anterior LEC layer and using optic materials with high fibrogenetic potential enhance the strength and permanence of the barrier by maximising fibrotic sealing of the capsular leaves along the optic rim
- While capsular polishing, therefore, is counterproductive, performing a primary posterior capsulorhexis is a safe and effective adjunctive method that creates a "second line of defence" against LECs that may overcome the optic edge barrier
- Though we do have methods at our disposal that effectively prevent after-cataract formation, these have been shown to fail in cases (e.g. deficient capsular bag sealing, delayed barrier failures; posterior optic ongrowth), which nourishes the quest for still more effective alternative approaches

6.1
Definition, Types and Natural Behaviour of "After-Cataract"

The term "after-cataract" describes growth of lens epithelial cells (LECs) left behind on the lens capsule following cataract removal [23]. These cells proliferate and migrate and finally may cause visual impairment due to pearl formation on, or whitening and shrinkage of the capsule. The term "after-cataract" should be preferred over "capsule opacification", since the capsule itself remains transparent [23]. Nevertheless, the term "posterior capsule opacification", or "PCO" has become widespread and its use generally accepted also in literature. More recently, the term "ACO" has also been widely used as an abbreviation of "anterior capsule opacification". Therefore, both terms will be applied in the following.

PCO and ACO not only describe different locations, but also different entities of after-cataract, as they are caused by different subpopulations of LECs [28], (Figs. 6.1, 6.2).

PCO is mainly caused by the "equatorial LECs", or "E-cells" that reside in the capsular bag equator. E-cells have an exquisite potential to migrate and may encroach upon the centre of the posterior capsule if not hindered to do so. As they tend to form globular structures called "pearls", the term "pearl after-cataract" has also been used.

When an intraocular lens (IOL) has been placed in the capsular bag, the rim of the optic acts as a mechanical barrier against centripetal cell migration. If the extended posterior capsule is firmly attached to the posterior optic surface, the capsule-optic interface will remain clear

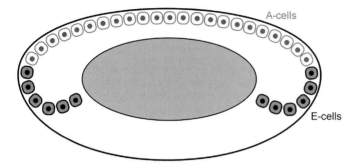

Fig. 6.1. Residual LECs belonging to two different subpopulations

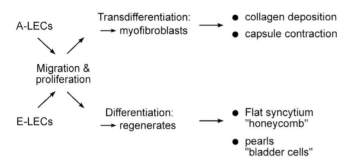

Fig. 6.2. Lens epithelial cell (LEC) population. Properties of E- and A-LECs

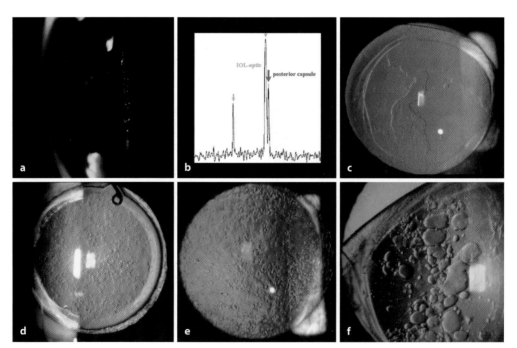

Fig. 6.3 a–f. "Regeneratory after-cataract" derived from E-LECs. Optic–capsule interspace as visualised by high-intensity slit-beam illumination (**a**); as measured by partial coherence laser interferometry (**b**); illdefined syncytial LEC layer (**c**); pearl monolayer (**d**); pearl multilayer (**e**); huge pearls ("bladder cells") (**f**)

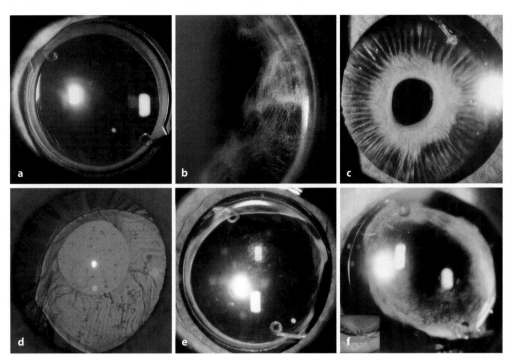

Fig. 6.4 a–f. "Fibrotic after-cataract" derived from A-LECs. Circumferential rhexis-optic overlap with consecutive fibrosis ("full in-the-bag") (**a**); peripheral posterior capsule fibrosis with round edge optic (**b**); excessive rhexis contraction ("rhexis phimosis") (**c**); asymmetric rhexis contraction with consecutive optic decentration (**d**); partial rhexis retraction ("buttonholing") (**e**); complete rhexis retraction (full "buttonholing", "haptics in – optic out") with consecutive central posterior capsule fibrosis (**f**)

("no space – no cells"). If, however, the posterior capsule stays at a distance to the optic surface, cells may eventually gain access to this interspace. Once arrived there, E-cells tend to undergo swelling the morphological result of which depends upon the width of the capsule-optic interspace. In a narrow interspace, these cells form flat structures with a honeycomb-like appearance which may finally end up in a contiguous syncytial cell layer. These optically homogeneous structures do not significantly interfere with the patient's vision. With a wider interspace, however, the E-cells turn into globular structures, or "pearls", the borders of which become apparent with retroillumination. With a still wider interspace, these pearls may become multilayered or huge (Fig. 6.3). These entities are termed "regeneratory" after-cataract. Pearls may significantly interfere with the patient's vision especially when forward-scattered light

causes glare and veiling and frequently require Nd:YAG capsulotomy.

ACO (Fig. 6.4), in contrast, derives from the "anterior LECs", or "A-cells" that reside on the anterior capsular leaf left back following capsulorhexis (rhexis). Though these cells also exhibit some potential to migrate, their characteristic is the exquisite potential to turn into myofibroblasts ("myofibroblastic transdifferentiation") where traumatised (rhexis edge) or establishing contact with IOL material (peripheral optic, haptic). These cells then tend to contract and deposit collagen, which leads to shrinkage and whitening of the anterior capsule. This entity is addressed as "fibrotic" after-cataract, "capsular fibrosis", or simply "fibrosis". Fibrosis typically forms in the area of contact between the anterior capsule leaf adjacent to the rhexis (rhexis leaf) and the IOL optic, but also on the posterior capsule central to the rhexis edge in a collapsed (e.g. aphakic) capsular bag.

If fibrosis is excessive, significant contraction of the rhexis opening ("rhexis phimosis") may result. Shrinkage of the anterior capsular leaf may be asymmetric, resulting in sometimes significant secondary decentration of the IOL optic despite a centred rhexis opening (Fig. 6.4 d). As A-cells also migrate, they may gain access to the anterior optic central to the rhexis edge ("LEC ongrowth") to there form transient and sometimes permanent LEC membranes. Also, A-cells may migrate peripherally to access the posterior capsule. Once arrived there, these cells loose their capability to migrate, but contract and deposit collagen as a result of transdifferentiation ("posterior capsule fibrosis"). Biomicroscopically, contraction (focal, "wrinkling"; or concentric, "sand-duning") and whitening of the peripheral posterior capsule is seen. With a larger optic, posterior capsule fibrosis usually does not approach the visual axis.

If contraction of the posterior capsule behind the optic periphery exceeds that of the anterior capsule, the rhexis edge may be retracted to finally be flipped over and around the optic to then establish contact with the posterior capsule behind the IOL optic. This leaves the optic partly or even totally captured, or "button-holed" [18,31] (Fig. 6.4 e,f). This is less seen with thinner high-refractive silicone and acrylic IOLs featuring a smaller optic thickness and a less convex anterior optic surface, or a reduced fibrogenetic potential [30]. A-cells then migrate centrally from the rhexis edge unto the posterior capsule where they undergo transdifferentiation. Though migration again is thus limited, the resulting capsular fibrosis may significantly narrow the free optical zone especially with small-optic IOLs (Fig. 6.4 f).

The severity of ACO resulting from contact between rhexis leaf and IOL optic is material dependent, the latter varying in its potential to "catalyse" transdifferentiation. Some materials (e.g. silicones) induce more fibrosis than others (e.g. some hydrophilic acrylics). With a small optic diameter and an optic material that strongly triggers A-LEC transdifferentiation, the risk of central encroachment of the posteri-

or capsule by fibrosis increases. This is true for any amount and extent of rhexis-optic overlap (lacking or incomplete overlap; full in-the-bag, partly or fully buttonholed optic).

Fibrosis of the central posterior capsule interferes less with visual acuity and contrast vision than pearl formation [9], but may also require Nd:YAG capsulotomy. When necessary, however, performing the Nd:YAG capsulotomy may be difficult: With regeneratory after-cataract, the capsule is thin and vulnerable, and at a distance to the optic, which usually allows for posterior defocus and requires only low laser energy, thus posing a low risk of optic damage. With vision-impairing fibrotic after-cataract, however, the capsule is thickened and tough. As capsular whitening hinders posterior laser defocus and as the capsule is usually firmly attached to the optic, considerable damage of the optic may be unavoidable.

Fibrotic after-cataract formation usually ceases after 3 to 6 months, while regeneratory after-cataract develops over a much longer time to become visually disturbing after 1–3 years. In a 1998 meta-analysis, the reported PCO rates of after extracapsular cataract surgery with IOL implantation were 11.8% at 1 year, 20.7% after 3 years, and 28.4% after 5 years [3].

Summary for the Clinician

- Visual disturbance is mainly caused by equatorial LECs that gain access to the posterior optic-capsule interspace and form pearls
- Anterior LECs tend to cause capsular whitening and shrinkage following myofibroblastic transdifferentiation upon contact to the IOL
- "Regeneratory after-cataract of the posterior capsule", and "fibrotic after-cataract of the anterior or peripheral posterior capsule" more appropriately describe what has been generally termed "PCO" and "ACO"
- Fibrotic after-cataract formation mainly occurs during the first 3 months, while regeneratory after-cataract formation starts later, culminating between the years 2 and 3, and occasionally lasting up to 5 years

6.2
Quantification of After-Cataract

Efforts have been made to create methods to quantify the extent and severity of after-cataract. Different approaches are necessary for PCO and ACO.

For regeneratory PCO, retroillumination images are currently used for evaluation. Subjective grading, which is largely based on intuition, has been replaced by three methods: (1) Manually outlining areas of different severity and then multiplying area by severity (EPCO) [51]; (2) automatically calculating the total area of opacification (POCO-A) [2]; and (3) automatically calculating a score for area and severity by either: (a) implementing an additional mathematical algorithm into the POCO-A system (POCO-S, so far unpublished), or (b) by applying a fully-automated mathematical algorithm based on the evaluation of pixel entropy of the image (AQUA) [14]. The latter was developed in Vienna and is used as our standard evaluation method since it has shown a very high reproducibility and correlation with subjective grading and EPCO scoring while the POCO-A system was not adopted because it exhibited too early saturation and thus overestimation of low-grade and intermediate PCO [14].

Any evaluation method can only pick up the variability displayed by the image. Thus efforts have been made to devise a photographic set-up optimising sagittal alignment [44]. Inherently, reflected-light images better display morphological details than retroillumination images [8]. However, full area coverage is impractical, and evaluation software is not available. Thus, assessment of retroillumination images has become the standard. As an alternative, area densitometry with the Scheimpflug camera system has been used, and has been shown to correlate well with the patient's visual acuity [19].

For ACO, reflected-light images are mandatory, as only these accordingly display the degree of whitening and wrinkling, or fibrosis. Apart from subjective grading, an automated evaluation method has been developed by applying the Photoshop software on standardised reflected-light images [47].

Summary for the Clinician

- Current methods of PCO quantification rely on retroilluminated imaging
- The subjective EPCO system and the objective AQUA system correlate well with each other, while both also do so with subjective grading
- For ACO grading the degree of whitening is assessed either subjectively or using standard image analysis software (Photoshop)
- Future technologies may focus on reflected-light image evaluation which better display morphological details

6.3
Prevention of After-Cataract

6.3.1
Removing LEC from the Equator to Reduce the Proliferative Potential

A logical approach is to selectively target those LECs that finally interfere with the patient's vision, i.e. the equatorial LEC population with its exquisite potential to migrate centrally and to then form pearls within the retro-optical interspace. However, these cells cannot be directly removed as they are remote in the flaccid equatorial capsule and cannot be directly visualised. Thus, direct and complete aspiration is not feasible. However, reducing the number of E-LECs may at least retard and mitigate after-cataract formation though it will not totally preclude it. Therefore, efforts should be made to remove as many of these cells as possible during surgery. Direct abrasion of E-cells using dusted curettes, and ultrasound or diathermy probes has been attempted. However, these procedures are poorly controlled, and E-LEC removal is inherently incomplete. Damage to the capsule, zonules, and ciliary tissue cannot be excluded.

Lens fibres are derived from LECs in the lens bow which have differentiated to build up the lens. Incomplete removal may result in proliferation of these cells known as Soemmering's ring formation. Therefore, every effort should be made to indirectly reduce the amount of cellular material in the capsular equator by aiming at the complete removal of all lens fibres, using a method that may be termed *cortical fibre stripping*: Following aspiration of the cortical masses left behind after phacoemulsification, residual lens fibres may be detected adhering to the posterior capsule when focussing it at higher magnification. When jetting water through a thin cannula, the central end of these fibres is detached from the capsule to then float freely. Using an aspiration cannula, the ends of these cells can be aspirated and occlusion attained by additionally engaging the underlying capsule. Thus, the residual lens fibre bundles may be efficiently stripped off towards the periphery. With appropriate instrumentation and flow/vacuum settings (e.g. Brauweiler cannula by Geuder: 7 ml/min, 100 mmHg), this has been routinely performed by the author without a single case of posterior capsule damage. The goal is: (a) to completely remove all lens fibre material, thus precluding Soemmering's ring formation, and (b) to potentially also catch hold of contiguous E-cells of the capsular bag equator, which my also reduce their proliferative potential.

Summary for the Clinician

- Complete removal of all LECs from the capsular equator by "capsule polishing" techniques is impracticable

- Thorough cortical clean-up using "hydrodissection" and "lens fibre stripping" may prevent Soemmering's ring and PCO formation by reducing the number and thus the proliferative potential of the equatorial LEC population

6.3.2
Erecting Mechanical Barriers to Prevent LEC Migration

Since complete mechanical E-LEC removal cannot be achieved, efforts must be made to prevent LECs from migrating centrally and reaching the visual axis. The rim of the IOL optic is known to form a mechanical barrier. The importance of the rim shape, however, became obvious only more recently when a sharp sharp-edged IOL (Acrysof MA60BM) was shown to allow for significantly less PCO than IOLs with round edges. Meanwhile, the sharp posterior optic edge design has been implemented into essentially all new lenses on the market with the effect of significantly lower Nd:YAG capsulotomy rates (Fig. 6.5).

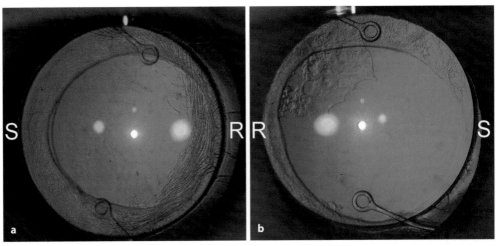

Fig. 6.5 a, b. "Hybrid IOLs" with round (sharp) optic edge oriented nasally (temporally). Note fibrotic/regeneratory after-cataract trespassing round optic edge

6.3.2.1
Mechanism of Optic Edge Barrier Effect

Apart from its sharpness, the efficacy of the posterior optic edge to permanently prevent LEC migration is strongly dependent upon the optic overlap by the rhexis leaf. Without such overlap, the barrier effect generally is only weak and transient. This is understood when looking at the postoperative changes of the capsular bag following IOL implantation as discussed in the following sections.

Capsular Bag Closure

"*Capsular fusion*": Within days after the evacuation of the lens contents, the capsular bag starts shrinking. Setting out from the bag equator, the anterior and posterior capsule leaves progressively fuse. Depending upon the design of the IOL, this fusion process is more or less asymmetric and incomplete, as the haptics variably distort the contour of the capsular bag and the IOL interferes with the approximation of the capsular leaves. With a three-piece open-loop IOL and a circumferential rhexis-optic overlap, however, this generally ends up with the two capsule leaves tightly fused around the optic rim, with the rhexis leaf stretched out and settled down on the optic in the area of overlap, and with the posterior capsule pulled up around the posterior edge of the optic to then join the anterior capsule (Fig. 6.6a–c)

"*Capsular sealing*": When during the course of capsular bag closure the rhexis leaf settles down on the optic surface, the anterior LECs take up contact with the optic material and transform into myofibroblasts, which contract

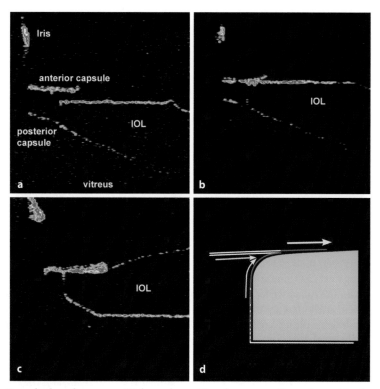

Fig. 6.6 a–d. Capsular bag closure. **a–c** High-resolution OCT imaging of capsular fusion process. **a** Day 1: capsular bag widely open. Note pronounced distance of rhexis leaf to optic surface and posterior capsule. **b** Week 1: capsular fusion in progress: rhexis leaf settling down on optic surface. **c** Month 1: capsular fusion finalised; posterior capsule wrapped around posterior optic edge. **d** Capsular sealing: fibrosis providing strong and permanent "shrink wrapping"

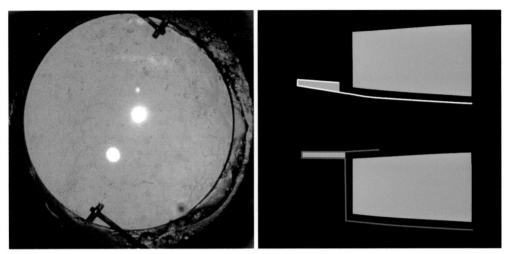

Fig. 6.7. Absent rhexis–optic overlap resulting in "primary barrier failure"

and deposit collagen. The collagen deposited along the optic rim seals the two capsular leaves together, thus creating a strong and permanent sealing line (Fig. 6.6 d).

The *speed and completeness of capsular fusion* varies and is influenced by the design and material characteristics of the implant [21, 42]. The *firmness of capsular sealing* is determined by the catalysing potential of the optic material and the extensiveness and intensity of contact between optic and capsule. Its potential strength may be experienced when trying to surgically reopen a well-sealed capsular bag.

Capsular Bending

During the course of capsular closure the posterior capsule is distended and pulled around the optic rim. This has been shown to result in a mechanical barrier against LEC migration. There is still controversy on the causative factor for this effect. It has been attributed to the capsular bending itself and the resulting "contact inhibition" [39], or to the mechanical pressure building up along the line of capsular apposition [4, 5, 34]. Both factors may most likely be involved [36]. The strength of the barrier depends upon the tension of the capsule and the angle of the posterior optic edge, and is greatest with a tense capsule and a sharp optic edge. As the A-cell-mediated contraction of the anterior and adjacent posterior capsule tightly wraps the capsular bag around the implant ("shrink-wrapping"), the posterior capsule is tightly pulled around the posterior optic edge, thus creating a sharp bend and maximising the pressure exerted along the contact line between the sharp posterior optic edge and posterior capsule. With a lacking capsular overlap, however, such a bend cannot form. Though collagenous attachment may also form along the contact line between rhexis edge not overlapping the optic rim and the posterior capsule [23], this barrier is more easily overcome by migrating LECs, as is the optic rim when not overlapped by the rhexis leaf (Fig. 6.7).

6.3.2.2
Clinical Evidence
for Sharp Optic Edge Efficacy

The role of a sharp implant edge as a migration inhibiting factor and the mechanism of capsular bending was for the first time realised in the mid-1990s. Before, the reduced PCO formation observed with the Acrysof MA60BM three-piece IOL was thought to reflect a specific inhibitory material property. However, attention was drawn to the edge design when it became apparent that most of the PCO inhibitory effect was lost with a lacking rhexis/optic overlap (Fig. 6.7). Thus, the formation of a capsular bend along the sharp posterior optic edge of the Acrysof when circumferentially overlapped by the rhexis leaf was isolated as the cardinal factor explaining for the PCO inhibiting effect of this IOL. In a number of pertinent animal studies, Nishi corroborated the effectiveness of the sharp posterior edge for various optic materials. Conversely, he was able to show that most of the PCO-inhibiting effect of the Acrysof IOL was lost when the edge was blunted or rounded [40]. This was experimental proof that the preventive effect of the Acrysof IOL on PCO was essentially the effect of its rectangular, sharp-edged design rather than the adhesiveness or bioactivity of the specific acrylic material as forwarded by others [26, 43].

Once having realised the importance of the sharp optic edge design, clinical studies were initiated to confirm this for, and to isolate possible differences between the various IOL optic materials. Most of these studies, however, investigated IOLs differing in the material *and* the optic edge design *and/or* the haptic construction [1, 20, 53]. At the University of Vienna, the author and his group (Vienna IOL Study Group) started conducting a series of prospective clinical implant studies systematically evaluating the influence of the IOL design and material, and that of surgical measures by only varying one single parameter in each study. The eyes were randomised and compared intraindividually, since LEC proliferation rates and confluence times have been shown to be age dependent and to correlate closely between pairs of eyes [12]. One series compared lenses of a specific IOL material [poly(methyl methacrylate) (PMMA), silicone, hydrophobic acrylic] that differed solely in the design of the optic edge. The sharp-edged PMMA and silicone IOLs used in the early series were custom-made IOLs provided by Dr. Schmidt Intraokularlinsen (St. Augustin, Germany). The acrylic and silicone IOLs investigated later were provided by Allergan (now AMO, Irvine, CA). All IOLs were investigational IOL models now marketed by Dr. Schmidt Intraokularlinsen as MicroPlex MC220 (PMMA) and MicroSeal MS 612 (silicone), and by AMO as Sensar AR40e (hydrophobic acrylic) and ClariFlex CLFLX B (silicone). The edge design of the two companies differed in that those

provided by Dr. Schmidt Intraokularlinsen featured both a posterior and an anterior sharp edge (truncated edge), while those by Allergan/AMO had a squared posterior edge while the side edge was sloping and the anterior edge round (patented "OptiEdge" design).

Meanwhile, 3- to 5-year follow-up data are available for all three materials (MicroPlex MC220, MicroSil MS612, Sensar AR40e; Table 6.1). The fact that with all IOL materials the sharp-edged models showed significantly lower PCO rates unanimously supports the concept that the sharp optic edge, at least with the materials and designs (open-loop) used, is *the* dominating PCO inhibiting factor. The crucial role of a sharp posterior edge is evidenced by the fact that IOLs with a sharp posterior and a rounded anterior edge profile performed comparably well as those with a truncated edge [6, 7]. The subordinate though well-evidenced role of the IOL optic material has been demonstrated by the above-mentioned animal experiment conducted by Nishi, where blunting or rounding off the edges of optic resulted in a loss of the PCO inhibiting effect of the Acrysof IOL [40].

A sharp posterior optic edge and a circumferential rhexis overlap as the prerequisite to allow for posterior capsule bending have thus been isolated as the causative factors for effectively inhibiting LEC migration at the optic rim.

Summary for the Clinician

- The formation of a capsular bend at the posterior optic edge is the substrate of the barrier effect observed at the optic rim
- Full circumferential rhexis-optic overlap is a prerequisite for capsular bend and thus barrier formation along the posterior optic edge
- The barrier effect is attributed to the mechanical pressure and/or the contact inhibition caused by the capsular bend
- The influence of IOL design and optic material characteristics, and the surgical technique has been isolated in prospective randomised bilateral clinical studies with only one single varying parameter

Table 6.1. PCO and YAG rates with different IOL styles, materials and surgical procedures

Follow-up Parameter	1 Year Subj[a] AQUA[b]	YAG	2 Years Subj AQUA	YAG	3 Years Subj AQUA	YAG	4 Years Subj AQUA	YAG	p Values[c]
PMMA[d] Truncated-edge/round					2.0/4.2	2/6 (n=16)			<0.001
Silicone[e] Truncated-edge/round					-----		1.0/2.6	0/4 (n=25)	<0.001
Silicone[f] OptiEdge/round	0.3/1.3 0.7/1.4	0/1 (n=40)			1.2/3.2 1.8/3.1	1/12 (n=31)			<0.001 <0.001
Acrylic[g] OptiEdge/round	0.4/1.5 1.0/2.2	0/1 (n=31)							<0.001 <0.001
Truncated Silicone[h] vs acrylic[i] [subj,ACO-score:]					0.7/1.4 1.9/2.2 [1.4/1.1]				0.051 0.28
Capsular bending ring: CBR/Control					----- 2.0/4.4	1/11 (n=28)			<0.001
Round-edge silicone[k] Polish/non-polish	----- 1.8/1.6 p=0.79	9/2 (n=33)			----- 3.7/3.3 p=0.1	18/11 (n=33)			
Truncated-edge silicone[h] Polish vs non-polish			----- 1.5/1.2	1/0 (n=43) No YAG					0.052
Truncated acrylic 1-piece[i] vs 3-piece[l]	(0.1/0.6) (0.9/1.3) p<0.05		0.7/1.1 1.3/1.5 p>0.05						
PPCCC round-edge IOL Silicone[k] vs Hydrogel[m]			----- 2.3/3.2[n] (4.3/4.7)[o]	2/2 (YAG or AVE)					0.03 (0.25)

[a]Subjective PCO score [11]; [b]Objective PCO score (AQUA [11]); [c]P-value for PCO scores at last follow-up; [d]MicroPlexMC220 (Dr. Schmidt Intraokularlinsen, St. Augustin, Germany); [e]MicroSil MS612 (Dr. Schmidt Intraokularlinsen); [f]ClariFlex (AMO, Irvine, CA); [g]Sensar (AMO); [h]CeeOn Edge 911A (Pharmacia, Groningen, The Netherlands); [i]Acrysof SA60AT (Alcon); [j]Capsular Bending Ring Type 14E (Morcher, Stuttgart, Germany); [k]SI40 (AMO), Silens6 (Domilens, Lyon, France); [l]Acrysof MA60BM (Alcon, Fort Worth, TX); [m]Hydroview (Storz Ophthalmics, St Louis, MO); [n]Inside PCCC; [o]Capsule outside PCCC.

6.4
Rationale for Investigating Alternatives: "Optic Edge Barrier Failures"

When thinking about alternatives to the "sharp posterior optic edge concept", one question may immediately arise: "If a sharp posterior optic edge so effectively prevents migrating LECs from entering the retro-optical space, why then should we search for alternatives?" Much more so, as the technology can be implemented in almost any IOL style and does not require additional surgical skills or implant devices. The answer is: "To explore even more effective or adjunctive approaches, as a sharp posterior optic edge does not completely and permanently prevent PCO in all eyes, especially over longer time periods (1–2 years and thereafter)". This becomes obvious when not only looking at statistical differences between sharp and round IOLs, but when analysing the unfavourable cases in the sharp-edged cohort.

6.4.3.1
Primary Barrier Failures

Additional to the circumferential overlap of the optic by the rhexis leaf, centripetal fusion of the two capsular leaves resulting in capsular bag closure during the first weeks postoperatively is another prerequisite for capsular bend and thus barrier formation at the posterior optic edge. However, in some cases, this process of capsular closure may been incomplete, or even lacking. This may be termed "primary barrier failure". LECs then are only temporarily, if at all, withheld at the optic edge to then invade the retrolental space (Fig. 6.8)

Incomplete
or Lacking Capsular Bag Closure

In some cases, the capsular bag fails to close without detectable reasons. In others, excessive stretch exerted by an oversized IOL may be isolated as the cause of symmetric barrier failures

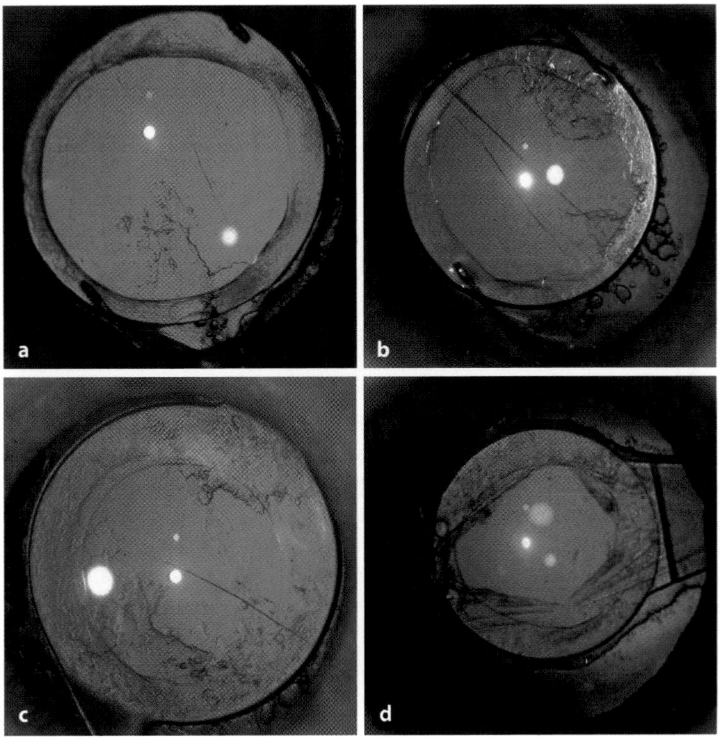

Fig. 6.8 a–d. Barrier failures. A long axial capsular stress lines (rigid oversized haptics) (**a, b**); at optic–haptic junction (one-piece IOLs) (**c, d**)

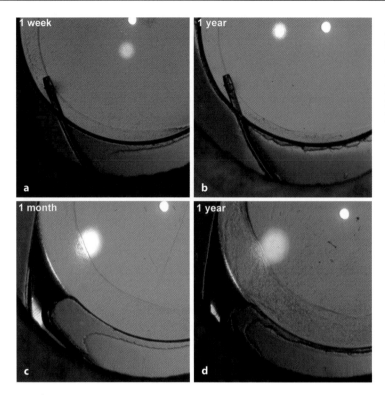

Fig. 6.9 a–d. "Junction phenomenon". Broad-based optic–haptic junction (*below*) interfering with capsular bending. Note "sealing line" detaching from optic rim at junction

occurring along the capsular stress lines (Fig. 6.8 a,b). Large optics also seem to hamper bag closure and bend formation [37].

"Junction Phenomenon"

Even at a slim haptic–optic junction, capsular fusion and consecutive bending is compromised (Fig. 6.9). Consequently, the barrier is partly interrupted or at least weakened at these sites. This is particularly true for any one-piece IOL featuring plate haptics, but also those with broad-based loops [37]. Capsular bending cannot occur even with the sharp optic edge continuing beneath the junction, thus allowing LECs to enter the retro-optical space (Fig. 6.8 c,d). This has been termed "junction phenomenon". The positive effect of looped haptics on capsular fusion may be partly neutralized if they are oversized and/or too rigid [49].

6.4.3.2
Secondary Barrier Failure

In cases with primarily complete capsular closure and bending around the optic, secondary reopening of the barrier with consecutive LEC invasion of the retro-optical space has been observed ("secondary barrier failure"). The reason for this is understood when considering the natural course of E-cell proliferation. Close consecutive in vivo observation of capsular bag closure and LEC migration suggests two phases of E-LEC migration and proliferation: In the first days and weeks postoperatively, and before the process of capsular bag fusion is finalised, early LEC migration can already be observed. Thus, E-LECs may already have reached the retro-optical capsule when capsular fusion has progressed far enough to implement capsular bending. E-LECs thus trapped in the retrolental space, supposedly due to the lack of nutrients, do not proliferate any further and seemingly undergo apoptosis. Such early LEC invasion of

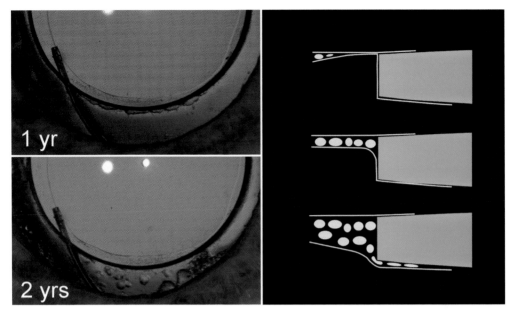

Fig. 6.10. "Secondary barrier failure" with reopening of fused capsules following weak fibrotic sealing

the retro-optical space seems to be influenced by the haptic–optic angulation, since angulated haptics provide for circular attachment of the sharp optic edge and induce capsular bending from the very beginning. In the months and years to follow, a second phase of E-LEC migration and proliferation can be observed: Partly amorphous and partly globular material forms in the capsular equator (Soemmering's ring [23]), which increases in volume and tends to mechanically reopen the once closed capsule bag. Once arrived at the optic, progression is halted by the collagenous sealing of the two capsule leaves along the anterior and lateral aspects of the lens optic and by the permanent posterior capsular bending thus induced (Fig. 6.6 d) which both resist the mechanical force exerted by the proliferating LEC masses. If collagenous sealing is weak relative to the proliferative pressure, however, the sealing line itself and/or the capsular bend thereby induced may break up secondarily, and LECs may enter the retrolental space (Fig. 6.10). As the collagenous sealing is mediated by the A-LECs that undergo myofibroblastic transdifferentiation upon optic contact, the optic material is an important determinant for the firmness and thus resistance of

capsular sealing. The various IOL materials differ in their inherent ability to catalyse myofibroblastic transdifferentiation leading to collagen deposition and capsular contraction. Silicones exhibit the highest and hydrophilic acrylics the lowest catalysing effect, while that of hydrophobic acrylics is labelled intermediate. Thus, the PCO score of IOLs that show relatively low PCO rates during the first 1–2 years may increase thereafter due to secondary barrier failure (e.g. hydrophobic acrylics), while such decay of PCO performance is less observed with other materials (e.g. silicones).

Summary for the Clinician

- A sharp posterior optic edge, though easy-to-implement and effective, does not completely and permanently prevent PCO in all eyes, especially over longer time periods
- Capsular bag closure is a prerequisite for capsular bend formation
- Primary disturbances of capsular bag closure are caused by capsular stress lines induced by oversized IOLs or at the optic–haptic junction of IOLs with a broad haptic base (primary barrier failure)

- A once closed capsular bag may be secondarily reopened by the mechanical pressure exerted by proliferating equatorial cells (secondary barrier failure)
- The material-dependent strength of collagenous sealing along the optic rim avoids secondary barrier failures as it resists the mechanical force exerted by LEC proliferation

6.34.4
Factors Influencing Fibrotic After-Cataract Formation

The extent and severity of ACO is influenced by the extent and intensity of the contact between the anterior capsule and the optic surface. Without such contact, the rhexis leaf remains clear, as the A-LECs do not transdifferentiate. This is best seen in eyes where a capsular bending ring (CBR) keeps the rhexis leaf at a pronounced distance to the optic surface.

Certain pathologies predispose to excessive fibrotic shrinkage ("phimosis") which may end up in total closure of the rhexis opening, especially with an extensive primary rhexis–optic overlap. The causative factor is either zonular weakness (e.g. pseudoexfoliation syndrome, uveitis, pars planitis, high myopia, retinitis pigmentosa) and/or abnormal myofibroblastic activity (e.g. myotonic dystrophy [35]). The lens style determines the type of capsular fibrosis: Slim-looped IOLs, especially those with silicone optics [18, 31], often provoke half- or even full-circumference buttonholing, while the broad junction of plate-lenses inherently reduces this risk. On the other hand, silicone plate-lenses show a strong tendency to induce rhexis phimosis [11], while this is much less the case with open-looped silicone IOLs. The optic edge profile also influences ACO: IOLs with a sharp posterior optic edge hinder A-LECs from "escaping" into the retrolental space. As a result, fibrosis of the peripheral posterior capsule decreases, while anterior capsule fibrosis increases, as evidenced by the enhanced whitening and shrinkage observed [48]. As mentioned above, fibrosis also strongly depends upon the IOL material. There are significant differences in the ability to catalyse myofibroblastic transdifferentiation upon contact [52], with silicones being the most potent ones. In conjunction with a sharp-edged open-loop IOL and symmetrical rhexis-optic overlap, however, this property of the silicone material provides the desired capsular wrapping and sealing of the optic addressed above. The pressure thus created between the posterior capsule and optic edge provides a strong and permanent barrier against (early) A-cell as well as (delayed) E-cell immigration and prevents fibrotic and regeneratory after-cataract formation behind the optic.

How can excessive fibrosis and its negative sequelae be counteracted? Apart from hindering the rhexis leaf to establish contact with the IOL optic by inserting a capsular bending, or distance ring, fibrotic capsular opacification can be avoided by anterior capsule polishing, thereby removing the A-LEC layer as the substrate of myofibroblastic transdifferentiation. In cases predisposed for excessive anterior capsule fibrosis and shrinkage, this protective effect of anterior capsule polishing may outweigh the disadvantages of a compromised barrier formation at the optic edge (see Sects. 6.3.7.2, 6.3.7.4).

Summary for the Clinician

- The extent and severity of ACO is influenced by the extent and intensity of the contact between the anterior capsule and the optic surface
- Certain pathologies predispose to excessive fibrotic shrinkage of the rhexis leaf ("rhexis phimosis")
- IOL determinants of ACO type and intensity are material, but also lens style and optic edge profile
- Use of a capsular bending ring and anterior capsule polishing effectively counteract rhexis whitening and shrinkage, but weaken the barrier at the optic edge

6.4.5
The Role of Optic Material

Originally, the PCO inhibitory effect was attributed to the IOL material. Conversely, when the sharp posterior edge was recognised as a key factor, it became widespread to underestimate or even ignore the influence of the material. Theoretically, the optic material may influence PCO development at three different stages: (1) capsular bag closure (bend formation), (2) fibrotic edge sealing (bend maintenance), and (3) LEC migration and proliferation in the optic–capsule interspace. Most clinical studies comparing IOLs with regard to PCO performance have been using IOLs that differed both in material *and* design. Considering these limitations, the following may be stated: (1) Speed of capsular bag closure is significantly faster with the silicone and acrylic IOL compared to the PMMA IOL, and significantly faster with the silicone IOL than with the acrylic IOL. This was demonstrated by observing capsular bend formation at the optic edge and apposition of capsule to the optic using the slit-lamp microscope [42] and Scheimpflug videophotography [21], respectively. (2) Firmness and thus permanence of fibrotic capsular sealing at the optic edge is significantly greater with silicone than with acrylics. This is evidenced by studies showing that round-edge silicone IOLs perform similarly well as sharp-edge acrylic, and significantly better than round-edge PMMA IOLs [20]. Differences in adhesiveness [43] and bioactive bonding [26] between optic and capsule have been attributed as factors inhibiting migration of LECs once arriving in the optic–capsule interspace. Others have described regression of PCO with specific IOL materials [22]. However, the clinical impact of these parameters remains to be established.

To clearly define the influence of each factor, however, IOLs have to be investigated that differ only in one single criterion [material, or optic (edge) design, or haptic design]. More recent intra- and inter-patient studies indicate that sharp-edge silicone IOL may outperform sharp-edge acrylic IOL in the long run [45] (Tables 6.1 and 6.2).

Table 6.2. Prerequisites for optimal optic edge barrier

Circumferential rhexis/optic overlap
Sharp posterior optic edge
Slim haptic/optic junction
Fibrosis-inducing optic material

Summary for the Clinician

- Speed of capsular bag closure is fastest with silicone IOLs, and faster with acrylic than with PMMA IOLs of similar design
- Firmness and thus permanence of fibrotic capsular sealing at the optic edge is significantly greater with silicone than with acrylic IOLs
- The clinical impact of material adhesiveness and bioactive bonding on after-cataract formation remains to be established

6.4.6
The Role of Patient Age

Organ culture experiments with human LECs have revealed an age dependency between proliferation rates and confluence times [12]. Accordingly, children exhibit high LEC proliferation rates. The proliferative pressure is strong enough to regularly break open and breach the capsular sealing line. A primary posterior capsulorhexis (PPCCC) as a second line of defence is also easily overrun by exuberantly proliferating LECs which use the anterior hyaloid surface as a scaffold. Regarding preventive surgical measures there is general consensus with regard to the necessity of performing a PPCCC in infants and children. However, there is controversy on the need and type of additional measures. According to Koch and Kohnen a PPCCC must be combined with anterior vitrectomy (AVE) to be an effective method of preventing or delaying secondary cataract formation in these patients [24]. For children younger than 7 years the necessity of additionally performing a AVE has been confirmed for the sharp-edge three-piece acrylic IOL Acrysof [25]. The efficacy of capturing the IOL optic through the PPCCC opening

Table 6.3. Indications for alternatives to sharp-edge optic

Primary posterior capsulorhexis
Primary posterior capsule fibrosis (thick plaque: HF-diathermy)
Non-availability of patient (non-compliant, immobile, remote)
Multifocal IOLs (early loss of contrast)
Synchysis scintillans (trans-rhexis AVE)
Children (combined with AVE up to at least school-age)
High myopes (weakened barrier effect at implant edge)
Capsular bending ring
In children (in addition to PPCCC)
Possible/planned vitreoretinal surgery
Capsule polishing
Risk for rhexis phimosis (pseudoexfoliation, uveitis, pars planitis, high myopia, retinitis pigmentosa; myotonic dystrophy)

as a sole measure without AVE has been controversially valued [17, 24, 55]. It may be considered as a simple and potentially useful additive measure against after-cataract formation which also improves optic centration, though lens deposits and posterior synechiae may more often form. In children older than 7 years, AVE may not be necessary with modern sharp-edge IOLs [25], while others consider an additional AVE as a mandatory procedure for children up to 12 years even with posterior optic capture [55] (Table 6.3).

Summary for the Clinician

- Children exhibit high LEC proliferation rates
- There is general consensus with regard to the necessity of performing a PPCCC in infants and children, but controversy on the need and type of additional measures
- Combining the PPCCC with anterior vitrectomy up to an age of at least 7 years has been strongly recommended
- Capturing the IOL optic through the PPCCC opening may be considered as a simple and potentially useful additive measure against after-cataract formation, and also improves optic centration

6.4.7
Alternatives to the Sharp-Edged Optic

Several approaches have been investigated as possible alternative or adjunctive measures to prevent PCO formation. These are discussed in the following sections.

6.4.7.1
Posteriorly Vaulted Posterior–Convex Optic

The idea is highlighted by the "super-reversed optic" concept originally forwarded by Fechner [13]. It was aimed at maximising the posteriorly directed vector force of a posterior convex optic, thereby achieving tight attachment between optic and distended posterior capsule. In theory, no interspace would be left at all, or at least not wide enough to allow LECs to form out vision-disturbing pearls ("No space – no cells", or "small space – no pearls"). With current IOLs, such posterior vaulting characteristics can be implemented in three-piece IOLs with angulated loops made from permanent memory materials (e.g. polyimide), or in one-piece IOLs with angulated broad-based loop or plate haptics made from foldable acrylic or silicone. With plate-haptic IOLs, posterior haptic angulation is not a prerequisite, since posterior vaulting is initiated as the anterior capsule starts shrinking (e.g. STAAR AA4203) [10].

To prove the validity of this approach, we investigated the frequency and width of lens–capsule interspace as detectable with high-intensity slitlamp illumination and/or partial coherence laser interferometry with different IOL styles [15]. Interestingly, no statistically significant difference was found. Notably, the IOLs with the strongest permanent backward vault (Corneal ACR6D SE, STAAR AA4203) exhibited the widest mean space (160 µm) of all lenses investigated. Also, we have seen significant regeneratory PCO formation with a posteriorly vaulted plate IOL (IOGEL) [29]. In conclusion, this concept must be considered ineffective.

6.4.7.2
Capsular Bending Ring

The capsular bending ring (CBR) was conceived and first investigated in rabbit eyes by Nishi [38]. After having proven the safety and short term efficacy in a human pilot study, trials were initiated at the Nishi and University Eye Hospitals in Osaka and Vienna intraindividually comparing the effect of a CBR (Morcher Type 14E; Morcher, Stuttgart, Germany) on after-cataract formation. The device was conceived to act in two ways. Firstly, to keep the entire posterior capsule clear up to the very periphery by inducing a capsular bend at the equator. Secondly, to also keep the anterior capsule clear by keeping it at a pronounced distance to the posterior capsule and the anterior optic surface ("capsular distance ring", or "CDR"). In fact, the CBR showed effectiveness in both aspects during a 2-year follow-up period [32, 41]. However, in a small number of CBR eyes some amount of regeneratory LEC invasion was still observed. Some of these failures could be explained by the gap between the ring eyelets in a large bag allowing LECs to gain access to the posterior capsule. This was remedied by modifying the design of the ring (injectable CBR Morcher Type 14F after Menapace and Nishi). This still left us with some cases of regeneratory after-cataract formation without a detectable cause. Our only explanation is that in these cases E-cells may still be residing central to the posterior bending line. These small numbers of "fenced in" LECs would eventually also invade the posterior capsule. Since with a CBR in place capsular bending at the optic rim can no longer occur, LECs can easily access the space between the tense posterior capsule and the periphery of a posteriorly convex optic, though they cannot readily access the very centre of the optic as the apex of such an optic is firmly attached to the capsule. Nevertheless, in our randomised study, differences in PCO were highly significant: After 1 year, the EPCO PCO score within the 6 mm zone was 0.4 in the CBR as opposed to 0.8 in the control group. After 3 years, the AQUA score was 2.4 in the CBR versus 4.4 in the control group. Of the 28 patients, only one patient had required Nd:YAG capsulotomy in the CTR eye, as opposed to 11 patients with a YAG capsulotomy in the control eye. In conclusion, the CBR concept does work, but (at least with the IOL styles currently available) not efficiently enough to justify the routine use of such an additional implant.

6.4.7.3
Primary Posterior Capsulorhexis (PPCCC)

LECs use the posterior capsule as a scaffold when migrating centrally. Consequently, vision-disturbing after-cataract should be excluded when the central posterior capsule is removed. Even though, cases with vision-disturbing after-cataract formation have been reported with PPCCC. In children, the hyaloid surface is known to serve as an alternative scaffold for E-LEC migration. Despite the differences in hyaloid anatomy, such failures have also been reported in adults. Our theory was that in adults the posterior optic surface may alternatively serve as a scaffold. We conducted a randomised prospective clinical trial intraindividually comparing the efficacy of PPCCC with different optic materials (silicone as a hydrophobic versus hydrogel as a hydrophilic material) using IOLs with a similar design [16]. The main outcome measure was LEC ongrowth within the PPCCC opening in cases with optic edge barrier failure. A capsular tension ring was additionally used in this series to provide for a fully distended posterior capsule and thus circular attachment of the PPCCC margin to the optic. In our study, PPCCC was demonstrated to be safe with no case of associated retinal complication, as also demonstrated by others [54]. In 58 eyes of 29 patients completing the 2-year follow-up, the PPCCC opening remained clear with 66% of the silicone IOLs as opposed to only 41% of the hydrogel IOLs. Partial closure of the PPCCC was observed with 55% of the hydrogel IOLs but with only 28% of the silicone IOLs. Total closure of the PCCC occurred in three eyes, two in the hydrogel group and one in the silicone group. PCO score within the PPCCC opening was significantly lower with silicone IOLs as compared to hydrogel IOLs (AQUA-score 2.3 versus 3.2, $p=0.03$; Table 6.1). Biomicroscopy, and the dependency on optic material confirmed that it was the optic surface that had served as a scaffold in these cases. In conclusion, PPCCC is effective but, as it requires additional surgical skills, may be reserved to supplement the use of a sharp-edged optic in cases with a higher PCO risk (children and young patients, high myopes) or those who are difficult to follow-up or treat (non-compliant or remote patients). In adults silicone optics should be preferred at least over hydrophilic acrylic IOLs because of greater PPCCC efficacy while no retinal complications have been observed so far.

6.4.7.4
"Capsule Polishing"

In theory, the most straight-forward and effective way to exclude any form of after-cataract would be to completely remove all LECs during cataract surgery. In principle, this may be achieved by the application of chemicals or immunotoxins selectively targeting LECs. This, however, has so far not been possible, postoperative uveitis with clinically effective doses constituting the main problem. So far, no method has been shown to be safe for clinical use [27].

Alternatively, efforts have been made to mechanically abrade the lens epithelium. Rentsch developed a ring curette to be entered through the cataract incision ("Ring curettes", Geuder). However, a set of three differently angulated curettes is required to cope with the varying angles of approach. Also, the efficiency of the polishing procedure itself is low as the curettes have to be actively pressed against the flaccid and slippery capsule in a bag expanded with viscoelastic. In general, 5 min under bright coaxial illumination are usually required. Inherently equatorial LEC removal and its completeness cannot be assured. Thus, in an uncontrolled retrospective study conducted by Rentsch [46], 12 % of the eyes that had undergone full circumferential polishing using this method still required Nd:YAG capsulotomy within 3 years.

Therefore, an alternative instrument was developed by Menapace before embarking on a controlled prospective bilateral study to elucidate the efficacy of capsule polishing ("aspiration curette", Geuder). Since mechanical polishing of the equator is inherently uncontrolled

and incomplete, this instrument was specifically designed for efficient polishing of anterior capsule only. Thus, the A-LEC and those E-LECs that reside on the peripheral anterior capsular are targeted. The cannula features an upward-facing slit-like opening with sharp edges on both flanks and rounded edges at the flexes. The uniplanar configuration of the entry allows for firm occlusion when brought into contact with the back surface of the anterior capsular leaf. A bypass hole allows for smooth vacuum build-up. The cannula is compatible with the bimanual cortex aspiration set designed by Brauweiler (Geuder). The cannula is consecutively entered through three paracentesis openings each 120° apart and the slit-like opening lifted up against the contralateral rhexis leaf to allow for occlusion and vacuum build-up. When the cannula is then moved from one side to the other like a windshield wiper, the sharp slit edges efficiently shear off the anterior lens epithelium. Through each paracentesis, one third of the contralateral rhexis circumference is thus deepithelialized. The procedure is visually controlled, and in several hundred cases the cannula has proven to be safe (no case of capsular or zonular damage) and efficient (mean cleaning time 1.5 min).

A prospective study was carried out intraindividually comparing the efficacy of anterior capsule polishing with regard to after-cataract prevention. On a randomised basis one eye underwent extensive polishing using the aspiration curette described above, while the other eye was left unpolished. Round-edge open-loop silicone IOLs were implanted. Main outcome measures were: (a) PCO scores and YAG capsulotomy rates after 1 and 3 years, and (b) ACO and fibrotic PCO after 3 years.

The study produced the following results: (a) Fibrotic after-cataract [50]: ACO in the polished eyes was significantly reduced, with almost no whitening and contraction of the rhexis leaf as opposed to the non-polished eyes. Mean ACO was 17 % for the polished eyes and 26 % for the unpolished eyes ($p<0.01$). Mean fibrotic PCO score was 0.5 and 1.0, respectively ($p<0.01$). Efficacy with regard to fibrotic ACO and PCO prevention thus was very satisfactory. (b) Regeneratory after-cataract [56] (Table 6.1).

At year 1, the polished eyes did not show significantly lower PCO scores than the unpolished eyes. When sorting the eyes according to PCO severity, the worst cases were predominantly found in the polished group. At year 1, no capsulotomy was required in either group. At between 1 and 3 years, nine of the polished and two of the unpolished eyes required Nd:YAG capsulotomy. After 3 years, nine additional eyes in each group needed KT. Thus, the cumulative KT rate was 18 in the polished eyes and 11 in the unpolished group. AQUA scores, however, did not differ significantly. This discrepancy may be explained by an obvious morphological difference: PCO in polished eyes tended to be more homogeneous, while in unpolished eyes it exhibited greater propensity to form well-defined pearls. This layer of poorly delineated PCO after polishing is not adequately depicted on photographs retroilluminated by reflected or backward scattered light. Any evaluation based on retroilluminated images may largely underscore PCO, while the patient's vision is significantly degraded by glare and blur due to forward scattered light.

In conclusion, polishing was effective in preventing fibrotic, but ineffective in reducing regeneratory after-cataract. Nd:YAG capsulotomies had to be performed more often (18 vs 11 out of 33 eyes) and at an earlier time (nine vs two during years 1–3).

Unfavorable results of capsule polishing with regard to regeneratory after-cataract have also been reported by another study using the "ring curettes": In a large study comprising over 1200 eyes, Miller et al. reported a cumulative Nd:YAG capsulotomy rate of 46% in the polished group versus 20% in non-polished eyes in the not polished group ($p=0.0001$) [33]. This strongly supports the concept of capsular fibrosis as a crucial factor for the barrier formation at the optic edge: Without capsule polishing, both the A- and E-cell population are left untouched. Following capsular closure, the A-cells cause fibrosis, thereby firmly sealing the capsular leaves together along the optic circumference. This forms a strong barrier against the delayed migration and proliferation of E-cells. Following capsule polishing, the A-cells and the more anteriorly located E-cells are removed. However, the more remote equatorial portion of E-cells is left at least partly in situ and viable. Though reduced in number, these residual E-cells will also migrate and proliferate, and finally get numerous enough to reach the optic rim. Since no fibrotic sealing of the capsules at the optic rim has occurred, the fusion line is easily overcome, thus allowing the migrating LECs to gain access to the retro-optical space along the whole circumference. Preliminary data from a more recent study indicate that polishing also compromises the barrier effect of sharp-edged optics, though seemingly to a lesser extent (Table 6.1).

Summary for the Clinician

- The concept of avoiding PCO by creating a strong and permanent posterior optic vault has failed
- The capsular bending ring significantly reduces regeneratory after-cataract, while at the same time it avoids ACO (distance effect); however, its limited efficacy with currently available IOLs and the need for an additional implant limits its application
- Primary posterior capsulorhexis is safe and effective, and supplements the efficacy of a sharp-edge optic IOL forming a "second line of defence"; however, the surgical skill required limits its widespread use
- "Capsular polishing" is counterproductive, as it interferes with fibrotic sealing of the capsular leaves along the optic rim, predisposing for secondary barrier failures and, consequently, unimpeded access of E-cells to the retro-optical space

Acknowledgements. The author wishes to express his gratitude to his co-workers at the Vienna IOL Study Group who helped compile the data on which this chapter is based.

References

1. Abhilakh Missier KA, Nuijts RM, Tjia KF (2003) Posterior capsule opacification: silicone plate-haptic versus AcrySof intraocular lenses. J Cataract Refract Surg 29:1569–1574
2. Barman SA, Hollick EJ, Boyce JF et al (2000) Quantification of posterior capsular opacification in digital images after cataract surgery. Invest Ophthalmol Vis Sci 41:3882–3892
3. Bertelmann E, Kojetinsky C (2001) Posterior capsule opacification and anterior capsule opacification. Curr Opin Ophthalmol 12:35–40
4. Bhermi GS, Spalton DJ, El-Osta AA, Marshall J (2002) Failure of a discontinuous bend to prevent lens epithelial cell migration in vitro. J Cataract Refract Surg 28:1256–1261
5. Boyce JF, Bhermi GS, Spalton DJ, El-Osta AR (2002) Mathematical modeling of the forces between an intraocular lens and the capsule. J Cataract Refract Surg 28:1853–1859
6. Buehl W, Findl O, Menapace R et al (2002) Effect of an acrylic intraocular lens with a sharp posterior optic edge on posterior capsule opacification. J Cataract Refract Surg 28:1105–1111
7. Buehl W, Menapace R, Findl O (in press) Effect of a silicone intraocular lens with a sharp posterior optic edge on posterior capsule opacification. J Cataract Refract Surg
8. Camparini M, Macaluso C, Reggiani L, Maraini G (2000) Retroillumination versus reflected-light images in the photographic assessment of posterior capsule opacification. Invest Ophthalmol Vis Sci 41:3074–3079
9. Cheng CY, Yen MY, Chen SJ, Kao SC, Hsu WM, Liu JH (2001) Visual acuity and contrast sensitivity in different types of posterior capsule opacification. J Cataract Refract Surg 27:1055–1060
10. Cumming JS (1993) Postoperative complications and uncorrected acuities after implantation of plate haptic silicone and three-piece silicone intraocular lenses. J Cataract Refract Surg 19:263–274
11. Dahlhauser KF, Wroblewski KJ, Mader TH (1998) Anterior capsule contraction with foldable silicone intraocular lenses. J Cataract Refract Surg 24:1216–1219
12. El-Osta AA, Spalton DJ, Marshall J (2003) In vitro model for the study of human posterior capsule opacification. J Cataract Refract Surg 29:1593–1600
13. Fechner PU, Trier HG (1990) Super-reversed intraocular lens. J Cataract Refract Surg 16:471–476
14. Findl O, Buehl W, Menapace R et al (2003) Comparison of 4 methods for quantifying posterior capsule opacification. J Cataract Refract Surg. 29:106–111
15. Findl O, Drexler W, Menapace R et al (1998) Accurate determination of effective lens position and lens-capsule distance with 4 intraocular lenses. J Cataract Refract Surg 24:1094–1098
16. Georgopoulos M, Menapace R, Findl O et al (2003) After-cataract in adults with primary posterior capsulorhexis: comparison of hydrogel and silicone intraocular lenses with round edges after 2 years. J Cataract Refract Surg 29:955–960
17. Gimbel HV (1997) Posterior continuous curvilinear capsulorhexis and optic capture of the intraocular lens to prevent secondary opacification in pediatric cataract surgery. J Cataract Refract Surg. 1997:652–656
18. Hayashi K, Hayashi H, Nakao F, Hayashi F (1996) Capsular capture of silicone intraocular lenses. J Cataract Refract Surg 22[Suppl 2]:1267–1271
19. Hayashi K, Hayashi H, Nakao F, Hayashi F (1998) In vivo quantitative measurement of posterior capsule opacification after extracapsular cataract surgery. Am J Ophthalmol 125:837–843
20. Hayashi H, Hayashi K, Nakao F, Hayashi F (1998) Quantitative comparison of posterior capsule opacification after polymethylmethacrylate, silicone, and soft acrylic intraocular lens implantation. Arch Ophthalmol 116:1579–1582
21. Hayashi H, Hayashi K, Nakao F, Hayashi F (2002) Elapsed time for capsular apposition to intraocular lens after cataract surgery. Ophthalmology 109:1427–1431
22. Hollick EJ, Spalton DJ, Ursell PG, Pande MV (1998) Lens epithelial cell regression on the posterior capsule with different intraocular lens materials. Br J Ophthalmol 82:1102–1103
23. Kappelhof JP, Vrensen GF (1992) The pathology of after-cataract. A minireview. Acta Ophthalmol Suppl 205:13–24
24. Koch DD, Kohnen T (1997) Retrospective comparison of techniques to prevent secondary cataract formation after posterior chamber intraocular lens implantation in infants and children. J Cataract Refract Surg 23:657–663
25. Kugelberg M, Zetterstrom C (2002) Pediatric cataract surgery with or without anterior vitrectomy. J Cataract Refract Surg 28:1770–1773
26. Linnola RJ (1997) Sandwich theory: bioactivity-based explanation for posterior capsule opacification. J Cataract Refract Surg 23:1539–1542
27. Meacock WR, Spalton DJ, Hollick EJ et al (2000) Double-masked prospective ocular safety study of a lens epithelial cell antibody to prevent posterior capsule opacification. J Cataract Refract Surg 26:716–721

28. Marcantonio JM, Vrensen GF (1999) Cell biology of posterior capsular opacification. Eye 13:484–488

29. Menapace R (1996) Posterior capsule opacification and capsulotomy rates with taco-style hydrogel intraocular lenses. J Cataract Refract Surg 22[Suppl 2]:1318–1330

30. Menapace R (1995) Evaluation of 35 consecutive SI-30 PhacoFlex lenses with high-refractive silicone optic implanted in the capsulorhexis bag. J Cataract Refract Surg 21:339–347

31. Menapace R, Amon M, Papapanos P, Radax U (1994) Evaluation of the first 100 consecutive PhacoFlex silicone lenses implanted in the bag through a self-sealing tunnel incision using the Prodigy inserter. J Cataract Refract Surg 20:299–309

32. Menapace R, Findl O, Georgopoulos M et al (2000) The capsular tension ring: designs, applications, and techniques. J Cataract Refract Surg 26:898–912

33. Miller, KM, Farzad S, Grusha Y (2000) Anterior capsule polishing and the need for laser posterior capsulotomy. Abstract Symposium on Cataract, IOL and refractive surgery, May, Boston

34. Nagamoto T, Fujiwara T (2003) Inhibition of lens epithelial cell migration at the intraocular lens optic edge: role of capsule bending and contact pressure. J Cataract Refract Surg 29:1605–1612

35. Newman DK (1998) Severe capsulorhexis contracture after cataract surgery in myotonic dystrophy. J Cataract Refract Surg 24:1410–1412

36. Nishi O (2003) Effect of a discontinuous capsule bend. J Cataract Refract Surg 29:1051–1052

37. Nishi O, Nishi K (2003) Effect of the optic size of a single-piece acrylic intraocular lens on posterior capsule opacification. J Cataract Refract Surg 29:348–353

38. Nishi O, Nishi K, Mano C et al (1998) The inhibition of lens epithelial cell migration by a discontinuous capsular bend created by a band-shaped circular loop or a capsule-bending ring. Ophthalmic Surg Lasers 29:119–125

39. Nishi O, Nishi K, Sakanishi K (1998) Inhibition of migrating lens epithelial cells at the capsular bend created by the rectangular optic edge of a posterior chamber intraocular lens. Ophthalmic Surg Lasers 29:587–594

40. Nishi O, Nishi K, Akura J, Nagata T (2001) Effect of round-edged acrylic intraocular lenses on preventing posterior capsule opacification. J Cataract Refract Surg 27:608–613

41. Nishi O, Nishi K, Menapace R, Akura J (2001) Capsular bending ring to prevent posterior capsule opacification: 2 year follow-up. J Cataract Refract Surg 27:1359–1365

42. Nishi O, Nishi K, Akura J (2002) Speed of capsular bend formation at the optic edge of acrylic, silicone, and poly(methyl methacrylate) lenses. J Cataract Refract Surg 28: 431–437

43. Oshika T, Nagata T, Ishii Y (1998) Adhesion of lens capsule to intraocular lenses of polymethylmethacrylate, silicone, and acrylic foldable materials: an experimental study. Br J Ophthalmol 82: 549–553

44. Pande MV, Ursell PG, Spalton DJ et al (1997) High-resolution digital retroillumination imaging of the posterior lens capsule after cataract surgery. J Cataract Refract Surg 23:1521–1527

45. Prosdocimo G, Tassinari G, Sala M et al (2003) Posterior capsule opacification after phacoemulsification: silicone CeeOn Edge versus arylate AcrySof intraocular lens. J Cataract Refract Surg 29:1551–1555

46. Rentsch FJ, Bauer W (1996) Langzeitergebnisse nach Entfernung des Linsenepithels bei der extrakapsulären Kataraktoperation mit Phakoemulsifikation. In: Rochels R, Duncker G, Hartmann C (eds) 9. Kongress der Deutschsprachigen Gesellschaft für Intraokularlinsen-Implantation. Springer, Berlin Heidelberg New York, pp 399–407

47. Sacu S, Findl O, Menapace R et al (2002) Assessment of ACO: photographic technique and quantification. J Cataract Refract Surg 28:271–275

48. Sacu S, Findl O, Menapace R et al (2003) Effect of IOL design on fibrotic after-cataract. Abstract, XXI Congress of the ESCRS, September, Munich

49. Sacu S, Findl O, Menapace R (in press) Comparison of PCO between 1-piece and 3-piece Acrysof IOL: 2-year results of a randomized prospective trial. Ophthalmology, in press

50. Sacu S, Menapace R, Wirtitsch M et al (in press) Effect of anterior capsule polishing on fibrotic after-cataract: three-year results. J Cataract Refract Surg

51. Tetz MR, Auffarth GU, Sperker M et al (1997) Photographic image analysis system of posterior capsule opacification. J Cataract Refract Surg 23:1515–1520

52. Tognetto D, Toto L, Sanguinetti G et al (2003) Lens epithelial cell reaction after implantation of different intraocular lens materials: two-year results of a randomised prospective trial. Ophthalmology 110:1935–1941

53. Ursell PG, Spalton DJ, Pande MV et al (1998) Relationship between intraocular lens biomaterials and posterior capsule opacification. J Cataract Refract Surg 24:352–360

54. Van Cauwenberge F, Rakic JM, Galand A (1997) Complicated posterior capsulorhexis: aetiology, management, and outcome. Br J Ophthalmol 81: 195–198

55. Vasavada AR, Trivedi RH, Singh R (2001) Necessity of vitrectomy when optic capture is performed in children older than 5 years. J Cataract Refract Surg 27:1185–1193

56. Wirtitsch M, Menapace R, Findl O et al (2003) Effect of anterior capsule polishing on PCO and Nd:YAG capsulotomy rates: a 3-year follow-up study. Abstract, XXI Congress of the ESCRS, September, Munich

Management of the Mature Cataract

Samuel Masket

7.1
Introduction

The mature cataract may represent one or both of two clinical entities. The cortical mature cataract (Fig. 7.1) has opaque, milky white, (potentially) liquefied cortex that, at surgery, obscures the red reflex and the nature of the underlying lens nucleus. The nuclear mature cataract (Fig. 7.2 a,b) contains an ultra-firm and visibly dark lens nucleus in which an epinucleus cannot be easily delineated and little to no cortex remains; it may consist virtually of "rock-hard" nuclear lens material and lens capsule. Given that a very dark cataract can obscure the red reflex and that a white cataract may harbour an ultra-dense nucleus, there may be crossover between the two entities.

Mature cataracts pose certain challenges to the surgeon and add surgical outcome risks to patients. Because phacoemulsification may be anything but routine in these cases, ophthalmologists have historically considered alterna-

Fig. 7.1. Cortical mature white cataract. Note the white lens. Additionally, an iridodialysis can be noted to the *left* indicating the traumatic nature of this cataract

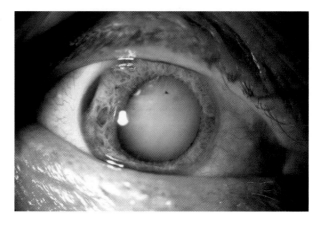

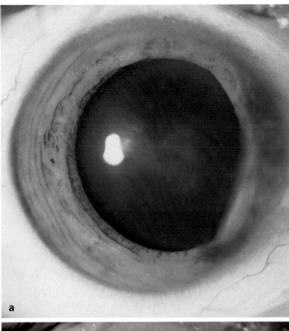

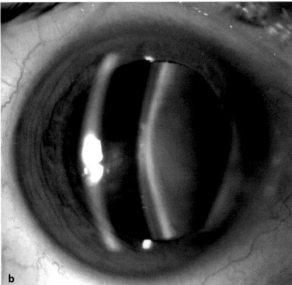

Fig. 7.2. a Nuclear mature cataract. Note the *deep brown colour* of the nuclear cataract. Also visible is a defect in the iris and a corneal scar inferonasally following penetrating trauma earlier in life. **b** Nuclear mature cataract in slit view. Note the deep colour of the cataract and presence of a thin layer under the anterior capsule. No epinucleus is visible

tive surgical methods when faced with mature cataract of either type. Nevertheless, observant presurgical evaluation, careful surgical planning, and skilful and diligent surgical technique can combine to afford the patient the opportunity for rapid visual and physical recovery by means of small incision cataract surgery. Patients contemplating surgery for a mature cataract should be counselled regarding the likelihood for increase surgical time, a slower recovery of vision postoperatively, and an increased risk for intraoperative complications. Likewise, the surgeon must be properly prepared for the increased demands necessary for successful small incision surgery in these cases.

Fig. 7.3. Phacomorphic glaucoma in an eye with a mature white cataract and induced acute and marked elevation of IOP. Note the scleral injection, suggestive of significant inflammation

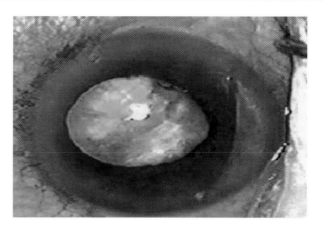

7.2
Cortical (Intumescent) Mature Cataracts

The aetiology of the cortically mature cataract is generally unknown, but the condition is characterised by hydration of lens cortex sufficient for the cortical lens fibres to become swollen and opaque milky white. In the extreme case the lens cortex becomes fully liquefied, leaving only a small firm floating nucleus within a sac of white fluid; this special condition is referred to as a "morgagnian cataract". It is uncertain why some cataracts become cortically mature unless a specific rent in the capsule can be identified. However, the likely final common pathway is the mixture of aqueous humour with lens material. Cases without demonstrable trauma or physical openings in the lens capsule have, most likely, imbibed aqueous through the ordinarily semi-permeable lens capsule. In these cases the lens generally swells, inducing an increased hydrostatic or "intralenticular pressure". Lens swelling may be sufficient to cause narrowing of the chamber angle and the potential for phacomorphic glaucoma (Fig. 7.3).

Raised pressure within the capsule bag (or the eye) is but one factor that can complicate surgery in this group of patients. Capsulorhexis can be very difficult, given that the capsule may be very friable and readily tear to the equator. Furthermore, the surgeon is hindered by the absence of the red reflex, making capsulorhexis

even more challenging. Finally, these case types may be problematic since the density of the nucleus is obscured and cannot be evaluated until after the anterior capsule has been opened. Should the nucleus be very hard, phacoemulsification presents added risks since no epinucleus is present and the milky cortex may tend to wash out, leaving no protective cushion for the posterior capsule during the emulsification process.

The surgical approach to the cortically mature cataract begins with the preoperative evaluation. Gross presurgical vision testing can be assessed with two-point white light discrimination, perception of colour with bright light, and entoptic phenomena. Additionally, the condition of the corneal endothelium should be evaluated with specular microscopy or slit lamp examination, since it may be necessary to elevate the nucleus into the anterior chamber during surgery, should the capsulorhexis fail, the posterior capsule rupture, etc. If the nucleus is very firm and the endothelium poor, emulsification in the anterior chamber may be contraindicated. Lastly, the preoperative evaluation should rule out phacolysis with lens-induced inflammation and secondary elevation of intraocular pressure. In that case intensive topical steroids and/or ocular hypotensive agents may be necessary prior to surgery. Phacomorphic angle closure from an intumescent white lens may require laser iridotomy prior to surgery.

Anterior capsulorhexis remains the most important and the most challenging aspect of the surgery. Generally, if one can complete the capsulorhexis, all else is likely to succeed. The factors that make the capsulorhexis difficult, as discussed above, include poor visibility and the friable nature of the capsule, particularly if it is under tension from increased hydrostatic pressure within the capsular bag. The surgical "game plan" must consider these issues.

Table 7.1 lists the presently available options for increasing visibility during the capsulorhexis. The surgeon should alter the parameters of the microscope, increasing magnification and slowing the motorised changes in magnification, zoom, and X-Y position. In that manner the cut edge of the capsule may be kept in the surgeon's view. Additionally, reducing the ambient room lighting will eliminate glare and improve the visibility of the events occurring in the anterior chamber. Another commonly encountered problem of visibility may occur when the capsule is first punctured, as liquefied cortex may escape from the capsular bag and mix with the aqueous or the viscoagent. This may be prevented by "overfilling" the anterior chamber with a highly retentive viscoagent prior to initiating the capsule tear. This also helps to avoid peripheralisation. Should cortex enter the chamber during capsulorhexis, and preclude an adequate view, it may be necessary to move it out of the way with additional viscoelastic or evacuate with the I/A handpiece or cannula.

Viscoelastic agents vary in their clinical behaviour according to their chemical composition. Although individual stages of the surgery may require different visco-characteristics, the optical clarity, cohesiveness and high viscosity of Healon 5 (Pfizer, New York, NY) at zero shear make it an excellent agent for capsulorhexis in cases with white cataract. However, once the emulsification process is initiated, a dispersive visco-agent may be useful to protect the endothelium and capsule if the nucleus is firm; Viscoat (Alcon) performs well under these circumstances, but might reduce visibility as it traps bubbles and liquefied lens cortex.

The key factor in determining successful completion of a circular anterior capsulotomy (capsulorhexis) in cases with white mature cataracts is visualisation of the anterior capsule and the advancing torn edge of the capsule. Previously, use of a retinal endoilluminator, held tangential to the limbus, had been helpful in aiding the capsule tear [1]. Nevertheless, in my own experience, the endoilluminator method succeeds in less than 100 % of cases. Presently, vital staining of the anterior capsule with either indocyanine green (ICG) or trypan blue has been popularised; this method is virtually always successful. ICG is readily available as an intravenous agent for retinal angiography and renal and hepatic imaging. Horiguchi et al. [2] have developed a system for its dilution, preparation and use in cataract surgery. It is essential to follow the prescribed method, as ICG can be modestly toxic to the corneal endothelium. As initially reported by Melles et al. [3], trypan blue is an excellent stain for the anterior capsule in cases of mature cataract. It is commercially available as a liquid in sterilised unit dose vials, is less costly than ICG, safe with respect to the endothelium and provides excellent contrast between the stained capsule and the underlying opaque or milky white cortex, as can be noted in Fig. 7.4. Given its advantages, trypan blue has become the method of choice for management of cortically mature cataracts. Nonetheless, it is presently unavailable in the USA, as the FDA has not evaluated it or approved its use. Other dyes for capsule staining (Table 7.1) are either more toxic or less efficacious.

Following capsule staining, the capsule tear should be initiated under a retentive viscoelastic in the centre of the anterior lens capsule in order to prevent peripheralisation at the outset of the capsulotomy. Furthermore, if liquefied cortex escapes from the lens and obscures an adequate view, it is wise to aspirate the material or push it aside with additional visco-agent. In rare situations, all of the liquefied cortex may exude from the capsule bag and require removal before the capsulotomy can be completed; in such cases, after evacuating the cortex, the capsule can be filled with viscoelastic, making the surgery technically feasible.

Hydrodissection is often unnecessary in cases of white cataracts, as the liquefaction process may have sufficiently eliminated cortical-capsular adhesions. The surgeon should attempt to

Fig. 7.4. Intraoperative view of capsulorhexis after staining of the anterior capsule with trypan blue. Note that the capsule is easily visualised and contrasts well with the underlying white cortex

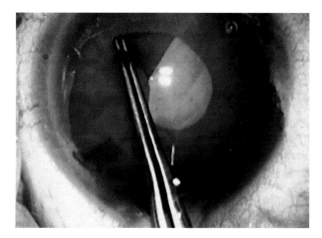

Fig. 7.5. Following capsulorhexis, careful hydrodissection may be performed with a blunt cannula to avoid tearing the fragile anterior capsule

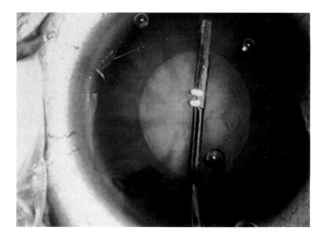

rotate the nucleus after capsulorhexis; if the nucleus is immobile, cautious hydrodissection is necessary (Fig. 7.5). Given the friable nature of the capsule in these cases, hydrodissection must be approached with great care in order to prevent rupture of the capsule; small aliquots of balanced salt solution (BSS) should be injected very slowly to prevent elevation of lens hydrostatic pressure. Furthermore, cases with recent trauma are likely to have a capsule rent which may be extended with aggressive hydrodissection; posterior lens dislocation is an unfortunate, but possible sequel. On the other hand, a case of old trauma may demonstrate a fibrotic lens capsule (membranous cataract) and partially absorbed lens cortex. Hydrodissection may be impossible in cases of this nature.

Table 7.1. Methods to enhance visibility during capsulorhexis

Alter microscope parameters
Increase magnification
Reduce focus speed
Reduce zoom speed
Reduce X-Y speed
Turn off room lights
Liberal use of visco-agent
Side lighting – retinal endoilluminator
Stain the anterior capsule
Trypan blue
Indocyanine green (ICG)
Flourescein sodium
Methylene blue
Gentian violet
Brilliant green
Autologous blood

Nuclear emulsification may be carried out with the most appropriate strategy for the given case; nuclear chopping methods reduce the total amount of ultrasound necessary for lens disassembly. Care must be taken to avoid damage to the anterior capsule rim, the equatorial capsule, and the posterior capsule. Occasional addition of viscoelastic during the emulsification process can be very protective. Also, the nuclear fragments and sharp edges should be brought away from the posterior capsule and into the central aspect of the chamber before emulsification; the centre offers the furthest distance from both the posterior capsule and the corneal endothelium. If the lens nucleus is particularly dense and no cortex remains, anterior chamber or iris plane emulsification should be considered, although the presurgical status of the corneal endothelium must be factored. In very rare circumstances, it might be safest to remove the nucleus manually, particularly if capsular integrity is compromised. Recent forms of ultrasound energy modulation have helped to reduce total energy exposure and have resulted in clearer corneas early after surgery and a more rapid return to normal visual function.

Cortex removal following nuclear emulsification is rarely challenging in cases with white cataracts. Nevertheless, it is common to encounter resistant fibrotic plaques on the posterior capsule. These may be left alone, or, in rare circumstances, a posterior capsulorhexis may be performed. Following "cortical clean-up", lens implantation can be performed routinely. Postoperative management should present no unusual hurdles unless preoperative lens induced inflammation or elevation of IOP continue after surgery.

7.3
What to Do When Things Go Wrong

The most frequent complication, as it were, is failure to complete a smooth-edged continuous tear anterior capsulotomy. The capsulotomy may be completed by the "can-opener" method or by starting another capsulorhexis in the opposite direction, if possible. Added care must be taken when carrying out nuclear emulsification in cases without continuous capsulotomy. Given generally poor visibility, a friable capsule, little to no cortical or epinuclear cushion, my preference is to bring the nucleus into the anterior chamber with a "tire-iron" manoeuvre, using the viscoelastic agent with its cannula. Anterior chamber emulsification is performed unless the lens is extraordinarily dense and/or the endothelium significantly compromised preoperatively. Under those circumstances, manual removal of the nucleus is a safer option. In that case, it may be wise to abandon the temporal clear corneal incision and prepare a sclerocorneal incision superiorly for best wound and astigmatism management. Also, removal of the nucleus, in this situation, is properly managed with a vectis, loop, or spoon rather than by expression since the firm, large nucleus may tear the capsule or rupture zonules during the expression manoeuvre. In fact, cases of this nature are at added risk for posterior dislocation of the nucleus during attempted expression.

Summary for the Clinician

- Successful completion of capsulorhexis is the key to surgical outcome in cases with cortically mature (white) cataracts
- Capsule staining significantly enhances the surgeon's view, but great care must be taken to manage the friable capsule, particularly if the lens is intumescent with high "intralenticular" pressure
- Given the potential need to emulsify a dense nucleus in the anterior chamber, the surgeon should carefully evaluate the health of the cornea as part of the preoperative evaluation

7.4
The Nuclear Mature (Brunescent) Cataract

Brunescent nuclear cataracts (see Fig. 7.2 a, b) can progress to very advanced stages while producing little apparent loss of visual function. Most patients with nuclear cataract experience reduced distance vision, notice difficulty seeing at night and complain of glare symptoms. These cases generally have increased nuclear opalescence mixed with other forms of cataract. However, in some eyes the nucleus changes very gradually from clear to dark brown or black, passing through stages of yellow to deep red. In some of these cases, particularly those without nuclear opalescence, there is little distortion, glare, or relative loss of night vision; the patients are often tolerant of the slowly evanescent reduction in contrast sensitivity and colour perception associated with this cataract type. The net result is that the surgeon may be confronted with the paradox of a very advanced cataract and a relatively asymptomatic patient. On one hand, cataract extraction should be performed before the surgery becomes extraordinarily risky, while on the other the patient may perceive little need for the proposed surgery, even though visual function may be significantly reduced.

A nuclear cataract may be considered as mature when an epinucleus cannot be defined with routine hydrodelineation. Additionally, the maturation process may advance to where lens cortex is minimal, or nearly non-existent. These cases present added challenges intraoperatively with regard to the capsulorhexis, hydrodissection, and lens emulsification in particular. Furthermore, even in cases without surgical complication, there is the potential for prolonged recovery of vision postoperatively, owing to an increased likelihood for transient corneal oedema following prolonged phacoemulsification.

Summary for the Clinician

- Nuclear mature cataracts require significantly greater energy for emulsification
- There may be no protective epinucleus to act as a cushion for the posterior capsule
- Chopping techniques may not be feasible. As a result, nuclear emulsification will require greater caution, time, and diligence
- Generous use of viscosurgical devices can be of significant benefit

7.5
Surgical Management

Surgical treatment for cases with nuclear mature cataracts begins with careful presurgical evaluation and planning. Certain factors must be considered. These include the depth of the anterior chamber and the preoperative condition of the corneal endothelium. Prolonged emulsification time, almost unavoidable with advanced brunescent cataracts, will place a significant burden on the survival of corneal clarity, should the chamber be shallow or the endothelium already compromised. Likewise, lengthy emulsification might be accompanied by significant zonular traction with an attendant potential for long-term complications, particularly if the presurgical condition of the zonules is compromised, as in some cases with pseudoexfoliation. Therefore, in light of these few examples alone, preoperative examination should be considered as an integral part of the surgical management of nuclear mature cataracts.

Capsulorhexis can be challenging should the red reflex be obscured by the extraordinary density of the lens nucleus. In this case, it is advisable to consider any or all of the "tricks" for enhanced visibility of the capsulotomy in cases with white mature cataracts (see Table 7.1). The capsulotomy should be generous in size, perhaps larger than usual in order to avoid damage to the anterior capsule rim during emulsification and to facilitate removal of the nucleus from the capsule bag should it be necessary for any reason (ruptured posterior capsule, etc.). I generally aim for a centred anterior circular capsulorhexis of 6.0 mm or more with these cases, whereas in the routine situation I prefer the capsulotomy to be roughly 5.0–5.5 mm.

Hydrodissection must be carried out with great caution. In the "garden variety" cataract case, the epinucleus and cortex can act as a reservoir for the injected fluid during the hydrodissection. However, in the situation of a mature nuclear cataract, there is little more than a thin lens capsule and a firm nucleus. As a result, there is no cushion or "sponge" to absorb excess fluid as it is injected during hydrodissection; a bolus of BSS, having no opportunity to be absorbed, can "blow out" the thin posterior capsule. Alternatively, if the BSS is injected slowly and in judicious amounts, the fluid can cleave the nucleus from the cortex and capsule without incident.

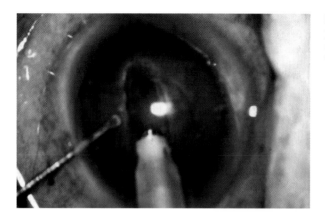

Fig. 7.6. A deep groove is dissected by phacoemulsification, allowing nuclear division if the cataract is judged to be too dense for routine chopping methods

Nuclear emulsification will take added time, care, and patience when compared with the routine situation. When planning the surgical day, one should recognise that phacoemulsification of mature cataracts potentially takes longer than for typical cases. Recognising and planning for the needed extra time will relieve, to some extent, the added stress of dealing with cases of this nature. As mentioned above, modulation of emulsification energy through recent technologic advances may spare endothelial damage.

While there has been a general trend toward nuclear chopping and away from traditional "divide and conquer" sculpting methods for nuclear disassembly, chopping of very dense nuclear cataracts can be difficult and potentially dangerous, given that most chopping instruments are not sharp enough or long enough to adequately penetrate a very dense nucleus. Furthermore, the added toque needed to chop a large "rock-hard" nucleus is likely to add undesirable stress on the zonules. Therefore, in certain cases, I prefer to sculpt and hemi-divide nuclear mature cataracts before chopping the segments (Fig. 7.6). Sculpting is facilitated by using a tip with an increased cutting angle for greater efficiency. Also, use of increased emulsification energy will facilitate the sculpting process which should be carried out deeply into the central nucleus. The latter manoeuvre allows the nucleus to be "cracked" for disassembly. Furthermore, when sculpting a firm nucleus, only a small amount of tissue should be removed with each pass in order to avoid zonu-

lar stress. A worthwhile adage suggests that "nuclear tissue should be removed rather than moved" during sculpting. Finally, I generally add a highly retentive dispersive visco-agent (Viscoat, Alcon, Forth Worth, TX) or a visco-adaptive agent (Healon 5, Pfizer) to the chamber on several occasions during the emulsification process. This technique yields added protection to the cornea and capsule during surgery, but increases the risks for incisional burns.

During nuclear sculpting I partially de-bulk the centre of the lens and create a central trough which is used for the initial crack, creating two hemi-nuclei. Should the nucleus fail to crack, it is generally necessary to sculpt deeper. Hard cataracts are notoriously difficult to divide as the lens is noted to have "leathery" posterior bridges and adhesions when cracking is attempted. Surgeons attempt a variety of personal tricks when confronted with a "non-cracking" nucleus.

Following successful hemi-division of the nucleus, the two pieces may be sculpted and divided or chopped, varying with conditions, equipment, and surgeon experience. For very dense cataracts I prefer to sculpt and divide into four or more equal size pieces before removing any of the segments, since it is easier to rotate the lens as a single unit. Prior to removing the fragments I add viscoelastic to the chamber. The segments are brought forward with a spatulated instrument through a paracentesis. I attempt to raise the sharp angulated portion of the nuclear piece away from the posterior capsule rather than have it sweep against the capsule and risk capsule rupture. I employ high vacuum fluidics to facilitate aspiration and I bring the free nuclear piece into the centre of the chamber, so that emulsification can be carried out in the deepest portion of the chamber, giving the greatest possible protection to the cornea and the posterior capsule. In order to prevent wound burn during this case type, it is necessary to work with an incision of adequate width, allow adequate BSS (chilled) exchange, clear a path through the visco-agent (with irrigation and aspiration) prior to emulsification, and avoid (prolonged) tip occlusion by using modulated phacoemulsification energy when removing the quadrants. As a rule, newer, reduced dimension micro-tips are not ideal for emulsification of cases of this type since the diameter of the tip prolongs removal of the bulky, dense cataract. Following nuclear emulsification, cortex removal and lens implantation should be routine.

Small incision cataract surgery provides rapid and stable optical recovery [4]. Advantages accrue to the patient, to the surgeon, and to society. Fortunately, by adhering to the above guidelines and suggestions, patients with mature cataract of both types may, in many cases,

be managed as routine and can expect excellent return of visual function after surgery.

References

1. Mansour AM (1993) Anterior capsulorhexis in hypermature cataracts (letter). J Cataract Refract Surg 189:116–117
2. Horiguchi M, Miyake K, Ohta I, Ito Y (1998) Staining of the lens capsule for circular continuous capsulorhexis in eyes with white cataract. Arch Opthalmol 116:553–537
3. Melles GRJ, de Waard PWT, Pameyer JH, Beekhuis WH (1999) Trypan blue capsule staining to visualize the capsulorhexis in cataract surgery. J Cataract Refract Surg 25:7–9
4. Masket S, Tennen DG (1996) Astigmatism stabilization of 3.0 mm temporal clear corneal cataract incisions. J Cataract Refract Surg 22:1451–1455

Core Messages

- Preoperative specification of uveitis aetiology is mandatory for surgical success
- Any of the decisions on cataract surgery, including surgical technique, IOL implantation and perioperative medication, rely on proper patient selection
- Complete quiescence of inflammation must be obtained before cataract surgery
- The most important general principle for the surgery is to minimise the surgical trauma
- While IOL implantation is safe in many of the uveitis patients, it is not recommended in patients of less than 2 years of age, or with active uveitis of any aetiology, aggressive course of inflammation in spite of high-dose immunosuppression and in uncertain uveitis course
- The postoperative anti-inflammatory treatment must be adjusted according to the surgical manoeuvres and the inflammatory activity
- Although several complications may occur in the postoperative course, reported functional results are generally encouraging
- A major goal in the care of uveitis patients is the prevention of inflammatory relapses and of cataract formation

8.1 Introduction

Cataract formation is an especially common complication resulting from uveitis. It is rare in posterior uveitis, but occurs in up to 50% of patients with anterior and intermediate uveitis [21], and in nearly 80% of patients with Fuchs heterochromic iridocyclitis (FHC). Duration and intensity of inflammation, and treatment, e.g. corticosteroids and previous vitrectomy, are critical determinants for cataract formation. Compared with the general population, cataract formation occurs at an earlier age in uveitis patients [36].

The common prejudices concerning cataract surgery in uveitis patients are that the surgery has a poor final outcome, induces severe postoperative recurrence of uveitis, has a high rate of ocular hypotony and phthisis and that intraocular lens (IOL) implantation is absolutely contraindicated. Although a number of typical intra- and postoperative problems must be considered with regard to patient selection for surgery, for the surgical technique and the pre- and postoperative care of the patients, the results after cataract surgery are generally quite good [16].

8.2 Basics for Cataract Formation in Uveitis

Cataract may appear in various clinical forms. Posterior synechiae are often seen with focal areas of anterior capsule necrosis and underlying lens opacities. Fibrin membranes overlying the lens are often accompanied by an opacification

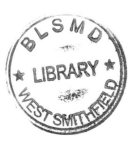

under the anterior capsule. Nevertheless, the typical form of complicated cataract seen in patients with uveitis is posterior subcapsular cataract formation. In rare cases, an anterior subcapsular opacity can be observed primarily. Cataract formation at the posterior pole of the lens can be explained by a missing epithelial barrier and by the thinnest part of the lens capsule. Inflammatory stimuli or degeneration might induce proliferation of lens epithelial cells (LEC). These abnormal cells produce extracellular basal membrane material and extracellular matrix before they degenerate in combination with surrounding lens fibres [44]. The typical progression of cataract depends on the severity of inflammation. In older uveitic patients, the proliferation potential of LEC is reduced and, therefore, it is difficult to distinguish from senile subcapsular opacity.

8.3
Basics for the Consideration of IOL Implantation

The outcome of cataract extraction with IOL implantation in uveitis patients depends largely on the biocompatibility of the lens material used. Uniformly, any implanted material acts as an artificial surface that may lead to foreign body reaction. Reactions on the lens surfaces were taken as a marker for the degree of biocompatibility of the implanted lens material. Uveal biocompatibility refers to the relationship to the vascular tissue of eye while capsular biocompatibility generally refers to the contact with the remnant lens epithelial cells [3]. Due to the different parameters investigated for uveal and capsular biocompatibility one might be excellent and the other might be poor.

8.3.1
Uveal Biocompatibility

The breakdown of the blood–aqueous barrier (BAB) is the first striking event during or directly after surgery. The average time to re-establish the BAB is 3 months [42]. The increase of cells and cytokines in the anterior chamber (AC) in-

fluences the degree of uveal and also of capsular biocompatibility. Activation of the complement cascade (primarily the alternative pathway) initiates the inflammatory response to the artificial material. Fragments of C3 bind to the surface of the implant and C5 is released into the aqueous [24]. Chemotactic C5 derived peptides support polymorphonuclear leukocyte (PMN) influx into the AC. PMNs adhere to the surface-bound C3 fragments and amplify the adhesion and aggregation of further cells. Other groups proposed that IOLs might not alter the complement levels significantly [30].

Some degree of foreign body reaction occurs in all eyes after cataract surgery in order to clear debris from the IOL surface. The first cells noted on the surface are small and spindle-shaped macrophages. Epithelioid or giant cells, resembling uni- or multinucleated macrophages, are found at the end of the first week. While most of these cells usually disappear, few cells can be found on IOLs years later. An early giant cell reaction with few cells occurs within the first month in many patients. The cells clear after some weeks without any clinical significance. The late reaction is regarded as a foreign-body reaction to the IOL. Groups of multi-nucleated cells appear usually after the first month and are often located at the pupillary border. Cells most probably originate from the anterior segment vessels or from synechiae.

The aqueous humour in uveitis patients after cataract surgery shows abundance of macrophages. While the expressions of the typical macrophage cytokines IL-1 and IL-12 are low or absent, respectively, a shift towards a T helper cell type 1 cytokine expression (IL-2 and IFN-γ) is found. The data suggested that the long-standing immunosuppressive therapy or the chronicity of the uveitis suppressed or switched off macrophages function [33]. It has been speculated that the alteration of macrophage functions and the modified cytokines in the aqueous fluid of uveitis patients may delay the clearing of cells from the AC or may even turn it in the opposite direction.

Other studies have shown that the surface of foreign bodies absorbs proteins within seconds or minutes after AC implantation. These include fibrinogen, albumin, γ-globulin and small amounts of fibronectin and coagulation factors [4]. The consistence of this initial layer appears to differ with the IOL material and may, therefore, explain why uveal and capsular biocompatibility depends on the lens material [27].

8.3.2
Capsular Biocompatibility

The capsular biocompatibility is characterised by lens epithelial cell (LEC) migration, by anterior capsule opacification (ACO) and posterior capsule opacification (PCO). These parameters also depend on the above mentioned mechanism of BAB breakdown and protein absorption of the IOL. Absorption patterns differ extremely between the lens materials. Linnola and coauthors [27] showed that fibronectin is responsible for the IOL attachment to the capsular bag. This bioactive bond between lens and capsule may reduce lens epithelial cell migration, being one reason for a lower PCO rate. Due to a severely damaged BAB and changed cytokines in uveitic eyes, LEC may loose their ability to attach to the lens surface [27]. Therefore, the capsular biocompatibility of one IOL material also depends on the intraocular environment.

Summary for the Clinician

- Any IOL material may lead to a foreign body reaction
- Uveal biocompatibility influences the degree of cell deposits on the IOLs
- Capsular biocompatibility influences the opacification of the anterior and posterior capsule

8.4
Patient Selection

Any of the decisions on cataract surgery (e.g. surgical technique, IOL implantation, perioperative medication) rely on a meticulous evaluation. Patient selection is of the utmost importance for surgical success. For example, the surgical techniques and success rates after cataract surgery differ profoundly between patients with FHC and juvenile idiopathic arthritis (JIA)-associated uveitis.

The preoperative evaluation is indicated in order to specify the aetiology of uveitis. The ophthalmological examination should always include visual acuity tests, slit-lamp evaluation, tonometry, and ophthalmoscopy. Additional tests may be indicated, such as interferometry, sonography, fluorescence angiography, visual field assessment or electrophysiological tests. A comprehensive review of systems, clinical evaluations by consulting physicians, laboratory and radiological investigations must be included.

8.4.1
Aetiology of Uveitis

The management of uveitic cataract is principally dependent on the underlying aetiology of uveitis, since the diverse types of uveitis differ extremely in their typical postoperative complications and courses of visual loss. The recommendations and evidence that are published must be considered when selecting the surgical method for the individual patient. For example, while IOL implantation can be recommended in patients suffering from FHC, it is generally contraindicated in patients with JIA uveitis.

8.4.2
Indications and Contraindications
in Cataract Surgery

The indications for the treatment of uveitic cataracts differ profoundly between the patients:

1. The major cause for surgery is mostly poor vision. However, the contribution of cataract to visual deterioration must be distinguished from other factors, such as vitreitis, cystoid macular oedema (CME) or amblyopia in children.
2. The fundus exploration may be impaired due to the cataract. Cataract extraction may be indicated to judge the abnormalities that are critical for the configuration of the treatment plan, e.g. CME, neovascularisation of retinal

vessels, CNV, retinal detachment or uveal effusion.

3. Vitreous or macular surgery may be necessary, but it may not be safely performed because of dense cataract.

4. In the rare cases of phacoantigenic uveitis, in which the leakage of lens proteins is the cause of inflammation, removal of the lens cures the uveitis.

There is a short list of contraindications against cataract surgery. The presence of active inflammation in the anterior chamber is an absolute contraindication against the operation. Young patient's age, relatively good vision and the advantages of accommodation must be considered.

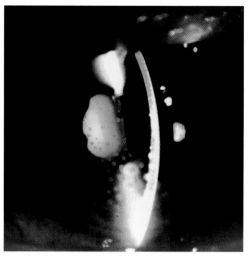

Fig. 8.1. Iridocyclitis, active inflammation, posterior synechiae and cataract

Summary for the Clinician

- Careful patient selection is important for surgical success
- Preoperative evaluation is mandatory in order to specify the aetiology of uveitis
- Presence of active inflammation is a contraindication to surgery

8.5
Timing of Surgery and Preoperative Management

8.5.1
Timing of Surgery

Most authorities agree to the notion that complete quiescence of inflammation, e.g. 10 cells or less in the slit-lamp high-power field in the anterior chamber (1+, according to previously published classification [7]), must first be obtained before cataract surgery can be planned. At least 8 weeks of remission of inflammation before surgery are commonly recommended [36]. Surgery should be deferred, if inflammation persists or frequently recurs (Fig. 8.1). The experience of ocular attacks during the previous year may indicate the postoperative course, as has been observed in Behçet's disease [28], sarcoidosis and JIA-associated uveitis. In these cases, appropriate anti-inflammatory medication must be adjusted first before proceeding

with surgery. Low intraocular pressure (IOP), cells in the vitreous and thickening of the choroid may also demonstrate ongoing inflammation.

The issue of amblyopia is further complicating the timing of surgery in children, as the surgical success may be negotiated by irreversible amblyopia, if surgery is delayed too long. However, lens removal with the consequence of loss of accommodation has great impact in young children.

8.5.2
Preoperative Anti-inflammatory Medication

Anti-inflammatory medication is commonly instituted prior to surgical intervention. Usually, the application of topical corticosteroids, such as prednisolone acetate 1% or dexamethasone 0.1% five times daily for 1 week in addition to the individual treatment regiment is generally sufficient. Transseptal injections of dexamethasone 4 mg or triamcinolone acetonide 40 mg may also be used in patients with a known high degree of postoperative fibrin formation.

A systemic corticosteroid application is indicated in selected cases with previous or current

CME, with intermediate or posterior uveitis or with known attacks of severe inflammation after previous intraocular surgery. Although the optimal preoperative dosages are not well defined, prednisone 1 mg/kg body weight given for 3 days or intravenous methyl prednisone injections on the day before surgery may be effective.

Patients suffering from an endogenous uveitis with a devastating chronic course with vision threatening complications should be set on immunosuppression in advance. Most of the drugs must be given 1–3 months before they achieve sufficient anti-inflammatory effects.

The value of topical and/or systemic nonsteroidal anti-inflammatory drugs (NSAID) for the preoperative management of inflammation is not well known. Systemic NSAID cannot be recommended as they can increase the intraoperative bleeding rate.

There is common consent that glaucoma should be stabilised before surgery. The use of miotic drugs before surgery is strongly discouraged. This is because of their tendency to disrupt the blood–aqueous barrier resulting in an increased rate of postoperative fibrin formation and because of the small pupil size that main makes surgery more difficult and that may increase the bleeding rate.

Since many of the uveitis patients are under long-term immunosuppressive treatment, perioperative prevention of postcataract surgery infections must be considered. Since the rate of reactivation of toxoplasmosis is increased after cataract surgery, prophylactic use of antiparasitic drugs may be started in selected patients during surgery [9].

Summary for the Clinician

- At least 8 weeks of remission of inflammation are required before surgery
- The experience of ocular attacks during the previous course may indicate the postoperative course of uveitis
- Application of topical prednisolone acetate 1 % five times daily for 1 week in addition to the individual treatment regiment is generally sufficient

- Patients with a devastating chronic course of uveitis and with vision threatening complications should be set on immunosuppression in advance
- Glaucoma must be stabilised before surgery

8.6
Surgery

8.6.1
Intraoperative Medication

In the hour before surgery, phenylephrine-, tropicamide- and cyclopentolate hydrochloride are repeatedly instilled onto the eye. The topical application of non-steroidals, e. g. ketorolac 0.5 %, flurbiprofen 0.03 % or diclofenac 0.1 %, improves intraoperative pupil dilation.

At the end of surgery, a transseptal injection of dexamethasone 4 mg is applied. In patients with uveitis that respond with severe postoperative fibrin formation or frequent development of CME, methylprednisolone 500–1000 mg may be injected intravenously. Alternatively, triamcinolone 2 mg may be injected into the anterior chamber.

8.6.2
Approaches to Cataract Surgery

While topical- or retrobulbar anaesthesia is the preferred technique for many cataract surgeons, general anaesthesia may be chosen for children and for cases with surgically challenging conditions, such as with marked anterior synechiae, fibrovascular membranes or with vitreitis. The application of Hanons' balloon before surgery is recommended in children and in cases with a complicated anatomy.

The most important general principle for the surgery of uveitic cataract is to minimise the surgical trauma. A short duration of surgery leads to less inflammation. It is impossible to standardise the surgical method in uveitis patients. While the choice of the optimal surgical procedure depends largely on the aetiology and course of uveitis, it is also dependent on the preference of the surgeon. A recent multi-centre study suggested that phacoemulsification with in the bag IOL implantation should be the preferred surgical technique for the majority of uveitis patients [2]. Compared with ECCE and IOL implantation, patients after phacoemulsification and IOL implantation had lower incidences of CME, epiretinal membranes and synechiae [11, 15]. However, the surgical approach must be reconsidered in every individual patient.

Summary for the Clinician

- General anaesthesia may be chosen for children or in cases with surgically challenging conditions

8.7
Extracapsular Cataract Extraction

Careful extracapsular cataract extraction (ECCE) and complete removal of cortex can be achieved with iris retraction and capsule inspection. The initial study on ECCE and IOL implantation in patients with uveitis reported that visual acuity was 20/40 or better in 87% of the patients after a mean of 43 months of follow up [13, 15]. However, further studies indicated that phacoemulsification with continuous curvilinear capsulorhexis (CCC) induced less surgical trauma and postoperative inflammation than ECCE operation with linear capsulotomy [16, 37, 39].

8.8
Phacoemulsification

For the majority of adults with uveitis and cataract formation, an anterior scleral or corneal incision can be recommended [2, 13]. It has been shown previously that small incisions induce a lower grade of inflammation than do longer incisions, and corneal may be better than scleral incisions. The fact that the high dosages of corticosteroids given in uveitis patients may interfere with wound healing further supports the use of small tunnels. Corneal incisions are advantageous in patients who may require filtrating glaucoma surgery.

The anterior capsulotomy should be obtained with CCC. An intact, well-centred CCC that is overlapping the optic edge reduces the development of PCO as compared to the can-opener technique, and minimises IOL decentration. Fibrous capsular bands can be excised with a cutter or fine scissors.

On the other hand, CCC may lead to a fibrotic opacification of the anterior capsule, which may obscure visualisation of the peripheral fundus. Compared with a 4-mm CCC, the 5.5-mm opening allows the removal of nearly twice as many epithelial cells. The number of epithelial cells and capsular fibrosis can be reduced by aspiration of the posterior surface of the anterior capsule [34], which is highly recommended in children. Capsule contraction syndrome is more often seen with a small CCC and in patients with uveitis than in others [1].

In cases with pre-existing fibrosis of the posterior capsule or a high risk of rapid PCO development, a central opening of the posterior capsule should be performed with the use of Utrata forceps, cutter or fine intraocular scissors.

Phacoemulsification is currently the preferred technique for nucleus removal in most of the uveitis patients. Compared with senile cataracts, considerably less uveitis patients have hard nuclear opacities, as after pars plana vitrectomy. The remaining cortex is carefully removed by irrigation/aspiration. It has been shown that cortical remnants induce a higher degree of postoperative inflammation, capsule shrinkage and fibrosis from the residual epithelial cells. Therefore, a complete cortical removal is highly recommended. Polishing of the posterior capsule may additionally reduce PCO. A peripheral iridectomy should be performed, when extensive sphincter manipulations are indispensable.

Summary for the Clinician

- Phacoemulsification with in the bag IOL implantation should be the preferred surgical technique for the majority of uveitis patients
- Small incisions induce a lower grade of inflammation than longer incisions

- An intact, well-centred CCC that overlaps the optic edge reduces the development of capsule fibrosis
- Capsule contraction syndrome is more often seen with a small CCC and in patients with uveitis than in others

8.9
Lensectomy

8.9.1
Pars Plana Approach to Lensectomy – Anterior Vitrectomy

Eyes with cataracts and minimal posterior segment involvement often do well with anterior segment surgery alone. If vitreous opacification or another vitreoretinal complication exists, several approaches are possible. Pars plana lensectomy – vitrectomy – has been historically the procedure of choice. With recent developments in microsurgical instruments and techniques in cataract- and vitreoretinal surgery, other techniques are rarely performed nowadays. However, it is still the preferred surgical approach for treating cataracts in children with JIA-associated iridocyclitis.

The combination of phacoemulsification with PPV in uveitis patients appears to be advantageous, when IOL implantation is desired. Firstly, it reduces the rate of lens fragment loss into the vitreous, as compared to pars plana lensectomy and vitrectomy [12]. Secondly, patients with Behçet's disease who underwent ECCE or phacoemulsification had better visual outcome and less phthisis than patients who had PPV combined with lensectomy [46].

Indications for vitrectomy include persistent, dense vitreous inflammation, vitreous haemorrhage, traction retinal detachment, and epiretinal membrane formation. CME refractory to medical therapy may be a relative indication, especially when other vitreoretinal complications coexist. The visual outcome in patients who underwent pars plana vitrectomy with or without lensectomy was in cases excellent [29]. The average improvement in visual acuity was five Snellen lines. A total of 50% of eyes attained a final visual acuity of 20/40 or

better. The principal limiting factor in visual recovery was persistent CME.

8.9.2
Limbal Approach to Lensectomy – Anterior Vitrectomy

Intracapsular cataract extraction via a limbal incision was recommended for patients with subluxation or dislocation of the lens and for patients with phacoantigenic uveitis. However, subluxated or dislocated lenses may preferably be treated by three-port pars plana lensectomy. Phacoemulsification with meticulous removal of all cortical remnants or lensectomy is a safe surgical method for phacoantigenic uveitis.

Cataract surgery in children with JIA-associated uveitis may be followed by vigourous inflammation and loss of vision. Some evidence indicated that the intact posterior capsule, anterior hyaloid membrane and vitreous are associated with an increased probability of cyclitic membrane formation with subsequent hypotony and phthisis. Inflammatory membranes may be very dense, enveloping the IOL in a "cocoon". Iris capture and iris bombé with glaucoma can develop. Unexpectedly, these changes also occur in the absence of clinically obvious inflammation.

As a consequence, complete removal of the lens, capsule and anterior vitreous is recommended for treating uveitic cataract in JIA patients [22]. Usually, a small scleral incision is used in these children. After an incision in the capsule, the nucleus is removed by endocapsular phacoemulsification and the cortex is then aspirated as completely as possible. Large diameter capsulotomies of the anterior and posterior lens capsule are made with Utrata forceps or cutters. Anterior vitrectomy is then performed. A peripheral iridectomy should be made. No IOL is implanted in patients with uveitis associated with JIA [19, 22]. The tunnel incisions in children should always be secured with sutures.

Kanski [22] reported that visual acuity improved in 77% of the patients after lensectomy-vitrectomy, and this was superior to the results seen after ECCE. The main causes of vision of 6/60 or less were glaucoma, amblyopia and phthisis. It is not yet clear whether pars plana lensectomy, phacoemulsification, a combination of both or a single or two-step approach should be preferred.

Summary for the Clinician

- In JIA-associated uveitis, the intact posterior capsule, anterior hyaloid membrane and vitreous are associated with an increased probability of cyclitic membrane formation with subsequent hypotony and phthisis
- Lensectomy with anterior vitrectomy is the preferred surgical approach for treating cataracts in children with JIA-associated iridocyclitis

8.10
IOL Implantation

8.10.1
General Concerns

The best available means of achieving visual rehabilitation after cataract surgery is IOL implantation. In general, the rate of complications associated with the implantation of an IOL has been low to date in the adult population. However, many patients with uveitis are young and have severe inflammation, and long-term follow-up clinical trials are still needed. The issue of whether or not IOL implantation in uveitis patients can be recommended is discussed controversially.

It has been suggested in the past that implantation of IOL aggravates inflammation and encourages the formation of membranes in the anterior chamber. There is no doubt that concerns regarding the IOL implantation in inflamed eyes are justified. However, recent studies have shown that the results after cataract surgery and IOL implantation in patients with certain uveitis types can be very satisfying. When patients with chronic uveitis were randomly assigned for cataract extraction with or without IOL implantation, no significant differences in the final vision and complications were found between the two groups [47].

8.10.2
Indications and Contraindications

The uveitis conditions in which IOL implantation may be performed include burned-out uveitis of any aetiology, intermediate uveitis, sarcoidosis, FHC, inactive infectious uveitis (e.g. toxoplasmosis, herpetic uveitis, tuberculosis and borreliosis), and endogenous posterior uveitis without active iridocyclitis. On the contrary, IOL implantation is not recommended in patients less than 2 years of age, active uveitis of any aetiology, aggressive course of inflammation although on high-dose immunosuppression and in uncertain uveitis courses.

There is a general agreement that IOLs should not be implanted as a routine in patients with JIA-associated uveitis. These patients, however, constitute a heterogeneous population. They differ in age, in intensity and duration of inflammation, response to treatment and complications. It has been noted previously that a subgroup of adult JIA patients with burned-out disease tolerated the implantation of an IOL very well [40]. Furthermore, it has been suggested more recently that IOL implantation under the meticulous control of inflammation with immunosuppression may even be a reasonable option in the group of JIA children [25]. However, care must be taken, and IOLs should only be placed in patients whose inflammation can be controlled for an extended period of time before surgery [13].

8.10.3
Placement of the Intraocular Lenses

Generally, in the bag fixation of IOLs should be anticipated in uveitis patients. When rapid PCO is expected, the IOL haptics should be fixed in the bag and optic capture through a primary posterior CCC may be chosen [48]. A sulcus fixation may be required if the capsule ruptures. However, the degree of inflammation was slightly higher when IOL haptics were placed into the sulcus and not in the bag; the final vision and complication rate did not differ between the groups.

Contact between the IOL haptic and the iris is inadvisable, as permanent rubbing of the haptic against the uveal tissue may increase inflammation. Therefore, iris-claw IOLs are contraindicated in patients with uveitis. Also, angle-supported IOLs should be avoided because of the risk of uveitis, glaucoma and hyphema (UGH) syndrome.

The safety of trans-sclerally sutured IOLs in uveitis is unproven. If secondary IOL implantation is requested from the patients, implantation of a large-optic IOL into the ciliary sulcus may be considered.

8.10.4
IOL Material

Chronic postoperative smouldering inflammation may also result from the IOL material. The biocompatibility of the IOLs can be assessed by the degree of postoperative aqueous cells and flare, and the cell and pigment deposition on the lens surface.

Lower laser-flare levels and cellular deposits on the IOLs were observed with heparin-surface-modified (HSM) poly(methyl methacrylate) (PMMA) IOLs than with unmodified PMMA IOLs [8, 26]. More recently, the most frequently used IOL materials have been evaluated in a prospective study among a group of patients with uveitis [2]. Compared to other IOL materials, reduced PCO rates and postoperative inflammation were seen with acrylic IOLs. In contrast, silicone IOLs were associated with increased inflammation and PCO. Less uveitis relapses occurred after HSM-PMMA lens implantation as compared to unmodified PMMA IOLs. In agreement with another study, silicone IOLs led to the highest incidence of relapses [2, 43].

The acrylic material of the AcrySof IOL ensures a firm contact between the IOL and posterior capsule due to adhesion to collagen IV, laminin and fibronectin, and this may prevent migration of the lens epithelial cells. Also, acrylic IOLs had the lowest grade of cell deposits [2, 20]. PCO was more severe in hydrophilic acrylic IOL than in hydrophobic acrylic IOLs. The greater the inflammation, however, the less the biocompatibility of acrylic material [1].

Although it has been previously noted that uveitis recurred more often in eyes that received three-piece IOLs with polypropylene haptics than in eyes that received all-PMMA IOLs, the relevance for uveitis patients must be proven by a further study [15].

8.10.5
IOL Design

It has been shown recently that a sharp, square optic edge of the posterior chamber (PC) IOL is capable of reducing the lens epithelial cell migration to the posterior capsule [35]. The sharp-edge design delayed PCO development in uveitic eyes [1]. In order to reduce the risk of IOL distortion and dislocation, IOLs with large optical zones, e.g. 6 mm or more, should be used in uveitis patients.

8.10.6
IOL Explantation

Numerous studies have provided clear evidence that under perioperative control of inflammation and careful patient selection, elective cataract extraction and IOL implantation is safe in uveitis patients. However, even when following these requirements and intensifying the anti-inflammatory medication, some of the patients do not tolerate IOLs (Fig. 8.2). This may be the consequence of the surgical trauma with prolonged breakdown of the blood–aqueous barrier or the sustained activity of the underlying inflammation. It was rather unexpected that the deposition of giant cells, fibrin and debris on the IOLs was commonly noticed in clinically quiet eyes. Patients with systemic diseases characterised by chronic inflammation (sarcoidosis and JIA), those with chronic inflammatory conditions and those with intermediate uveitis are at higher risk for this complication [14].

The IOL removal may be necessitated due to chronic uveitis unresponsive to inflammatory treatment, perilenticular membrane formation or cyclitic membrane formation with progres-

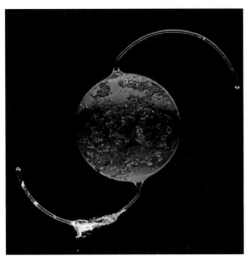

Fig. 8.2. Explanted poly(methyl methacrylate) intraocular lens with multiple cell deposits

sive hypotony [14]. Attempts at stabilisation, therefore, include control of inflammation or capsulectomy, membranectomy and vitrectomy. After IOL removal, in 74% of the patients the uveitis was controlled and vision improved [14].

Summary for the Clinician

- IOLs may be implanted in burned-out uveitis, intermediate uveitis, sarcoidosis, FHC, inactive infectious uveitis and endogenous posterior uveitis
- IOLs should not be implanted as routine in patients with JIA-associated uveitis
- In uveitis patients, in the bag fixation of IOLs should be anticipated and iris-claw IOLs are contraindicated
- Reduced PCO rates, postoperative inflammation and cell deposits were seen with acrylic and HSM-PMMA IOLs in uveitis patients
- The sharp-edge design may delay PCO development in uveitic eyes
- As a consequence of the surgical trauma with prolonged breakdown of the blood–aqueous barrier or the sustained activity of the underlying inflammation, some uveitis patients do not tolerate IOLs

8.11
Combined Vitrectomy

8.11.1
Anterior Vitrectomy

In patients with extensive opacities and membranes in the anterior part of the vitreous, excision of the posterior central capsule and subsequent vitrectomy via the limbal incision is indicated.

8.11.2
Pars Plana Vitrectomy (PPV)

The PPV is performed for therapeutic reasons (e.g. opacity removal) or for diagnostic purposes applying modern molecular biological tests, such as polymerase chain reaction (PCR).

Vitreous opacities are the main indication for therapeutic PPV, especially in patients with intermediate uveitis [17]. Patients with FHC generally show great benefit from early PPV [49].

There is no evidence to date that PPV in anterior or posterior uveitis without significant, steroid resistant vitreous inflammation exhibits any advantage over adequate immunosuppressive therapy. Immunosuppressive treatment may always be considered for the duration of months before and after PPV, although there is no clear evidence that this regimen reduces the risk of postoperative complications, e.g. CME.

It has been controversially discussed whether or not PPV can improve CME postoperatively. PPV may potentially reduce CME either by eliminating the contact of the inflamed vitreous body with the macula or by allowing better penetration or distribution of corticosteroids. The presence of vitreous traction to the macula, as detected by optical coherence tomography (OCT), is a clear indication for PPV in CME-patients. Since PPV can also induce a CME in uveitis patients, it is recommended to perform PPV only in those patients who do not respond sufficiently to a therapy with adequate immunosuppression and acetazolamide. Visual acuity may not improve after surgery, if secondary changes to the photoreceptors or an increased size of the foveal avascular zone are present.

Diagnostic PPV should be performed in atypical courses of uveitis, if standard immunosuppressive therapy does not match with the expected outcome, and in order to exclude infectious aetiology or malignant masquerade syndromes. An established collaboration with a microbiology department to test for infectious agents in vitreous fluid as well as an immediate transfer of vitreous cells to a pathology department to prevent rapid autolysis of the cells are prerequisites for diagnostic vitrectomies. Consequently, diagnostic PPV should only be performed in specialised centres.

A two-step approach to cataract extraction and PPV is suggested when a dense cataract does not allow the preoperative judgement of the pathology of the vitreous or fundus, and when heavy inflammation occurred after intraocular surgery in the past. Otherwise, simultaneous cataract extraction and PPV is a safe and effective approach for treating uveitis patients.

8.12
Typical Intraoperative Complications and Their Management

8.12.1
Band Keratopathy

The band keratopathy belongs to the group of very common complications from uveitis (Fig. 8.3). Dense opacities may require EDTA treatment before cataract surgery.

8.12.2
Synechiae

Anterior synechiae are most often associated with rubeosis iridis or may be the consequence of previous surgery. Dissecting the membranes from the cornea and the iris in the extremely flattened anterior chamber can be challenging. Visualisation of the iris or lens is sometimes ob-

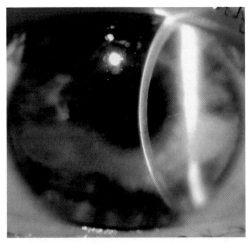

Fig. 8.3. Band keratopathy in a patient with chronic iridocyclitis

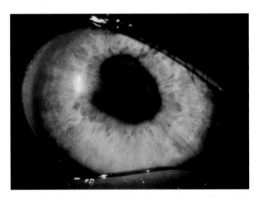

Fig. 8.4. Posterior synechiae in a patient with uveitis

scured due to corneal endothelial dysfunction. Blunt dissection with injecting ophthalmic viscoelastic devices (OVD) is preferred, and sharp dissection with fine scissors should be minimised.

Posterior synechiae are present in up to 80 % of uveitis patients (Fig. 8.4). Circumscribed posterior synechiae can easily be lysed with the injected high molecular weight OVD or with a spatula. Occasionally, the firmly fixed adhesions must be dissected with fine scissors.

Thin pupillary membranes are also common in uveitis patients. The lens may be completely occluded by a severe fibrin formation that may contract the pupil margins and fixes the iris to

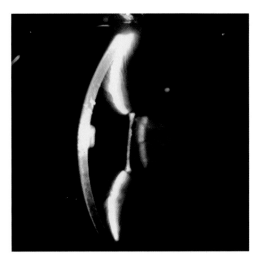

Fig. 8.5. Circular posterior synechiae, iris bombé, pupillary membrane and cataract in a patient with juvenile idiopathic arthritis-associated uveitis

the entire anterior lens capsule (Fig. 8.5). Typically, these fibrinous lens membranes cannot be simply peeled from the anterior surface of the capsule or from the pupil margin. First of all, an incision of the centre of the membrane may be obtained with a 27-gauge needle. After a blunt dissection from the lens capsule by injecting OVD between membrane and capsule, the membrane can be grasped with forceps and dissected with intraocular scissors or a cutter.

8.12.3
Miosis

Miosis is a very common finding in patients with uveitis. The pupil may be sufficiently dilated after synechiae are lysed or after the injection of suprarenin 1:1000 solution. The pupil margin can be gently dilated with a hook to allow perfect visualisation of the nucleus, cortex, capsule or IOL behind the pupil margin. This avoids additional disruption of the vessels within the pupil margin and subsequent bleeding or postoperative fibrin formation. However, sclerosis of the dilator muscle, circular membranes or diffuse adhesion of the posterior iris to the lens capsule may preclude sufficient dilation of the pupil. In these instances, a sufficient pupil size can be obtained with a gentle bimanual stretching of the iris sphincter with iris hooks. Some of the fibrovascular membranes can be gently pulled off the pupil margin. Others need to be disrupted by two or more incisions. Sometimes, 1- to 1.5-mm radial iridotomies of the sphincter muscle are required to obtain a symmetrically dilated pupil. Rarely, iris retractors may be inserted through additional limbal incisions.

8.12.4
Hyphema

Hyphema may appear from rubeotic vessels located in the chamber angle (e.g. in FHC) or at the pupil margin, or from the scleral tunnel incision. It also results from accidental iris disruption during phacoemulsification, from dissecting synechiae or fibrous membranes from the pupil margin or from the iridotomies. This complication is managed with the injection of OVD, increasing the IOD by raising the infusion bottle, or with the compression of the bleeding vessel with forceps. Rarely, wet-field cautery is required.

8.12.5
Vitreous Loss and Membranes

Compared with cataract surgery in elderly patients, due to synechiae, miosis, capsular fibrosis and vitreous opacities, the risk of capsule rupture and vitreous loss is increased in uveitis patients. The vitreous strands can be removed with a cutter via the anterior incisions. When the posterior capsule tears are small, in the bag haptic fixation with posterior optic placement can be recommended. Otherwise, IOL placement in the ciliary sulcus is also reasonable, as it is rarely complicated by inflammation. Transscleral IOL fixation in patients with uveitis may be complicated by inflammation and haemorrhages.

Summary for the Clinician

• Cataract surgery in uveitis patients may be particularly challenging due to band keratopathy, synechiae, miosis, fibrovascular membranes and hyphema

8.13
Typical Postoperative Complications and Their Management

8.13.1
Inflammation

It is not possible to completely standardise the postoperative treatment in uveitis patients, as it must be adjusted according to the surgical manoeuvres and the inflammatory activity. The recurrence rate in the early postoperative period is dependent on the underlying uveitis aetiology. Relapses may occur in up to 50 % in patients with anterior uveitis, while they are rare in infectious posterior uveitis [13, 15].

The golden standard is to increase the corticosteroid dosage postoperatively compared to the treatment level that the patients had before surgery. The dosages must be adapted to the inflammation. It is especially important that the increased dosages must be commonly continued for 8–12 weeks after surgery [1, 45].

Tapering off the dosages too early is followed by an increased risk for hypotony, posterior synechiae, IOL cell deposits or CME.

8.13.1.1
Topical Medication

Many of the patients with anterior uveitis do not need more than topical corticosteroids. During the first week, up to hourly applications may be necessary. The dosage can be tapered off subsequently, while the degree of cells in the anterior chamber should always be 1+ or less. Additional transseptal injections of dexamethasone may be useful in patients with a high degree of inflammation, and especially with fibrin formation. The topical application of non-steroidals has no proven additive effect when corticosteroids are used.

8.13.1.2
Systemic Medication

Many of the patients, and in particular those with intermediate or posterior uveitis, are treated with corticosteroids before surgery. All of the patients that required systemic corticosteroids in the past or that are at high risk of developing CME should be treated with systemic corticosteroids. Oral therapy may be started with 1 mg/kg, which can usually be tapered off within 6 weeks. Additional intravenous pulse treatment with methylprednisolone is helpful in patients with more severe inflammation.

If systemic immunosuppression has already been started before surgery, it should be maintained during the first 3 postoperative months. If the maintenance dosage of oral corticosteroids that is required for ensuring remission exceeds the Cushing level, the institution of immunosuppression or combined drug regiments are indicated. However, it must be kept in mind that it usually takes 2–3 months before a sufficient effect can be achieved with most of the immunosuppressive drugs.

8.13.2
Ocular Hypertension and Glaucoma

Open angle glaucoma is very common in uveitis patients. However, this is much more frequent in anterior than in posterior uveitis. The mechanisms that are involved in the postoperative rise in intraocular pressure (IOP) involve swelling of the trabecular meshwork, inflammatory cells or red blood cells that are trapped in the meshwork, neovascularisation or peripheral anterior synechiae.

As the elevated IOP in uveitis patients often returns to the normal level after inflammation subsides, the anti-inflammatory regiment should be optimised. The glaucoma medication is given as single or combination drug treatment as requested. Drugs that can be recommended for the treatment in uveitis patients include beta-blocking agents, brimonidine, dorzolamide, brinzolamide, latanoprost, bimatoprost or systemic acetazolamide.

Angle closure glaucoma after cataract surgery in uveitis patients is mostly the result of circular posterior synechiae with subsequent iris bombé and pupillary block. YAG laser iridotomy is the approach of first choice. Since the small iridotomies often occlude during ongoing inflammation, surgical peripheral iridectomy may be required afterwards.

8.13.3
Ocular Hypotony

Early hypotony is typically noted within the first postoperative weeks after cataract surgery. This may be the result from ciliary body detachment with and without uveal effusion, from remaining ciliary traction membranes or from the reduced secretion that is caused by active cyclitis. It must be managed promptly to avoid secondary complications, as CME, serous macular detachment, choroidal folds and phthisis. Firstly, wound leakage must be excluded. Since this is not uncommon in children and young adults, scleral tunnels may be superior to the corneal incisions and all incisions must be sutured. Secondly, topical and oral corticosteroids should be given at high dosages, or intravenous pulse methylprednisolone treatment may be given for 3 days. Cycloplegics are applied in all cases.

In some patients, ocular hypotony persists after quiescence from inflammation has been achieved. If this is a consequence of ciliary body destruction from inflammation, the rate of phthisis development is extremely high. However, ciliary body traction syndrome and detachment must be distinguished by the use of ultrasound bio-microscopy. Although persistent hypotony has been seen more often in eyes with preoperative hypotony [22], this is not an absolute contraindication to cataract surgery.

Management includes a course of high dosages of topical, transseptal or systemic corticosteroids, and immunosuppression must be adjusted individually in patients with persisting inflammation. The surgical removal of the membranes is technically very difficult and has a high complication rate, as postoperative bleeding, retinal detachment, uveal effusion and phthisis are very common. However, surgery may be the only therapeutic tool to prevent loss of vision. Permanent silicone oil tamponade to achieve a reattachment of the ciliary body is occasionally helpful to prevent phthisis or improve vision [32].

8.13.4
Retinal Detachment, Macular Pucker and Uveal Effusion

As is true for patients without uveitis, retinal detachment requires immediate surgery. However, due to an increased rate of PVR in uveitis patients, increased topical and systemic corticosteroids should be given, and this is also true for uveal effusion. Macular pucker may develop in patients with persisting active inflammation after cataract surgery. Early recognition and treatment is important, as CME and irreversible macular damage may account markedly for a poor visual outcome [17].

8.13.5
Synechiae

Synechiae between iris and IOL or lens capsule often occur with persistent or recurrent inflammation. Iris bombé and angle closure glaucoma may eventually result. In the chronic active uveitis patients (e.g. JIA-associated uveitis) pupillary capture of the iris that is pushing the IOL forward into the anterior chamber can develop (Fig. 8.6). Consequently, prevention of relapses and the use of short acting mydriatics are imperative.

Newly formed synechiae should immediately be treated with high dosages of topical and transseptal corticosteroids, and the injection of triamcinolone 5 mg into the anterior chamber may be helpful. Furthermore, the use of lytic cocktails (atropin, neosynephrine, phenylephrine, cocaine) may be indicated. The injection of tissue plasminogen activator into the anterior chamber has been suggested within the first few weeks after occurrence of severe synechiae formation [18]. However, compared with its capacity to fibrinolysis, this technique is less effective to achieve complete synechiolysis.

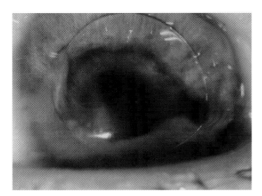

Fig. 8.6. Chronically active iridocyclitis with pupillary capture of the iris pushing the IOL forward into the anterior chamber

8.13.6
Hyphema and Rubeosis

Patients with FHC, herpes iridocyclitis or vasculitis have an increased risk of postoperative hyphema formation. Quiescence of inflammation must then be obtained with topical corticosteroids, and short-lasting mydriatics are given to avoid additional synechiae formation. The elevated IOP is treated with glaucoma medication. Anterior chamber injections of triamcinolone 5 mg can achieve regression of rubeosis and avoid re-bleeding.

Fundus neovascularisation must be ruled out, since ischemia may be present. The incidence of neovascularisation is increased after lensectomies. Regression of proliferation may then be obtained with antiinflammatory medication, and interferon-α or -β have been particularly helpful in this respect. Panretinal photocoagulation or peripheral retinal cryocoagulation may be indicated. If combined with vitreous haemorrhage, pars plana vitrectomy is required.

8.13.7
Posterior Capsule Opacification

Central posterior capsule opacification (PCO) is a consequence of the proliferation of lens epithelial cells onto the posterior capsule. Peripheral PCO is dependent on the quality and thoroughness of surgical cortical removal. The incidence of central PCO is lower when IOLs are fixated in the bag, and is higher when one or both haptics are out of the bag. Despite surgical aspects, PCO is more frequent in uveitis, as capsule opacification has been observed in up to 80 % of uveitis patients [36, 41]. The high PCO rate in distinct uveitis types must be considered in the decision of the appropriate surgical method. In children or adult patients with chronically active uveitis, lensectomy may be more suitable than phacoemulsification. Primary posterior capsule opening and IOL optic capture may be reasonable alternatives in selected patients. Furthermore, PCO rate in uveitis differed with IOL material, and has been the lowest with HSM-PMMA and acrylic lenses.

In many uveitis patients, multiple Nd:YAG laser capsulotomy treatment is necessary. In chronically active uveitis, the fibrotic membranes may need to be surgically disrupted with the use of a Sato knife or cutter. However, this does not necessarily prevent the later formation of retrolenticular membranes in children with uveitis.

8.13.8
Deposits of cells on the IOL

While few cells can be found on the surface of IOLs in the majority of otherwise healthy patients, the deposition of cells is more frequent in patients with uveitis. Higher grades of cells impair visual acuity and fundus visualisation.

A recent study [20] in patients with no history of uveitis showed that cell deposits are more frequent on silicone than on PMMA IOLs, and acrylic IOL had the lowest cell deposits. Lower incidence of giant cells was found on HSM-PMMA IOLs than on unmodified PMMA IOLs [8], and this notion has also been seen in uveitis patients [2]. The highest degree of cell deposition was found on silicone IOLs [2].

It is worthy not to implant an IOL in selected uveitis types that are known for their increased risk for cell deposition, e.g. patients with chronically persistent or recurrent disease. In order to prevent or minimise the cell deposition in uveitis patients, high dosages of topical corticosteroids should be given for 8–12 weeks after cataract surgery.

Cell deposits can be easily removed from the IOL surface by YAG laser polishing. A major drawback of this method is that giant cells frequently adhere to the IOL within a few weeks as soon as corticosteroids are tapered off [1]. As a consequence, long-term maintenance of topical corticosteroids may be required.

8.13.9
Contact Lenses and Amblyopia

In most cases, visual rehabilitation of aphakia can be obtained very well with rigid gas permeable contact lenses. Contact lens fitting and patching should be initiated early after surgery to avoid irreversible amblyopia. Poor compliance and intolerance can make visual rehabilitation in children with aphakia difficult. Contact lenses do permit continuation of topical therapy, although this increases the risk of infections. If band keratopathy is present, the use of unpreserved lubricants or EDTA treatment may be required.

8.13.10
Cystoid Macular Oedema

Cystoid macular oedema (CME) is a serious complication after cataract surgery in patients with uveitis. It has been observed in up to 50 % of cases, and it commonly occurs within the first postoperative weeks [15, 36]. In previous studies, CME has been the limiting factor in up to 80 % of cases with postoperative vision of 20/40 or less. There is no proof that the incidence of CME in uveitis patients increases with the implantation of IOLs [2, 6].

There is no consensus on the treatment of CME. In general, it is treated with high dosages of topical corticosteroids or transseptal steroid injections. Systemic steroids are added (initial oral dosage: prednisone 1 mg/kg), or the dosages are increased according to the inflammatory activity, the Amsler chart tests and visual acuity. Optical coherence tomography (OCT) and fluorescein angiography are helpful for management. Improvement of CME and functional recovery can be induced by intravitreal triamcinolone [5]. There is no proven effect of either additional topical or systemic nonsteroidal drugs.

Although the long-term benefit of acetazolamide in treating CME in uveitis patients is discussed controversially, it belongs to the primary tools of the treatment of post-cataract CME [10, 50]. A starting dosage of 500 mg daily is recommended, and the dosage is decreased thereafter according to the CME course. Pars plana vitrectomy should be considered if medical therapy proves ineffective.

Summary for the Clinician

- Since recurrence of uveitis occurs in up to 50 % of cases in the early postoperative period, the corticosteroid dosage should be increased postoperatively compared to the preoperative treatment level
- Many of the patients with anterior uveitis do not need more than topical corticosteroids. All of the patients that required systemic corticosteroids in the past or that are at high risk of developing CME should be treated with systemic corticosteroids
- Early hypotony that is typically noted within the first postoperative weeks after cataract surgery must be managed promptly in order to avoid secondary vision threatening complications
- Postoperative synechiae and pupillary capture may be prevented by the use of short acting mydriatics
- PCO rates can be reduced by thorough surgical cortical removal, by in the bag IOL fixation, and in selected patients by primary posterior capsule opening and IOL optic capture
- Long-term maintenance of topical corticosteroids may be required to reduce the IOL cell deposits
- CME commonly occurs within the first postoperative weeks after cataract surgery in uveitis patients and must be treated aggressively with corticosteroids and acetazolamide

8.14
Visual Outcome After Cataract Surgery in Patients with Uveitis

Although several complications may occur in the postoperative course, reported functional results are generally encouraging. Comparison of previous studies is difficult, as different uveitis types have been investigated [2, 13, 16, 36, 41].

In one previous report, 57 % had a visual acuity of 6/12 or better and 90 % had improved vision [36]. Another study showed that 73.3 % had visual acuity of 20/30 or better and 56.6 % had significantly improved vision [41]. In a further retrospective study, visual acuity improved in 95 %, and 87 % attained vision of 20/40 or better [11]. A recently published prospective study has noted that 88.6 % had improved vision and 46.3 % had visual acuity of 20/40 or better 1 year after surgery. It appeared that acrylic and PMMA lenses provided better vision than silicone lenses [2].

In the majority of studies, the predominant reasons for limited vision were preoperative macular pathologies and glaucoma [12, 15, 21, 23, 31]. It is surprising that the postoperative complications, such as CME, synechiae, pupillary membranes and cell deposits on the IOL were less commonly responsible for poor final vision.

However, the final outcomes differed markedly between the diverse uveitis aetiologies. Visual results were generally the best in FHC patients. Compared to the patients with anterior uveitis, those with intermediate or posterior uveitis had poor visual outcome after cataract surgery [36].

The worst long-term outcome has been found in children, and especially those with JIA-associated uveitis. However, lensectomy-vitrectomy followed by contact lens correction of aphakia appeared to be a safe technique with good functional results, as up to 75 % of the JIA patients achieved a vision of 20/40 or better after cataract surgery [12, 22, 38].

Summary for the Clinician

- Functional results after cataract surgery in uveitis patients are generally encouraging

8.15
Final Remarks

It is important to plan cataract surgery on a case-by-case basis, considering age, complications, aetiology and ease with which long-term control of inflammation is achieved. Since most of the problems after cataract extraction in uveitis patients are related to underlying inflammation, research is necessary to specify the pathogenesis of this disease in order to enable us to intervene much more specifically.

Research should also continue regarding the most suitable IOL material and design in order to improve uveal and capsular biocompatibility. When considering the no-space-no-cell theory, the combination of a material that firmly fixes the capsule to the IOL, combined with a lens design that avoids the bypassing of lens epithelial cells may prevent the development of PCO.

The major goals in the care of patients with uveitis are the prophylaxis of inflammatory relapses and the prevention of cataract formation. It is believed that the careful control of inflammation and limited use of corticosteroids may decrease the incidence of cataracts [12, 23]. Therefore, an increasing number of ophthalmologists are treating uveitis more aggressively and using immunosuppression perioperatively.

References

1. Abela-Formanek C, Amon M, Schauersberger J et al (2002) Uveal and capsular biocompatibility of 2 foldable acrylic lenses in patients with uveitis or pseudoexfoliation syndrome. Comparison to a control group. J Cataract Refract Surg 28:1160–1172
2. Alio JL, Chipont EC, BenEzra D et al (2002) Comparative performance of intraocular lenses in eyes with cataract and uveitis. J Cataract Refract Surg 28:2096–2108
3. Amon M (2001) Biocompatibility of intraocular lenses. J Cataract Refract Surg 27:178–179
4. Anderson JM, Kottke-Marchant K (1985) Platelet interactions with biomaterials and artificial devices. Crit Rev Biocomp 1:111–181

5. Antcliff RJ, Spalton DJ, Stanford MR et al (2001) Intravitreal triamcinolone for uveitic cystoid macular edema: an optical coherence tomography study. Ophthalmology 108:765–72

6. Belfort R Jr, Nussenblatt RB (1990) Surgical approaches to uveitis. Int Ophthalmol Clin 30: 314–317

7. BenEzra D, Forrester JV, Nussenblatt RB et al (1991) Uveitis scoring system. Springer, Berlin Heidelberg New York, pp 1–13

8. Borgioli M, Coster DJ, Fan FT et al (1992) Effect of heparin surface modification of polymethyl-methacrylate intraocular lenses on signs of postoperative inflammation after extracapsular cataract extraction. Ophthalmology 99:1248–1255

9. Bosch-Driessen LH, Plaisier MB, Stilma JS et al (2002) Reactivation of toxoplasmosis after cataract extraction. Ophthalmology 109:41–45

10. Cox SN, Hay E, Bird AC (1988) Treatment of macular edema with acetazolamide. Arch Ophthalmol 106:1190–1195

11. Estafanous MFG, Lowder CY, Meisler DM et al (2001) Phacoemulsification cataract extraction and posterior chamber lens implantation in patients with uveitis. Am J Ophthalmol 131:620–625

12. Foster CS, Barrett F (1993) Cataract development and cataract surgery in patients with juvenile rheumatoid arthritis-associated iridocyclitis. Ophthalmology 100:809–817

13. Foster CS, Fong LP, Singh G (1989) Cataract surgery and intraocular lens implantation in patients with uveitis. Ophthalmology 96:281–288

14. Foster CS, Havrou P, Zafirakis P et al (1999) Intraocular lens-explantation in patients with uveitis. Am J Ophthalmol 128:31–37

15. Foster RE, Lowder CY, Meisler DM, Zakov ZN (1992) Extracapsular cataract extraction and posterior chamber intraocular lens implantation in uveitis patients. Ophthalmology 99:1234–1241

16. Heger H, Drolsum L, Haaskjold E (1994) Cataract surgery with implantation of IOL in patients with uveitis. Acta Ophthalmol Copenh 72:478–482

17. Heiligenhaus A, Bornfeld N, Wessing A (1996) Longterm results of pars plana vitrectomy in the management of intermediate uveitis. Curr Opin Ophthalmol 7:77–79

18. Heiligenhaus A, Steinmetz B, Lapuente R et al (1998) Recombinant tissue plasminogen activator in cases with fibrin formation after cataract surgery: a prospective randomized multicentre study. Br J Ophthalmol 82:810–815

19. Holland GN (1996) Intraocular lens implantation in patients with juvenile rheumatoid arthritis-associated uveitis: an unsolved management issue. Am J Ophthalmol 122:255–257

20. Hollick EJ, Spalton DJ, Ursell PG, Pande MV (1998) Biocompatibility of poly (methyl methacrylate), silicone, and AcrySof intraocular lenses: randomized comparison of the cellular reaction on the anterior lens surface. J Cataract Refract Surg 24:361–366

21. Hooper PL, Rao NA, Smith RE (1990) Cataract extraction in uveitis patients. Surv Ophthalmol 35:120–144

22. Kanski JJ (1992) Lensectomy for complicated cataract in juvenile chronic iridocyclitis. Br J Ophthalmol 76:72–75

23. Kaufman AH, Foster CS (1993) Cataract extraction in patients with pars planitis. Ophthalmology 100:1210–1217

24. Kazatchkine MD, Carreno MP (1988) Activation of the complement system at the interface between blood and artificial surfaces. Biomaterials 9:30–35

25. Lam LA, Lowder CY, Baerveldt G et al (2003) Surgical management of cataracts in children with juvenile rheumatoid arthritis-associated uveitis. Am J Ophthalmol 135:772–778

26. Lin CL, Wang AG, Chou JCK et al (1994) Heparin-surface-modified intraocular lens implantation in patients with glaucoma, diabetes, or uveitis. J Cataract Refract Surg 20:550–553

27. Linnola RJ, Werner L, Pandey SK et al (2000) Adhesion of fibronectin, vitronectin, laminin, and collagen type IV to intraocular lens materials in pseudophakic human autopsy eyes. Part 1: histological sections. J Cataract Refract Surg 26:1792–1806

28. Matsuo T, Takahashi M, Inoue Y et al (2001) Ocular attacks after phacoemulsification and intraocular lens implantation in patients with Behçet disease. Ophthalmologica 215:179–182

29. Mieler WF, Will BR, Lewis H, Aaberg TM (1988) Vitrectomy in the management of peripheral uveitis. Ophthalmology 95:859–864

30. Mondino BJ, Rao H (1983) Hemolytic complement activity in aqueous humor. Arch Ophthalmol 101:465–468

31. Moorthy RS, Rajeev B, Smith RE, Rao NA (1994) Incidence and management of cataracts in Vogt-Koyanagi-Harada syndrome. Am J Ophthalmol 118:197–204

32. Morse LS, McCuen BW (1991) The use of silicone oil in uveitis and hypotony. Retina 11:399–404

33. Murray PI, Clay CD, Mappin C et al (1999) Molecular analysis of resolving immune responses in uveitis. Clin Exp Immunol 117:455–461

34. Nishi O (1989) Intercapsular cataract surgery with lens epithelial cell removal: part II. Effect on prevention of fibrous reaction. J Cataract Refract Surg 15:301–303

35. Nishi O, Nishi K, Sakanishi K (1998) Inhibition of migrating lens epithelial cells at the capsular bend created by the rectangular optic edge of a posterior chamber intraocular lens. Ophthalmic Surg Lasers 29:587–594

36. Okhravi N, Lightman SL, Towler HMA (1999) Assessment of visual outcome after cataract surgery in patients with uveitis. Ophthalmology 106:710–722

37. Oshika T, Yoshimura K, Miyata N (1992) Post-surgical inflammation after phacoemulsification and extracapsular extraction with soft or conventional intraocular lens implantation. J Cataract Refract Surg 18:356–361

38. Paikos P, Fotopoulou M, Papathanassiou M et al (2001) Cataract surgery in children with uveitis. J Pediatr Ophthalmol Strabismus 38:16–20

39. Pande MV, Spalton DJ, Kerr-Muir MG, Marshall J (1996) Postoperative inflammatory response to phacoemulsification and extracapsular cataract surgery: aqueous flare and cells. J Cataract Refract Surg 22:770–774

40. Probst LE, Holland EJ (1996) Intraocular lens implantation in patients with juvenile rheumatoid arthritis. Am J Ophthalmol 122:161–170

41. Rauz S, Stavrou P, Murray PI (2000) Evaluation of foldable intraocular lenses in patients with uveitis. Ophthalmology 107:909–919

42. Sanders DR, Kraff MC, Lieberman HL et al (1982) Breakdown and reestablishment of blood–aqueous barrier with implant surgery. Arch Ophthalmol 100:588–590

43. Schauersberger J, Kruger A, Abela C et al (1999) Course of postoperative inflammation after implantation of 4 types of foldable intraocular lenses. J Cataract Refract Surg 25:1116–1120

44. Scott JD (1982) Lens epithelial proliferation in retinal detachment. Trans Ophthalmol Soc UK 102:385–389

45. Suresh PS, Jones NP (2001) Phacoemulsification with intraocluar lens implantation in patients with uveitis. Eye 15:621–628

46. Tabbara KF, Chavis PS (1995) Cataract extraction in patients with chronic posterior uveitis. Int Ophthalmol Clin 35:121–131

47. Tessler AH, Farber MD (1992) Intraocular lens implantation versus no intraocular lens implantation in patients with chronic iridocyclitis and pars planitis. Ophthalmology 100:1206–1209

48. Vasavada AR, Trivedi RH, Singh R (2001) Necessity of vitrectomy when optic capture is performed in children older than 5 years. J Cataract Refract Surg 27:1185–93

49. Waters F, Goodall K, Jones N et al (2000) Vitrectomy for vitreous opacification in Fuchs' heterochromic uveitis. Eye 14:216–218

50. Whitcup SM, Csaky KG, Podgor MJ, et al (1996) A randomized, masked, cross-over trial of acetazolamide for cystoid macular edema in patients with uveitis. Ophthalmology 103:1054–1062

Paediatric Cataract Surgery

Charlotta Zetterström

Core Messages

- It is important to detect cataract within the first weeks of life
- Life-long control is mandatory if operated on early, high risk for development of glaucoma
- Loss of accommodation, important to inform before surgery
- IOL implantation is safe and generally accepted over the age of 1 year
- After-cataract is problematic in children
- For lamellar cataract, surgery is often indicated before school start

9.1
Introduction

Bilateral congenital cataract is the most common cause of treatable childhood blindness. Unilateral congenital cataract is an important cause of amblyopia and strabismus.

Cataract surgery in children has changed and improved dramatically in recent decades. This is mainly a result of modern surgical techniques and improved intraocular lenses. Also, better knowledge of irreversible deprivation amblyopia and how to treat this has made an important contribution [13, 33].

9.1.1
Aetiology

In the developed world, the cause of most cases of bilateral congenital cataracts is idiopathic. About one third are hereditary without systemic disease. These are mostly autosomal dominant but autosomal recessive and X-linked traits occur. Rare causes of childhood cataracts are metabolic disorders such as galactosemia and hypocalcemia. Congenital cataracts can be combined with systemic abnormalities such as trisomy 21 and Turner's syndrome. Mental retardation is common in series of bilateral congenital cataract and there is a multitude of inherited syndromes with this combination associated with other abnormalities such as craniofacial or skeletal deformities, myopathy, spasticity or other neurological disturbances.

A number of intrauterine infections (toxoplasmosis, rubella, cytomegalic inclusion disease, herpes infection, varicella, and syphilis) may cause congenital cataracts. Of these, rubella is the most important. The rubella cataract is usually bilateral but may be unilateral.

Ocular conditions such as aniridia (Fig. 9.1) and iris coloboma (Fig. 9.2) are often seen together with cataract.

Unilateral congenital cataract is, as a rule, not associated with systemic disease, is rarely inherited and the cause is in the majority of cases idiopathic. About 10 % of cases are associated with lenticonus/lentiglobus and persistent foetal vasculature. It may also be masked bilateral cataract because of asymmetric lens involvement.

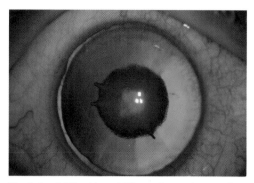

Fig. 9.1. Child with aniridia and complete nuclear cataract

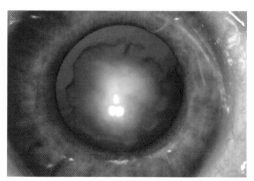

Fig. 9.3. New-born child with nuclear cataract dense in the centre

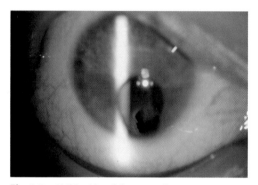

Fig. 9.2. Child with coloboma and cataract

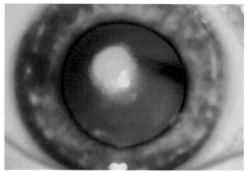

Fig. 9.4. Posterior cataract with persistent foetal vasculature

---

Summary for the Clinician

- In a clinically healthy child with one parent with the disease, and also in unilateral cases, an extensive preoperative investigation to establish a cause for the cataract is not necessary

---

9.1.2
Morphology

Nuclear cataract is usually present at birth and is non-progressive [30]. Dense cataracts present at birth, where early surgery is mandatory, are in most cases of nuclear type (Fig. 9.3). The opacification is located to the embryonic and foetal nuclei between the anterior and posterior Y sutures and is usually very dense in the centre. The eyes are almost always smaller than normal

eyes [18]. The cataract is bilateral in about 80% of cases. In cases with bilateral congenital nuclear cataract, inheritance can be demonstrated in 30%–50%. The inheritance is in most cases autosomal dominant.

Posterior unilateral cataracts in infants and children are in most cases associated with persistent foetal vasculature (PFV) and the affected eye is usually small (Fig. 9.4). The retrolental vascular structure in contact with the lens capsule may give way to blood vessels encircling the lens causing haemorrhage, particularly during surgery (Fig. 9.5). The fibrovascular stalk may cause tractional retinal detachment. After early surgery, secondary glaucoma is unfortunately a common complication in these eyes [26].

Cataract associated with posterior lenticonus or posterior lentiglobus usually develops

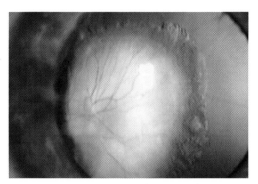

Fig. 9.5. Posterior persistent foetal vasculature

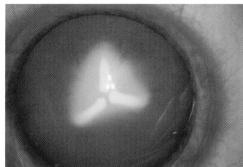

Fig. 9.7. Sutural cataract with little influence on vision

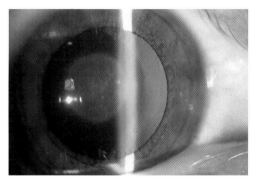

Fig. 9.6. Lamellar cataract in a 4-year-old child

after the critical period of visual development. It is mostly unilateral and occurs sporadically. The change in the lens develops as a small defect in the posterior lens capsule, which exhibits a progressive bowing resulting in a posterior bulging and disorganisation of the subcapsular lamellae and opacification. It is important to be aware of the weakness of the posterior capsule in these eyes during surgery and, if possible, avoid hydrodissection.

Lamellar cataract usually develops after establishment of fixation (Fig. 9.6). It is usually progressive and surgery is often performed before school age, but the cataract can remain subclinical for many years. The cataract involves the lamellae surrounding the foetal nucleus peripheral to the Y sutures [30]. Eyes with lamellar cataracts are usually of normal size with a normal-sized cornea. It is uniformly bilateral and

has commonly an autosomal dominant pattern of inheritance.

There are some other morphological types of congenital cataracts. Some are due to lenticular developmental defects present at birth. These may have only little influence on vision. Such defects are sutural cataract (Fig. 9.7), and anterior polar cataract, which usually do not progress.

Summary for the Clinician

- In the case of nuclear cataract, early surgery is often needed
- For lamellar cataract, surgery is often indicated before school start

9.1.3
Amblyopia and Congenital Cataracts

Amblyopia is caused by abnormal structural and functional evolution of the lateral geniculate nucleus and striate cortex due to the abnormal visual stimulation during the sensitive period of visual development.

Reversibility of amblyopia depends on the stage of maturity of the visual system at which abnormal visual experience began, the duration of deprivation and the age at which therapy was instituted. The most critical period is probably between 1 week and 2 months [40]. Disruption of vision during this period usually causes severe and permanent visual loss and permanent nystagmus if not managed. If visual deprivation

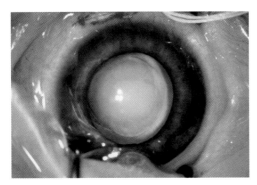

Fig. 9.8. Dense congenital cataract

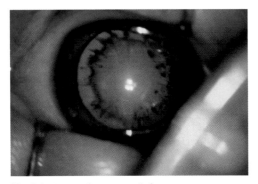

Fig. 9.9. Incomplete congenital cataract

occurs after the age of 2–3 months, the amblyopia is usually reversible. The sensitivity to amblyopia gradually decreases until the age of 6 or 7 years when the visual maturation is complete and the retinocortical pathway and the visual centres become immune to abnormal visual input [37]. It is thus essential that early treatment of dense congenital cataract is instituted in order to avoid irreversible amblyopia [9, 16, 31].

Visual loss and the development of amblyopia depend on the size and location of the cataract and particularly on the density. If the opacities are large enough to obscure the fundus view through an undilated pupil, amblyopia development can be expected (Fig. 9.8). If retinal details such as the larger vessels can be distinguished through the central portion of the cataract, conservative treatment can be considered (Fig. 9.9). Some infants with partial subclinical congenital cataract develop sufficient binocular interaction and form vision to allow a

normal maturity of the visual system. Thus, amblyopia might not be a problem for some children with partial congenital cataract. If surgery is considered in children with partial cataract it should, if possible, be postponed until the age at which the risk of post-operative complications diminishes. Children with partial cataract treated conservatively must be followed closely. Occlusion therapy is necessary in unilateral cases to prevent amblyopia. The clinical evaluation should entail evaluation of visual behaviour including monocular and binocular fixation patterns.

Unilateral congenital cataract, dense from birth, causes amblyopia with loss of binocular function and the development of secondary strabismus. In cases of dense bilateral congenital cataract, bilateral amblyopia and nystagmus will occur.

Summary for the Clinician

- To prevent irreversible amblyopia in infants with dense cataract from birth, the cataract extraction must be performed early
- Children with partial cataract must be followed closely

9.2
Congenital Dense Cataract

9.2.1
Pre-operative Examination

A careful pre-operative examination of the eyes is essential. The red reflex should first be assessed by direct ophthalmoscopy with the pupil undilated. The cataract is often most dense in the central part of the lens, after dilatation it seems to be less significant. It is important to examine both eyes and establish whether the cataract is bi- or unilateral. Unilateral congenital cataract presents a challenging problem, since even a mild cataract will cause irreversible deep amblyopia in one eye if not treated. In these children, vision in the affected eye is prevented from developing through active suppression by the non-affected eye [6]. While the newborn child is awake it is also important to assess visual function, if possible, with a clinical preferential looking grating acuity (Teller acuity card). It is also important to look at the ability to fix and follow and ask the parents if they have had any visual interaction with the child. Children with significant bilateral congenital cataracts may seem to have delayed development as well as obviously impaired visual behaviour. In contrast, children with monocular cataracts often present with strabismus, which may not develop until irreparable visual loss has occurred. Since their visual behaviour may be unaffected, children with monocular cataract are almost always detected much later than cases with bilateral cataract. Moreover, in most cases with monocular cataract, they have no family history and are otherwise healthy. The presence of manifest nystagmus at the age of 2–3 months or more generally indicates a poor visual prognosis. Complete examinations of infants often require sedation or general anaesthesia and can often be performed during the same anaesthesia as the surgery. Both eyes should be examined with dilated pupils because malformations in the non-cataractous eye are commonly found [24]. Anterior segment examination is carried out with measurements of the corneal diameter and intraocular pressure (IOP) by Tonopen or handheld Perkins tonometer. The IOP in the new-born is much lower than in the adult, often below 10 mmHg. If the clarity of the media permits so, indirect ophthalmoscopy may reveal persistent foetal vessels or any other posterior segment abnormalities that may have an impact on the visual outcome. Surgery for visually significant cataract should be carried out as soon as possible, preferably within the first weeks of life. If the cataract is unilateral it is even more important with early surgery to obtain some useful visual acuity in the affected eye. A treatment regime based on surgery within 2 months of life, prompt optical correction of the aphakia and aggressive occlusion therapy with frequent follow-up have been successful in several series [5, 7]. If the cataract is incomplete and not interfering with normal visual development, it is better to postpone surgery until the child is older with less post-operative complications. In these cases it is mandatory with close follow-ups by a well-trained paediatric ophthalmologist.

Summary for the Clinician

- An undilated pupil and no red reflex are indications for immediate surgery

9.2.2
Surgical Technique in Infants

In infants with bilateral cataracts it is advantageous to perform surgery in both eyes at the same surgical intervention. Most of the children are new-born, only a few weeks old, and these small children are extremely sensitive with regard to developing amblyopia. Surgery in one week on one eye while the other eye remains with dense cataract can cause irreversible amblyopia in the non-operated eye. If both eyes are operated at the same time sterility must be maintained during the whole procedure and changing all instruments and sterile clothing of the surgeon and nurse are advisable between the eyes.

Axial length and corneal curvature are essential measurements for contact lens fitting and IOL power calculation and could advantageously be performed immediately before surgery during the same anaesthesia. Eyes of infants with congenital cataract are shorter and have a smaller corneal diameter compared to controls.

Before surgery the pupil is dilated with a combination of 1.5% phenylephrine and 0.85% cyclopentolate. Rinsing of the conjunctiva with chlorhexidine solution 0.05% is performed 5 min before surgery.

The surgical intervention should be performed by a well-trained anterior segment surgeon to obtain the most advantageous outcome. Consequently most of the procedures are done with the anterior approach starting with a sclerocorneal tunnel, which ought to be rather long to minimise the risk for iris prolapse. High-viscosity ocular viscosurgical device (OVD) is used because the anterior chamber is shallow and a high vitreous pressure is found in these small eyes. If the pupil is small, which is rather common in eyes with congenital cataract, flexible iris retractors can be very helpful and four of them are placed in the pupil before the continuous anterior capsulorhexis is performed. There is no reason to open the pupil with the iris retractors more than necessary, since a damaged iris will cause more post-operative inflammation. If the cataract is very dense and grey, staining of the anterior capsule with dye makes the anterior capsulorhexis much easier and also safer to perform [32]. The dye can be administered with a blunt syringe under the OVD just above the anterior capsule and painted on the capsule with the end of the syringe. In this way a very small amount of the dye is needed and just the capsule and not the whole anterior segment is dyed. If an intraocular lens (IOL) is implanted the anterior capsulorhexis ought to be smaller than the optic, round and placed in the centre. Since the capsule is elastic and thick in the new-born it is important to re-grasp continuously when performing the rhexis. In contrast to the adult eye, one ought to aim for a small rhexis to achieve a good size. A complete rhexis without any tears is essential in cases when IOL implantation is planned.

Hydrodissection ought to be carried out with caution and sometimes avoided. In some eyes, often with very dense cataract, a defect in the posterior capsule, most often formed like an almond, could be found. Hydrodissection in these cases is of course not recommended because the high risk of loosing lens material into the vitreous during the procedure. These cases also have opacification with cells in the anterior part of the vitreous, looking like a fishtail in the anterior vitreous when moving the eye. The posterior capsule is thin and fragile in eyes with posterior lenticonus and hydrodissection ought to be performed carefully.

It is almost always possible to remove the nucleus and cortex with irrigation and aspiration. However, sometimes in very dense nuclear cataracts, and with white calcified parts in the nucleus, ultrasound has to be used. The new technique AquaLase liquefaction, which uses a warm-water stream, may prove very useful when removing these dense cataracts. It is important to remove all lens material to minimise post-operative inflammation, which is very pronounced in young patients. To reduce opacification of the visual axis removal of most lens epithelial cells is important; however, it is almost

impossible with the technique used routinely today. The most important cells concerning after-cataract are located at the lens equator and are impossible to see during surgery. When the capsular bag is empty of all lens material high-viscosity OVD is injected to fill the capsular bag and a posterior continuous capsulorhexis is performed: slightly smaller than the anterior rhexis. The posterior capsule is thinner than the anterior and not so elastic. Sometimes fibrotic parts are found in the posterior capsule which makes tearing impossible and scissors have to be used. It is wise to look for persistent foetal vasculatures, particularly in unilateral cases with posterior cataract. Persistent hyaloid artery is adherent to the posterior aspect of the lens and the optic disc. If present it ought to be cut with fine scissors; sometimes the vessel contains blood, but cautery is seldom indicated. Using this method it is possible to implant an IOL in the capsular bag during primary surgery or in the ciliary sulcus if a secondary implantation is scheduled for the future. Capsular fixation is preferred over ciliary sulcus placement because such complications such as pupillary capture and IOL decentration are more common with ciliary sulcus fixation [29].

Primary IOL implantation in the new-born eye is still debated [22, 39]. In unilateral cases the amblyopia is more severe, the occlusion therapy is very hard and the child has an otherwise healthy eye. Therefore it is easier to accept an IOL implantation in theses eyes today, even though there is no available IOL that really fits the small new-born eye. The bilateral cases are often easier concerning contact-lens wear and treatment of the amblyopia. If an IOL is to be implanted it ought to be in the bag with complete anterior and posterior capsulorhexes. A foldable one-piece hydrophobic IOL could be implanted with an injector through a 2.75-mm incision also in this age group. With high-viscosity OVD remaining in the anterior chamber and the IOL implanted in the bag, a dry anterior vitrectomy could safely be performed through the pupil and the two capsulorhexes. The OVD ought to be removed to avoid elevated IOP after surgery. The pupil is closed with acetylcholine (Miochol), and it is wise to ensure that no vitreous is present in the anterior part of the eye. The sclera is soft and elastic in children and it is hard to achieve a self-sealing incision in most cases. Thus the incision should be closed with a running or horizontal 10–0 nylon suture. Anterior synechia formation to the wound is rather often seen in the youngest. It is important at the end of the procedure to look for this and to have a stable and good anterior chamber. Iridectomy is not necessary in these eyes; this is true also if the eye is left aphakic. However, the lens capsule has to remain in the eye, otherwise it is wise to perform an iridectomy to avoid intra-ocular pressure spikes.

Endophthalmitis is one of the most serious complications after intraocular surgery and prophylactic antibiotics are recommended. Perioperatively, at the end of surgery, injection of 1 mg of cefuroxime (Zinacef) in 0.1 ml saline 0.9 % into the anterior chamber is an effective and safe method [27, 28] to avoid infection. In the new-born eye 0.5 mg of cefuroxime seems to be sufficient. This regime effectively prevents gram-positive bacteria species which is by far the most common bacteria. Prophylactic vancomycin in the irrigating solution during cataract surgery is not routinely recommended by the authors because of possible increased incidence of cystoid macular oedema [4] and the risk of emerging resistance to the antibiotic. The anti-inflammatory treatment should start early after surgery and a perioperative subconjunctival injection of 2 mg of steroids (Betapred) is recommended at the end of the surgical procedure. We have not used protective patches for any children after surgery for many years and have not seen any disadvantages with this regime. On the contrary, the child starts the amblyopia treatment immediately and the parents are very pleased when they are able to establish visual interaction with the child for the first time soon after surgery.

Summary for the Clinician

- Surgery ought to be centralised
- No patching after surgery
- Prophylactic antibiotic treatment should take the following forms:
  - Rinsing of conjunctiva with 0.05 % chlorhexidine solution or 5 % povidone iodine before surgery
  - 0.5–1.0 mg cefuroxime intracameral at the end of surgery

9.3
Cataracts in Older Children

9.3.1
Pre-operative Examination

If the cataract was incomplete at birth close follow-up by a paediatric ophthalmologist is advised. Visual acuity ought to be followed, if possible, with clinical preferential looking grating acuity (Teller acuity card). It is also important to look at the ability to fix and follow and ask the parents if they have visual interaction with the child. Examination of strabismus and binocular functions are also important. In older children visual acuity could be measured with greater reliability. Above the age of 4 years most children could be examined with letters and monocularly. In children not only the visual acuity has to be considered but also the development of amblyopia. If a child has unilateral cataract or a more dense cataract in one eye, occlusion therapy has to be considered. Most of the children with congenital cataract have small eyes and hyperopic glasses should be prescribed if needed.

Nowadays, surgery in children has almost the same indications as in grown-ups with one important exception, if the cataract is too dense, children below the age of 7 will develop amblyopia, which means it is not advisable to postpone the surgery.

In older children, both eyes could be operated during the same surgical intervention or in two sessions, while the development of amblyopia is not as quick as in the youngest. To wait 1–2 months between the eyes is in most cases acceptable. The child and the parents have to be informed before the intervention that accommodation is going to be lost after surgery and spectacles, often bifocal, are needed.

Summary for the Clinician

- Amblyopia can be avoided by performing surgery
- After surgery loss of accommodation is found and glasses are needed

9.3.2
Surgical Technique

The surgical technique used in children above the age of 1 year does not differ greatly from the technique used in the infant eye. The incision can be sclerocorneal or clear corneal and 12 o'-clock or temporally if preferred.

IOL implantation within the capsular bag is important to decrease after-cataract formation [42] and inflammation. Posterior capsulorhexis is regularly performed until at least the age of 15 years otherwise after-cataract will develop within a short time. Anterior dry vitrectomy ought to be performed at the primary surgery in pre-school children to avoid early after-cataract formation [15, 17, 35]. The authors prefer to perform the vitrectomy through the limbal incision, but others advocate a pars plana approach. With the pars plana approach, separate irrigation is provided anteriorly through a limbal paracentesis incision.

In children with cataract after trauma both the anterior and posterior capsule could be damaged. In cases with relatively immediate cataract development after a corneal wound the anterior capsule is often broken. The condition of the posterior capsule is unknown in most cases, and it is important to avoid hydrodissection, or performing it very carefully to avoid losing lens material into the vitreous. In some cases with blunt trauma, no perforation of the globe and rapid development of dense cataract one ought to consider a damaged posterior capsule. While the posterior capsule is much thinner and more fragile than the anterior one it could also break without perforation of the globe.

In cases with an incomplete anterior capsulorhexis as after trauma, and a broken anterior or posterior capsule, optic capture could be a good option to avoid late decentration of the IOL [10]. The optic is then pushed behind the posterior capsulorhexis, the haptics remaining in the bag. The capsulorhexis has to be in the centre and smaller than the optic, otherwise the IOL optic will escape from the capture. In these cases the lens epithelial cells may grow on the IOL surface forming after-cataract [36]. If performing optic capture in the posterior or anterior rhexis is considered, a three-piece IOL should be chosen rather than a one-piece design. The one-piece acrylic IOL cannot be pushed behind the capsulorhexis since the haptics and optic have to be in the same plane. Also, most of the three-piece lenses are posteriorly angulated and therefore suitable for this technique.

Summary for the Clinician

- Anterior and posterior capsulorhexis in all children
- Anterior dry vitrectomy in younger children below the age of 7 years
- IOL implantation is safe, including bilaterally, in children over the age of 1 year

9.4
IOL Power and Model

These days it is perfectly safe and acceptable to do a primary implant from the age of 1 year, even when both eyes are operated on [11, 41]. Primary implants in younger children is still controversial. In the unilateral cases operated on early, i.e. at only a few weeks of age, a possible option is a primary implant. It has been found that an implant in the capsular bag would decrease the total amount of proliferating lens epithelial cells [42]. The formation of after-cataract is particularly problematic in the youngest patients.

At least in the unilateral cases, implantation of an IOL could be an improvement in the treatment of aphakia, amblyopia, after-cataract and maybe also secondary glaucoma. In this age group the deprivation amblyopia is by far the greatest problem. Aiming for emmetropia at surgery is therefore most appropriate in this age group. Sometimes the desired IOL power is not available because of high hyperopia, in these cases a supplement of a contact lens for some time could be an option. The refraction will change considerably during the subsequent years and the eye will become highly myopic but hopefully not highly amblyopic. Corneal refractive surgery, piggyback implantation or implanted contact lenses are all different options in the future for correction of the myopia.

In bilateral cases the best solution is probably aiming for emmetropia when the child becomes an adult. Depending on the age at surgery the amount of hyperopia will differ. It is important to inform the child and parents before the surgery that the child will probably need bifocal glasses for the rest of his or her life.

Accurate axial length and corneal curvature measurements before surgery are necessary for IOL power calculation. In small children this could be performed during the same anaesthesia as the surgery and in older children it could be performed before the surgery. Eyes with congenital cataract are often shorter than normal eyes and most of the children do need higher IOL power than the average child of the same age.

The inflammatory reaction is more pronounced in children and it is very important to use an IOL with high biocompatibility and accurate clinical documentation.

Capsular bag growth does not continue after lensectomy, which is important when selecting lens implants [38].

A foldable acrylic lens with a sharp edge and an optic diameter of 6 mm is advantageous in decreasing or delaying after-cataract formation in the visual axis and minimising the incision size [12], which is advantageous because a smaller incision results in less post-operative inflammation [23]. By using a single-piece acrylic IOL and the Monarch injector, the incision size could be minimised to 2.75 mm [34].

This is also a very soft IOL and therefore probably suitable for the small eyes of the new-born baby when implanted in the capsular bag [20]. Problems such as breakage of the haptics and retarded ocular growth have been encountered with earlier generation IOLs implanted in the monkey and rabbit eye [19, 21]. The single-piece AcrySof is not recommended for sulcus fixation. Unlike the three-piece design, the haptics are thick and are not posteriorly angulated. Years after surgery decentration and iris chafing can occur. An IOL containing a filter removing the harmful blue light is most probably advantageous for the maculae in these eyes, which will have implants for many years.

Multifocal IOLs should not be considered in young children with a growing eye. The axial length increases during life from a mean of approximately 16.8 mm at birth to 23.6 mm in the adult with a very rapid growth during the first 18 months. The mean refractive power of the cornea decreases from about 51 dioptres at birth to 45 dioptres at 6 months of age and to 43.5 dioptres in adults. Consequently, the refraction will change dramatically during childhood.

Summary for the Clinician

- In unilateral cases aim for emmetropia at surgery
- In bilateral cases aim for emmetropia in adulthood

9.4.1
Post-operative Treatment

Post-operatively, the eye of a child will tend to react with much more inflammation than the adult eye, particularly in darkly pigmented eyes. Systemic treatment with glucocorticoids is most often not indicated, an exception to this rule being children with uveitis. It is however important to start the topical treatment with dexamethasone 0.1% or another potent topical corticosteroid immediately after surgery. The drops are tapered over 1 month starting with four to five times per day in the elderly. In the new-born the treatment has to be more intense starting with eight to ten times daily and tapered over 2–3 months. In the youngest eyes and in eyes with dark brown irides, mydriatic drops (tropicamide or cyclopentolate) are administered for several weeks after surgery. Following this treatment regime, synechia formation could more easily be avoided and retinoscopy would be easier to perform before glasses are prescribed.

Immediate correction of the aphakia is mandatory for the best possible visual outcome. There are different options and these days most of the children are implanted with an IOL during primary surgery. Some new-borns are implanted with an IOL; however, in most cases the IOL is not strong enough, leaving some uncorrected hyperopia in the beginning. In theses cases a contact lens is the best option, giving the opportunity to change the strength over time.

If no IOL is implanted contact lenses are best fitted already in the operating theatre for immediate optical correction, to prevent otherwise irreversible deprivation amblyopia. Several types of lenses are available. Rigid gas permeable lenses have a wide range of available strengths and have a great ability to correct large astigmatic errors. They are easy to insert and remove, but cause more foreign body sensation than soft lenses. The two major soft lenses are silicone and soft hydrogel lenses. Both are suitable but soft hydrogel lenses are less expensive which is an important consideration due to frequent lens loss. Loss of lenses and fast eye growth during infancy necessitate frequent lens replacements, especially during the first 2 years of life. Frequent retinoscopy must be performed to decide the power of the lens. Most authorities recommend an overcorrection of +2.0 to +3.0 D until bifocals can be tolerated, which occurs between the age of 2 and 3 years. The child should be provided with aphakic spectacles as an option if contact lenses are unsuitable.

In older children implanted with an IOL, bifocal glasses are prescribed after retinoscopy and the remaining hyperopia is corrected. This is often done at 1 month after surgery at the latest.

Occlusion therapy is started in unilateral cases as soon as the media is clear and the aphakia is corrected, and the therapy needs to be aggressive. Virtually all children with unilateral congenital cataract develop strabismus. In bilateral cases occlusion therapy is sometimes useful if one eye is more amblyopic than the other eye. The occlusion therapy in cases with bilateral cataract usually do not need to be as aggressive as in the unilateral cases.

Close follow-up by a paediatric ophthalmologist is mandatory until the patient is 7 years of age, while untreated amblyopia is soon irreversible. When surgery is performed during the first months of life, life-long follow-up is essential because of the high risk of developing secondary glaucoma.

Summary for the Clinician

- Intense topical treatment with a strong topical corticosteroid, e.g. dexamethasone, particularly in infants below age 2 years, is recommended
- Mydriatic drops in very young patients

9.4.2
Post-operative Complications

9.4.2.1
After-Cataract

Opacification of the visual axis is the most common complication found after cataract surgery, particularly in the youngest. Even when a posterior capsulorhexis has been performed, growth of lens epithelial cells on the vitreous surface or on the back of the optic can be found some months after surgery (Fig. 9.10). Performing posterior capsulorhexis and dry anterior vitrectomy seems to be one way to decrease opacifica-

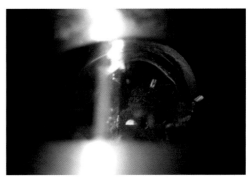

Fig. 9.10. After-cataract 2 years after surgery

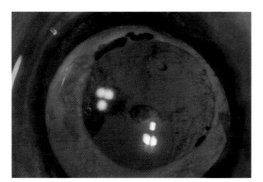

Fig. 9.11. Decentration of the posterior capsulorhexis

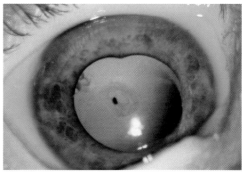

Fig. 9.12. Shrinkage of the capsule with phimosis of the rhexis

tion in the post-operative time [17]. In the very young patients, implanted during their first weeks of life, surgical intervention could be necessary several times, while the lens epithelial cells are growing over and over again on the back of the optic. An IOL implanted in the bag will decrease or prevent formation of Soemmering's ring and the epithelial cells can easier migrate from the periphery to the centre of the pupil. If opacification occurs in the pupil Nd:YAG laser treatment could be tried; however, this is often inadequate in children since reformation of the opacification can be found some months later in these highly reactive eyes. Surgical intervention is often necessary under general anaesthesia and has to be performed promptly to avoid amblyopia. Through a small limbal incision high-viscosity OVD is injected into the anterior chamber to keep it stable during the procedure. An incision in the pars plana and a sharp thin knife is inserted behind the iris and IOL and the membrane is divided. With dry anterior vitrectomy the lens epithelial cells growing in the pupil and also the anterior part of vitreous are removed. At the end of the surgery the pars plana incision is closed with a running suture and the OVD is removed from the anterior chamber to avoid a pressure peak postoperatively.

After the procedure, topical dexamethasone is needed for some weeks. Problems with the lens capsule after surgery, such as decentration (Fig. 9.11) of the anterior or posterior capsulorhexis or shrinkage of the capsular bag with phimosis (Fig. 9.12) of the capsulorhexis could make a secondary intervention necessary. Capsule contraction is more often found in eyes implanted with a silicone IOL [8].

9.4.2.2
Secondary Glaucoma

Secondary glaucoma is unfortunately a common complication and by far the most sight-threatening [2, 25]. The highest incidence is found when the surgery has been done early, that is below the age of 2 months, and a much lower incidence is found when surgery has been performed over the age of 1 year [25]. Eyes with small corneal size, nuclear cataract and persistent foetal vasculature are at greatest risk [30]. Implantation of an IOL into the capsular bag seems to inhibit the development of secondary glaucoma [3].

In the new-born eye a rise in the intraocular pressure will cause epithelial oedema of the cornea, a poor red reflex, photophobia and fast regression of hyperopia or growing eye. These children must be examined promptly under general anaesthesia. Corneal oedema in children wearing contact lenses could be due to hypoxia, and the contact lens must be removed immediately. The anaesthesia of choice is ketamine hydrochloride since it does not lower the IOP which most of the other anaesthetics do. During the evaluation under anaesthesia, IOP, corneal diameter, and axial length are measured and examination of the optic disc and retinoscopy are performed. Acute glaucoma may develop in cases with excessive inflammation leading to pupillary block and iris bombé. A peripheral iridectomy and an anterior vitrectomy are often sufficient to solve the problem. Later on, a more chronic type of glaucoma could develop probably due to the heavy inflammatory response after surgery leading to synechia formation in the chamber angle and a slow rise in IOP over time [14]. Some of the eyes with secondary glaucoma could be controlled with topical medication but many will need a trabeculectomy with mitomycin C. In some cases also a glaucoma shunt is required for pressure control.

It is important to remember that when cataract surgery has been performed during the first months of life the IOP and optic nerve have to be controlled life-long [1].

9.4.2.3
Fibrinoid Reaction

Because of the high degree of inflammation in children, fibrin in the pupil can be found even when an IOL with high biocompatibility has been implanted. Frequently administered topical steroids and mydriatics are helpful in these cases. In a few cases Nd:YAG laser treatment could be indicated to clear the visual axis. Posterior synechiae formation in the post-operative period is common, especially in the new-born when no IOL has been implanted.

9.4.2.4
Decentration of the Pupil

Incarceration of the iris in the wound is sometimes encountered. To avoid this complication a rather long tunnel is recommended during cataract extraction and suture ought to be used to close the wound. Careful surgery is also helpful leaving the iris without trauma and atrophy. If the visual axis is covered with iris it is important to promptly reposition the iris or make a new central pupil with surgical intervention or Nd:YAG laser treatment.

Summary for the Clinician

- Good red reflex is essential for favourable development of vision
- Rapid growth of the eye should arouse suspicion of secondary glaucoma
- Life-long follow-up in cases with surgery within the first months of life because of secondary glaucoma

9.5
Current Clinical Recommendations

Summarising the previously given information, the following recommendations can be made:
- Prompt surgery is performed in cases with dense congenital cataract – if nystagmus has developed, the amblyopia is irreversible
- Post-operative complications such as high rate of after-cataract and secondary glaucoma are matters of concern in the new-born and life-long follow-up is essential in these cases
- Occlusion therapy ought to be initiated if amblyopia is present in one eye
- IOL implantation could safely be performed above the age of one year
- Anterior dry vitrectomy ought to be performed in pre-school children to avoid after-cataract

References

1. Asrani SG, Wilensky JT (1995) Glaucoma after congenital cataract surgery. Ophthalmology 102:863–867
2. Asrani SG, Wilensky JT (1995) Glaucoma after congenital cataract surgery. Ophthalmology 102:863–867
3. Asrani, S, Freedman S, Hasselblad V, Buckley EG, Egbert J, Dahan E, Gimbel H, Johnson D, McClatchey S, Parks M, Plager D, Maselli E (2000) Does primary intraouclar lens implantation prevent "aphakic" glaucoma in children? J AAPOS 4:33–39
4. Axer-Siegel R, Stiebel-Kalish H, Rosenblatt I, Strassman E, Yassur Y, Weinberger D (1999) Cystoid macular edema after cataract surgery with intraocular vancomycin. Ophthalmology 106:1660–1664

5. Birch EE, Swanson WH, Stager DR, Woddy M, Everett M (1993) Outcome after very early treatment of dense congenital unilateral cataract. Invest Ophthalmol Vis Sci 34:3687–3699

6. Birch EE, Stager D, Leffler J, Weakley D (1998) Early treatment of congenital unilateral cataract minimizes unequal competition. Invest Ophthalmol Vis Sci 39:1560–1566

7. Cheng KP, Hiles DA, Biglan AW, Pettapiece MC (1991) Visual results after early surgical treatment of unilateral congenital cataracts. Ophthalmology 98:903–910

8. Cochener B, Jacq PL, Colin J (1999) Capsule contraction after continuous curvilinear capsulorhexis: Poly (methylmethacrylate) versus silicone intraocular lenses. J Cataract Refract Surg 25:1362–1369

9. Dutton JJ, Baker JD, Hiles DA et al (1990) Viewpoints: visual rehabilitation in aphakic children. Surv Ophthalmol 34:365–384

10. Gimbel HV (1997) Posterior continuous curvilinear capsulorhexis and optic capture of the intraocular lens to prevent secondary opacification in pediatric cataract surgery. J Cataract Refract Surg 23:652–656

11. Gimbel HV, Basti S, Ferensowicz M, DeBroff BM (1997) Results of bilateral cataract extraction with posterior chamber intraocular lens implantation in children. Ophthalmology 104:1737–1743

12. Hollick EJ, Spalton DJ, Ursell PG, Pande MV (1998) Lens epithelial cell regression on the posterior capsule with different intraocular lens materials. Br J Ophthalmol 82:1182–1188

13. Jacobson SG, Mohindra I, Held R (1981) Development of visual acuity in infants with congenital cataracts. Br J Ophthalmol 65: 727–735

14. Keech RV, Tongue AC, Scott WE (1989) Complications after surgery for congenital and infantile cataracts. Am J Ophthalmol 108: 136–141

15. Koch DD, Kohnen T (1997) Retrospective comparison of techniques to prevent secondary cataract formation after posterior chamber intraocular lens implantation in infants and children. J Cataract Refract Surg 23: 657–663

16. Kugelberg U (1992) Visual acuity following treatment of bilateral congenital cataracts. Doc Ophthalmol 82: 211–215

17. Kugelberg M, Zetterström C (2002) Pediatric cataract surgery with or without anterior vitrectomy. J Cataract Refract Surg 28: 1770–1773

18. Kugelberg U, Zetterström C, Syren-Nordqvist S (1996) Ocular axial length in children with unilateral congenital cataract. Acta Ophthalmol Scand 74: 220–223

19. Kugelberg U, Zetterström C, Lundgren B, Syrén-Nordqvist S (1996) Eye growth in the aphakic newborn rabbit. J Cataract Refract Surg 22: 337–341

20. Kugelberg M, Shafiei K, Zetterström C (2004) One-piece AcrySof in the newborn rabbit eye. J Cataract Refract Surg, in press

21. Lambert SR, Fernandes A, Grossniklaus HE (1995) Haptic breakage following neonatal IOL implantation in a non-human primate model. J Pediatr Ophthalmol Strabismus 32:219–224

22. Lambert SR, Buckley EG, Plager DA, Medow NB, Wilson ME (1999) Unilateral intraocular lens implantation during the first six months of life. J AAPOS 3:344–349

23. Laurell CG, Zetterström C, Lundgren B, Torngren L, Andersson K (1997) Inflammatory response in the rabbit after phacoemulsification and intraocular lens implantation using a 5.2 or 11.0 mm incision. J Cataract Refract Surg 23:126–131

24. Lewis TL, Maurer D, Tytla ME, Bowering ER, Brent HP (1992) Vision in the "good" eye of children for unilateral congenital cataract. Ophthalmology 99:1013–1017

25. Lundvall A, Zetterström C (1999) Complications after early surgery for congenital cataracts. Acta Ophthalmol Scand 77:677–680

26. Lundvall A, Kugelberg U (2002) Outcome after treatment of congenital unilateral cataract. Acta Ophthalmol Scand 80:588–592

27. Montan PG, Wejde G, Setterquist H, Rylander M, Setterström C (2002) Prophylactic intracameral cefuroxime. Evaluation of safety and kinetics in cataract surgery. J Cataract Refract Surg 28:982–987

28. Montan PG, Wejde G, Koranyi G, Rylander M (2002) Prophylactic intracameral cefuroxime. Efficacy in preventing endophthalmitis after cataract surgery. J Cataract Refract Surg 28:977–981

29. Pandey SK, Wilson ME, Trivedi RH, Izak AM, Macky TA, Werner L, Apple DJ (2001) Pediatric cataract surgery and intraocular lens implantation: current techniques, complications, and management. Int Ophthalmol Clin 41:175–196

30. Parks MM, Johnson DA, Reed GW (1993) Long-term visual results and complications in children with aphakia. A function of cataract type. Ophthalmology 100:826–841

31. Rogers GL, Tishler CL, Tsou BH, Hertle RW, Fellows RR (1981) Visual acuity in infants with congenital cataracts operated on prior to 6 months of age. Arch Ophthalmol 99:999–1003

32. Saini JS, Jain AK, Sukhija J, Gupta P, Saroha V (2003) Anterior and posterior capsulorhexis in pediatric cataract surgery with or without trypan blue dye: randomized prospective clinical study. J Cataract Refr Surg 29:1733–1737

33. Taylor D, Vaegan X, Morris JA, Rodgers JE, Warland J (1979) Amblyopia in bilateral infantile and juvenile cataract. Relationship to timing of treatment. Trans Ophthalmol Soc UK 99:170–175

34. Trivedi RH, Wilson EM (2003) Single-piece acrylic intraocular lens implantation in children 29:1738–1743

35. Vasavada A, Desai J (1997) Primary posterior capsulorhexis with and without anterior vitrectomy in congenital cataracts. J Cataract Refract Surg 23:645–651

36. Vasavada AR, Trivedi RH, Singh R (2001) Necessity of vitrectomy when optic capture is performed in children older than 5 years. J Cataract Refract Surg 27:1185–1193

37. von Noorden G (1978) Klinische Aspekte der Deprivationsamblyopie. Klin Mbl Augenheilk 173: 464–469

38. Wilson ME, Apple PJ, Bluestein EC, Wang XH (1994) Intraocular lenses for pediatric implantation: biomaterials, designs, and sizing. J Cataract Refract Surg 20:584–591

39. Wilson ME, Peterseim MW, Englert JA, Lall-Trail JK, Elliot LA (2001) Pseudophakia and polypseudophakia in the first year of life. J AAPOS 5:238–245

40. Wright K (1995) Visual development, amblyopia, and sensory adaptations. In: Wright KW (ed) Pediatric ophthalmology and strabismus. Mosby Year Book, St Louis

41. Zetterström C, Kugelberg U, Oskarsson C (1994) Cataract surgery in children with capsulorhexis of anterior and posterior capsules and heparin-surface-modified intraocular lenses. J Cataract Refract Surg 20:599–601

42. Zetterström C, Kugelberg U, Lundgren B, Syrén-Nordqvist S (1996) After-cataract formation in newborn rabbits implanted with intraocular lenses. J Cataract Refract Surg 22:85–88

Wolfgang Behrens-Baumann

10.1
Introduction

Post-cataract surgery infection presents as endophthalmitis – an eyeball-threatening situation. Johann Sebastian Bach and Georg Friedrich Händel both went blind following cataract surgery performed by John Taylor in 1750 and 1758, respectively [40]. Bach's eyes developed severe iridocyclitis [51] – probably an infection, as antisepsis had been unknown at that time. Over the subsequent 15 weeks he was acutely ill and died with a high fever and cerebral complications [*Schlagfluss* ("apoplexy") as his son Carl Philipp Emanuel reported in his necrology]. This may perhaps be interpreted as a brain abscess via the cavernous sinus.

10.1.1
Incidence

The incidence of post-cataract endophthalmitis is about 0.1% in industrial countries (Table 10.1). However, a study in Thailand reports a rate of 9.4% and demonstrates the value of hygienic measures.

There were only small differences of endophthalmitis rates when temporal clear cornea incision (CCI) were compared to superior corneal-scleral incision (CSI) in retrospective surveys: in Germany CCI 0.1% versus 0.07% CSI [89], and in Canada CCI 0.129% versus CSI 0.05% [27]. However, in a prospective randomised multi-centre study (11,595 eyes), the endophthalmitis risk was reduced five-fold in superior CSI (p=0.037) compared to temporal CCI [81]. This correlates with another recent study with a

Table 10.1. Incidence (%) of post-cataract endophthalmitis in industrial countries

Percentage	Country	Year	Reference
0.22	USA	1991	[72]
0.072	USA	1991	[58]
0.3	France	1992	[86]
0.148	Germany	1999	[89]
0.1	Netherlands	2000	[94]
0.1	Sweden	2002	[76]
0.198	Australia	2003	[79]
0.1	Norway	2003	[88]

three-fold higher risk associated with CCI than with CSI [28]. As many surgeons have now switched to posterior limbal tunnel incisions, which heal faster than CCI, the incidence has to be again evaluated for modern surgical techniques.

10.1.2
Sources of Contamination

In principle, there are four sources of intraocular contamination: (1) operating theatre including ventilation system, (2) medical personnel, (3) operating instruments, and (4) the patient him-/herself.

The latter source seems to be the most significant. Bacterial species dominate the resident flora of the outer eye [63]. Positive preoperative conjunctival smears range from 51% up to 76% (Table 10.2) [14, 16, 19, 35].

10.2
Prevention of Post-operative Endophthalmitis

10.2.1
Preoperative Prophylaxis

10.2.1.1
Topical Antibiotic Prophylaxis

Preoperative topical application of antibiotics appears rational to reduce the number of germs in the cul-de-sac [7, 14, 54, 67, 47]. A 3-day prophylaxis combined with a short-term application (1 h) is more effective than a short-term prophylaxis alone [93] in reducing conjunctival contamination. A 3-day preoperative administration of Neosporin followed by povidone-iodine 5% immediately before surgery was more effective for this purpose than the 3-day and preoperative application of povidone-iodine alone [7]. However, a reduction in intraocular contamination cannot be achieved [24, 43].

In a recent study on rabbit eyes it could be demonstrated that topical moxifloxacin hydrochloride 0.5% four times daily can prevent endophthalmitis in this model [61].

10.2.1.2
Antisepsis

To conform with general surgical principles, antisepsis is used to reduce the likelihood of wound infection by reducing bacterial counts in the wound area.

Table 10.2. Microbial findings from preoperative conjunctival smears

Positive smear (%)	Part (%) of germ in the bacterial spectrum	Reference
51	CNS (40), *S. aureus* (4), *Corynebacterium* spp. (3), *E. coli*, enterococci, *S. faecalis*, α-haemolytic Streptococci (each 1)	[14]
62	CNS (62), *S. aureus* (14), gram-negative bacteria (9)	[16]
75	CNS (66), *S. aureus* (9), anaerobes (11)	[19]
76	CNS (90), *P. acnes* (62), *Corynebacterium* spp. (18), Peptostreptococcus (3)	[35]

For *skin antisepsis,* a 10% povidone-iodine solution is widely used. In the periorbital region with its many sebaceous glands the antiseptic should be administered about 10 min before surgery to act sufficiently [31].

For *antisepsis of the conjunctiva* povidone-iodine may also be used. As little as 1% of the solution reduces conjunctival contamination [17, 18], as well as the 9% solution [50].

In a study involving 8,083 patients a significant difference (*p*<0,03) could be observed between the incidence of endophthalmitis with an antisepsis (2 of 3.489 or 0.06%) using 5% povidone-iodine and the control group (11 of 4,594 or 0.24%) using silver protein solution (Argyrol) [91]. The efficacy of povidone-iodine 5% in reducing conjunctival contamination is comparable to a 3-day course of topical antibiotics [6, 54].

10.2.2
Intraoperative Prophylaxis

According to surveys carried out in various countries antibiotics in the irrigation solution during phacoemulsification are used in varying percentages by the responding eye surgeons (Table 10.3).

In several publications and letters to the editor it has been suggested that the addition of antibiotics to the irrigation solution should have a protective effect, but this has not been confirmed yet by any prospective study, nor has it reduced the incidence of endophthalmitis. In addition, these suggestions have been based on retrospective data or on studies of antibiotic use without control groups [45, 46, 77].

Anterior chamber contamination following cataract surgery varies considerably (Table 10.4). No endophthalmitis occurred in these series except in two of Leong et al.'s cases 5 days postoperatively [64]. It should be noted that in his study no germs had been found in the anterior chamber at the end of surgery. In two studies a reduction of the contamination rate from 12/100 to 5/100 could be observed, when vancomycin was added to the irrigation solution [71] and from 22/110 to 3/110 with vancomycin/gentamicin [15]. In contrast, two other corresponding studies revealed no difference (8/190

Table 10.3. Number of eye surgeons (in percent), who add antibiotic to the irrigating solution during cataract surgery

Country	Number (%)	References
Australia	8.0	[78]
England	8.5	[33]Dinakaran and Crome 2002
New Zealand	16.0	[37]
USA	35.0	[69]
Germany	About 60.0	[89]

Table 10.4. Anterior chamber contamination (percentage and number of eyes) at the end of cataract surgery

Percentage	Number of eyes	References
43.0	13 of 30	[32]
26.0	29 of 110	[90]
13.7	98 of 700	[75]
6.0	12 of 200	[52]
4.9	5 of 103	[87]
0.3	1 of 346	[80]
0	0 of 98	[64]

control, 9/182 vancomycin [39] and 1/346 control, 2/353 gentamicin, *p*=0.57 [80]).

In any case, the effect of various antibiotics begins only after 3–4 h and full activity occurs after about 24 h [21, 48, 60, 59]. In this context it should be kept in mind that the aqueous humour flow rate is 2.75±0.63 µl/min (mean ± standard deviation) [20] and the anterior chamber is completely exchanged within 1–2 h. In an animal study for antibiotic prophylaxis in pars plana vitrectomy efficacy could only be established for low but not for moderate numbers of bacteria [65].

In addition, the risk of overdose (aminoglycoside retinal toxicity) should be considered. Moreover, resistance against antibiotics has been increased, especially against the reserve antibiotic vancomycin. Scientific organisations and authors, therefore, do not advise prophylactic antibiotics in the irrigating solutions, particularly since no benefit has yet been proven [2, 23, 70].

10.2.3
Postoperative Prophylaxis

The antimicrobial effect of antisepsis is superior to that mediated by an antibiotic for the first 24 h [8, 9]. Postoperatively, the application of 1.25 % povidone-iodine leads to a significant reduction in conjunctival contamination [55]. On the other hand, there are no studies confirming any benefit of post-operative antibiotics, especially after 24 h, although most surgeons use an antibiotic ointment or solution at the end of the procedure [66] and for several days post-operatively.

10.3
Treatment of Post-cataract Endophthalmitis

10.3.1
Diagnostic Measures

Prior to therapy, information should be gained relating to which germs are responsible for the infection. Material from the vitreous cavity should be sampled by the vitreous cutter before opening the infusion in the case of pars plana vitrectomy or as a puncture. Samples from the anterior chamber or the vitrectomy cassette are less successful [10, 74]. Within several minutes microscopy of the obtained specimen can give the required information: gram-positive or gram-negative germs or fungal infection.

In addition, results of microbiologic cultures are obtained after about 24 h and appropriate anti-infectives can be administered.

10.3.2
Anti-infective Therapy

10.3.2.1
Systemic Administration

According to the randomised multi-centre Endophthalmitis Vitrectomy Study (EVS), systemic antibiotics do not appear to have any effect on the course and outcome of endo-phthalmitis after cataract operations [38]. However, the study design using intravenous ceftazidime and intravenous amikacin for 5–10 days was not suitable to answer this question [36, 92]. In 38 % of the infective eyes gram-positive cocci were cultivated, in which ceftazidime is only slightly active, whereas vancomycin would have been significantly more effective. Until a suitable study becomes available, this author and others recommend intravenous antibiotic use [1, 36, 92].

If the causative organisms are not (yet) known, vancomycin can be used as a maximum therapy to cover gram-positive bacteria and also largely for methicillin-resistant staphylococci (MRSA), and ceftazidime to cover the gram-negative spectrum [12, 25]. These substances should be administered immediately after earning diagnostic samples and without waiting for the microbiologic results. Alternatively, imipenem in also suitable against gram-positive and ciprofloxacin against gram-negative species [4, 12, 13].

In endophthalmitis caused by *Propionibacterium acnes*, vancomycin, imipenem or clindamycin are effective [3, 95]. However, surgery often results [30], combined with intraocular antibiotic administration [5, 26] as the germs are typically located within the synechised capsular bag and hardly come in contact with the antibiotic.

If fungal infection is suspected, voriconazole or fluconazole (in case of *Candida albicans* infection) should be administered before considering amphotericin B [11, 44, 53, 82]. The latter drug has considerably more and severe side effects than the other antifungals.

Summary for the Clinician

- Maximal therapy may be the administration of intravitreal and systemic antibiotics and prednisolone combined with pars plana vitrectomy
- Intravenous drug therapy in acute endophthalmitis with unknown pathogens: vancomycin 1 g twice daily; ceftazidime 2 g three times daily; prednisolone 200 mg

Table 10.5. Intravitreal injection (Amikacin: cave macula infarction)

Substance	Dosage/0.1 ml
Vancomycin	1.0 mg
Ceftazidime	2.25 mg
(Amikacin)	(0.4 mg)
Amphotericin B	0.75 µg
Dexamethasone	0.4 mg

10.3.2.2
Intravitreal Administration

Using this route, the highest drug concentration can be achieved precisely at the target site. However, this concentration lasts only for a limited period, especially if pars plana vitrectomy has been performed. Injection alone may be successful [83], but is usually combined with vitrectomy. Vancomycin 1 mg/0.1 ml is suitable for gram-positive bacteria [38, 68] and is above the MIC_{90} of *Staphylococcus epidermidis* for >48 h [49]. Even vancomycin 0.2 mg/0.1 ml remains at a therapeutic level for 3–4 days [42]. Aminoglycosides are no longer recommended due to their retinal toxicity [41, 56] and should be replaced by ceftazidime 2 mg/0.1 ml to cover the gram-negative spectrum [22, 41, 56].

In fungal endophthalmitis 5–7.5 µg/0.1 ml amphotericin B is used [11, 84, 85]. Vancomycin is suitable in *Propionibacterium acnes* infection [5, 26]. The doses are summarised in Table 10.5.

10.3.2.3
Topical Administration

Antibiotic eye drops and ointment are only additionally indicated if the anterior segment of the eye is involved.

10.3.3
Anti-inflammatory Therapy

Corticosteroids should be administered to halt the self-destructive response of the host by leukocytes and toxic effects of cytokines [57] – in addition to antibiotic therapy, of course.

Moreover, the effect of antigens released by bacterial disintegration after antibiotic therapy should be hampered. Intravitreal dexamethasone (0.4 mg/0.1 ml) at the end of pars plana vitrectomy leads to rapid decrease of intraocular inflammation [29]. Oral administration (1 mg/kg body weight) 1 day after intravitreal antibiotic therapy has not shown any negative effect in the course of the infection [38] even when administered in mycotic endophthalmitis [57]. Parallel to intravenous antibiotics 200 mg prednisolone is often given systemically. However, no randomised studies are available on this subject.

10.3.4
Surgery

According to the prospective EVS [38], patients with *acute onset* of the infection after cataract surgery with an initial vision of hand movements or better should be treated by vitreous biopsy and intravitreal antibiotics. Immediate pars plana vitrectomy is only recommended in eyes with light perception. However, there has been some criticism of the EVS study design [25].

In addition, follow-up of the EVS patients revealed differences between diabetics and non-diabetics. Diabetics with a visual acuity of hand motion or better had a better visual outcome by vitrectomy (57%) than after biopsy (40%). Because of the low number of diabetic participants in the study, these results were not significant [34]. Due to the lack of more adequate studies, many ophthalmologists in tertiary centres perform early vitrectomy if necessary, especially since this type of surgery has become a routine procedure.

In the event of *late onset* of endophthalmitis following cataract surgery (about 2 weeks up to several months) the symptoms are milder and often recurrent after seemingly successful medical treatment. *Propionibacterium acnes* has been identified as the typical pathogen for this form of infection. As *P. acnes* is often enclosed in the synechised capsular bag, antibiotics may not affect the pathogen in concentrations high enough to be bactericidal. Consequently, surgery with posterior capsulectomy, vitrectomy or even intraocular lens and capsular sac explantation may be necessary. As a further advantage of surgery material for culturing can be obtained [73]. Therefore, pars plana vitrectomy may be advisable.

Summary for the Clinician

- Conjunctival antisepsis with povidone-iodine 5 % has been proven to significantly reduce the incidence of endophthalmitis
- Skin antisepsis with 10 % povidone-iodine solution, allow 10 min to act
- Conjunctiva antisepsis (twice) with at least 1.25 % povidone-iodine solution (up to 10 %) for 1 min. No substance should enter the anterior chamber

10.4
Conclusion

Endophthalmitis is still the most disastrous complication of cataract surgery since the other – explosive bleeding – has declined with the use of small incisions. Prevention with antiseptics (povidone-iodine) has reduced the incidence to 0.1 %. Maximal treatment of acute endophthalmitis with appropriate systemic and intravitreal antibiotics, corticosteroids and pars plana vitrectomy may improve the prognosis.

References

1. Aaberg TM, Sternberg P Jr (2001) Trauma: principles and techniques of treatment. In: Ryan SJ (ed) Retina. Mosby, St. Louis, pp 2400 – 2426
2. AAO-CDC Task Force (1999) The prophylactic use of vancomycin for intraocular surgery. Quality of Care Publications, Number 515, American Academy of Ophthalmology, San Francisco, www.aao.org
3. Abreu JA, Cordovés L (2001) Chronic or saccular endophthalmitis: diagnosis and management. J Cataract Refract Surg 27:650–651
4. Adenis JP, Mounier M, Salomon JL, Denis F (1994) Human vitreous penetration of imipenem. Eur J Ophthalmol 4:115–117
5. Aldave AJ, Stein JD, Deramo VA, Shah GK, Fischer DH, Maguire JI (1999) Treatment strategies for postoperative Propionibacterium acnes endophthalmitis. Ophthalmology 106:2395–2401
6. Apt L, Isenberg S, Yoshimori R (1984) Chemical preparation of the eye in ophthalmic surgery. III. Effect of povidone-iodine on the conjunctiva. Arch Ophthalmol 102:728–729
7. Apt L, Isenberg SJ, Yoshimori R, Spierer A (1989) Outpatient topical use of povidone-iodine in preparing the eye for surgery. Ophthalmology 96:289–292
8. Apt L, Isenberg S, Yoshimori R, Yoshimori CA, Lam G, Wachler B, Neumann D (1995) The effect of povidone-iodine solution applied at the conclusion of ophthalmic surgery. Am J Opthalmol 119:701–705
9. Apt L, Isenberg S (1995) The effect of povidone-iodine solution applied at the conclusion of ophthalmic surgery. Am J Ophthalmol 120:807–808
10. Barza M, Pavan PR, Doft BH, Wisniewski SR, Wilson LA, Han DP, Kelsey SF (1997) Evaluation of microbiological diagnostic techniques in postoperative endophthalmitis in the Endophthalmitis Vitrectomy Study. Arch Ophthalmol 115:1142–1150
11. Behrens-Baumann W (ed) (1999) Mycosis of the eye and its adnexa. Developments in ophthalmology, vol. 32. S. Karger, Basel (with a contribution by R. Rüchel)
12. Behrens-Baumann W (2004) Magdeburg plan for antibiotic prophylaxis and therapy. www.med.uni-magdeburg.de/augenklinik (1991–2004; regularly updated)
13. Behrens-Baumann W, Martell J (1987) Ciprofloxacin concentrations in human aqueous humor following intravenous administration. Chemoth 33:328–330
14. Behrens-Baumann W, Dobrinski B, Zimmermann O (1988) Bakterienflora der Lider nach präoperativer Desinfektion. Klin Mbl Augenheilkd 192:40–43
15. Beigi B, Westlake W, Chang B, Marsh C, Jacob J, Riordan T (1998) The effect of intracameral, peroperative antibiotics on microbial contamination of anterior chamber aspirates during phacoemulsification. Eye 12:390–394
16. Bialasiewicz AA, Welt R (1991) Präoperative mikrobiologische Diagnostik vor elektiven intraokuaren Eingriffen und Infektionsprophylaxe mit Tobramycin-Augentropfen. Klin Monatsbl Augenheilkd 198:87–93
17. Binder CA, Miño de Kaspar H, Engelbert M, Klauß V, Kampik A (1998) Bakterielle Keimbesiedelung der Konjunktiva mit Propionibacterium acnes vor und nach Polyvidon-Jod-Applikation vor intraokulären Eingriffen. Ophthalmologe 95:438–441

18. Binder CA, Miño de Kaspar H, Klauß V, Kampik A (1999) Präoperative Infektionsprophylaxe mit 1%-iger Polyvidon-Jod-Lösung am Beispiel von konjunktivalen Staphylokokken. Ophthalmologe 96:663–667

19. Boes D, Lindquist T, Fritsche T, Kalina R (1992) Effects of povidone-iodine chemical preparation and saline irrigation on the perilimbal flora. Ophthalmology 99:1569–1574

20. Brubaker RF (1991) Flow of aqueous humor in humans (The Friedenwald Lecture). Invest Ophthalmol Vis Sci 32:3145–3166

21. Caillon J, Juvin ME, Pirault JL, Drugeon HB (1989) Activité bactéricide de la Daptomycine (LY 146032) comparée à celle de la Vancomycine et de la Teicoplanine sur les bactéries à gram positif. Path Biol 37:540–548

22. Campochiaro PA, Lim JI (1994) Aminoglycoside Toxicity Study Group: aminoglycoside toxicity in the treatment of endophthalmitis. Arch Ophthalmol 112:48–53

23. Center of Disease Control (1995) Recommendations for preventing the spread of vancomycin resistance. Morb Mort Wkly Rep 44 (RR-12):1–13

24. Chitkara DK, Manners T, Chapman F, Stoddart MG, Hill D, Jenkins D (1994) Lack of effect of preoperative norfloxacin on bacterial contamination of anterior chamber aspirates after cataract surgery. Br J Ophthalmol 78:772–774

25. Ciulla TA (1999) Update on acute and chronic endophthalmitis. Ophthalmology 106:2237–2238

26. Clark WL, Kaiser PK, Flynn HW Jr, Belfort A, Miller D, Meisler DM (1999) Treatment strategies and visual acuity outcomes in chronic postoperative Propionibacterium acnes endophthalmitis. Ophthalmology 106:1665–1670

27. Colleaux KM, Hamilton WK (2000) Effect of prophylactic antibiotics and incision type on the incidence of endophthalmitis after cataract surgery. Can J Ophthalmol 35:373–378

28. Cooper BA, Holekamp NM, Bohigian G, Thompson PA (2003) Case-control study of endophthalmitis after cataract surgery comparing scleral tunnel and clear corneal wounds. Am J Ophthalmol 136:300–305

29. Das T, Jalali S, Gothwal VK, Sharma S, Naduvilath TJ (1999) Intravitreal dexamethasone in exogenous bacterial endophthalmitis: results of a prospective randomised study. Br J Ophthalmol 83:1050–1055

30. Deramo VA, Ting TD (2001) Treatment of Propionibacterium acnes endophthalmitis. Curr Opin Ophthalmol 12:225–229

31. Deutsche Gesellschaft für Hygiene und Mikrobiologie (German Society for Hygiene and Microbiology) (2002) List of disinfectives of the DGHM. mhp, Wiesbaden, Germany

32. Dickey JB, Thompson KD, Jay WM (1991) Anterior chamber aspirate cultures after uncomplicated cataract surgery. Am J Ophthalmol 112:278–282

33. Dinakaran S, Crome DA (2002) Prophylactic measures prevalent in the United Kingdom. J Cataract Refract Surg 28:387–388

34. Doft BH, Wisniewski SR, Kelsey SF, Fitzgerald SG (2001) Endophthalmitis Vitrectomy Study Group: diabetes and postoperative endophthalmitis in the Endophthalmitis Vitrectomy Study. Arch Ophthalmol 119:650–656

35. Doyle A, Beigi B, Early A, Blake A, Eustace P, Hone R (1995) Adherence of bacteria to intraocular lenses. A prospective study. Br J Ophthalmol 79:347–349

36. Durand ML (2002) The post-Endophthalmitis Vitrectomy Study era. Arch Ophthalmol 120:233–234

37. Elder M, Tarr K, Leaming D (2000) The New Zealand cataract and refractive surgery survey. Clin Exp Ophthalmol 28:89–96

38. Endophthalmitis Vitrectomy Study Group (1995) Results of the Endophthalmitis Vitrectomy Study. A randomized trial of immediate vitrectomy and of intravenous antibiotics for the treatment of postoperative bacterial endophthalmitis. Arch Ophthalmol 113:1479–1496

39. Feys J, Salvanet-Bouccara A, Emond J Ph, Dublanchet A (1997) Vancomycin prophylaxis and intraocular contamination during cataract surgery. J Cataract Refract Surg 23:894–897

40. Franken FH (1997) Die Krankheiten großer Komponisten. Florian Noetzel GmbH, Verlag der Heinrichshofen-Bücher, Wilhelmshaven

41. Galloway G, Ramsay A, Jordan K, Vivian A (2002) Macular infarction after intravitreal amikacin: mounting evidence against amikacin. Br J Ophthalmol 86:359–360

42. Gan IM, van Dissel JT, Beekhuis WH, Swart W, van Meurs JC (2001) Intravitreal vancomycin and gentamicin concentrations in patients with postoperative endophthalmitis. Br J Ophthalmol 85:1289–1293

43. Gelfand YA, Mezer E, Linn S, Miller B (1998) Lack of effect of prophylactic gentamicin treatment on intraocular and extraocular fluid cultures after pars plana vitrectomy. Ophthalmic Surg Lasers 29:497–501

44. Ghannoum MA, Kuhn DM (2002) Voriconazole – better chances for patients with invasive mycoses. Eur J Med Res 7:242–256

45. Gills JP (1991) Filters and antibiotics in irrigating solution for cataract surgery. J Cataract Refract Surg 17:385

46. Gimbel HV, Sun R, DeBrof BM (1994) Prophylactic intracameral antibiotics during cataract surgery: the incidence of endophthalmitis and corneal endothelial cell loss. Eur J Implant Ref Surg 6:280–285

47. Gray TB, Keenan JI, Clemett RS, Allardyce RA (1993) Fusidic acid prophylaxis before cataract surgery: patient self-administration. Aust N Z J Ophthalmol 21:99–103

48. Gritz DC, Cevallos AV, Smolin G, Whitcher JP Jr (1996) Antibiotic supplementation of intraocular irrigating solutions. Ophthalmology 103:1204–1209

49. Haider SA, Hassett P, Bron AJ (2001) Intraocular vancomycin levels after intravitreal injection in post cataract extraction endophthalmitis. Retina 21:210–213

50. Hara J, Yasuda F, Higashitsutsumi M (1997) Preoperative disinfection of the conjunctival sac in cataract surgery. Ophthalmologica 211[Suppl 1]: 62–67

51. Henning A (1992) Die Okulisten Joseph Hillmer und John Taylor in Leipzig. Aktuelle Augenheilkunde 17:204–214

52. Henry JC, Rozas D (1993) Bacterial growth from anterior chamber fluid aspirates using different irrigating solutions in phacoemulsification. Invest Ophthalmol 34:884

53. Holzheimer RG, Dralle H (2002) Management of mycosis in surgical patients – review of the literature. Eur J Med Res 7:200–226

54. Isenberg S, Apt L, Yoshimori R, Khwarg S (1985) Chemical preparation of the eye in ophthalmic surgery. IV. Comparison of povidone-iodine on the conjunctiva with a prophylactic antibiotic. Arch Ophthalmol 103:1340–1342

55. Isenberg S, Apt L, Yoshimori R, Pham C, Lam NK (1997) Efficacy of topical povidone-iodine during the first week after ophthalmic surgery. Am J Ophthalmol 124:31–35

56. Jackson TL, Williamson TH (1999) Amikacin retinal toxicity. Br J Ophthalmol 83:1199–1200

57. Kain HL (1997) Prinzipien in der Behandlung der Endophthalmitis. Klin Monatsbl Augenheilkd 210:274–288

58. Kattan HM, Flynn HW Jr, Pflugfelder SC, Robertson C, Forster RK (1991) Nosocomial endophthalmitis survey. Current incidence of infection after intraocular surgery. Ophthalmology 98:227–238

59. Keverline MR, Kowalski RP, Dhaliwal DK (2002) In vitro comparison of ciprofloxacin, ofloxacin, and povidone-iodine for surgical prophylaxis. J Cataract Refract Surg 28:915–916

60. Kowalski RP, Karenchak LM, Warren BB, Eller AW (1998) Time-kill profiles of Enterococcus to antibiotics used for intravitreal therapy. Ophthalmic Surg Lasers 29:295–299

61. Kowalski RP, Romanowski EG, Mah FS, Yates KA, Gordon YJ (2003) The prevention of bacterial endophthalmitis by topical moxifloxacin in a rabbit prophylaxis model. Abstract on www.arvo.org, presented May 04–09, Fort Lauderdale, USA

62. Kramer A, Below H, Behrens-Baumann W, Müller G, Rudolph P, Reimer K (2001) New aspects of the tolerance of the antiseptic povidone-iodine in different ex vivo models. Dermatol 204[Suppl 1]: 86–91

63. Kramer A, Behrens-Baumann W (2002) Microbial colonization of the eye as target for antiseptics. In: Kramer A, Behrens-Baumann W (eds) Antiseptic prophylaxis and therapy in ocular infections. S. Karger, Basel, pp 2–8

64. Leong JK, Shah R, McCluskey PJ, Benn RA, Taylor RF (2002) Bacterial contamination of the anterior chamber during phacoemulsification cataract surgery. J Cataract Refract Surg 28:826–833

65. Liang Ch, Peyman GA, Sonmez M, Molinari LC (1999) Experimental prophylaxis of staphylococcus aureus endophthalmitis after vitrectomy. The use of antibiotics in irrigating solution. Retina 19:223–229

66. Liesegang TJ (1999) Perioperative antibiotic prophylaxis in cataract surgery. Cornea 18:383–402

67. Maeck CR, Eckardt C, Höller C (1991) Comparison of bacterial growth on the conjunctiva after treatment with gentamicin or povidone-iodine. Fortschr Ophthalmol 88:848–851

68. Mamalis N, Kearsley L, Brinton E (2002) Postoperative endophthalmitis. Curr Opin Ophthalmol 13:14–18

69. Masket S (1998) Preventing, diagnosing, and treating endophthalmitis. J Cataract Refract Surg 24:725–726

70. May L, Navarro VB, Gottsch JD (2000) First do no harm: routine use of aminoglycosides in the operating room. Insight 25:77–80

71. Mendivil Soto A, Mendivil MP (2001) The effect of topical povidone-iodine, intraocular vancomycin, or both on aqueous humor cultures at the time of cataract surgery. Am J Ophthalmol 131:293–300

72. Menikoff JA, Speaker MG, Marmor M, Raskin EM (1991) A case-control study of risk factors for postoperative endophthalmitis. Ophthalmology 98:1761–1768

73. Meredith TA (2001) Vitrectomy for infectious endophthalmitis. In: Ryan SJ (ed) Retina, 3rd edn. Mosby Year Book, St. Louis, pp 2242–2263

74. Miño de Kaspar H, Grasbon T, Kampik A (2000) Automated surgical equipment requires routine disinfection of vacuum control manifold to prevent postoperative endophthalmitis. Ophthalmology 107:685–690

75. Mistlberger A, Ruckhofer J, Raithel E, Müller M, Alzner E, Egger St. F, Grabner G (1997) Anterior chamber contamination during cataract surgery with intraocular lens implantation. J Cataract Refract Surg 23:1064–1069.

76. Montan PG, Lundstrom M, Stenevi U, Thorburn W (2002) Endophthalmitis following cataract surgery in Sweden. The 1998 national prospective survey. Acta Ophthalmol Scand 80:258–261

77. Montan PG, Wejde G, Koranyi G, Rylander M (2002) Prophylactic intracameral cefuroxime. Efficacy in preventing endophthalmitis after cataract surgery. J Cataract Refract Surg 28:977–981

78. Morlet N, Gatus B, Coroneo M (1998) Patterns of peri-operative prophylaxis for cataract surgery: A survey of Australian ophthalmologists. Aust NZJ Ophthalmol 26:5–12

79. Morlet N, Li J, Semmers J, Ng J on behalf of the EPSWA team (2003) The endophthalmitis population study of Western Australia (EPSWA): first report. Brit J Ophthalmol 87:574–576

80. Motschmann M, Schmitz K, Lauf H, Schuster G, König W, Behrens-Baumann W (1998) Ist der Zusatz eines Antibiotikums zur Spüllösung bei der Kataraktoperation sinnvoll? In: Duncker G (ed) 12. Kongress der Deutschsprachigen Gesellschaft für Intraokularlinsen-Implantation und refraktive Chirurgie. Klin Monatsbl Augenheilkd 212:5

81. Nagaki Y, Hayasaka S, Kadoi C, Matsumoto M, Yanagisawa S, Watanabe Ka, Watanabe Ko, Hayasaka Y, Ikeda N, Sato S, Kataoka Y, Togashi M, Abe T (2003) Bacterial endophthalmitis after small-incision cataract surgery. Effect of incision placement and intraocular lens type. J Cataract Refract Surg 29:20–26

82. Narang S, Gupta A, Gupta V, Dogra MR, Ram J, Pandav SS, Chakrabarti A (2001) Fungal endophthalmitis following cataract surgery: clinical presentation, microbiological spectrum, and outcome. Am J Ophthalmol 132:609–617

83. Pavan PR, Oteiza EE, Hughes BA, Avni A (1994) Exogenous endophthalmitis initially treated without systemic antibiotics. Ophthalmology 101:1289–1297

84. Perraut LE Jr, Perraut LE, Bleiman B, Lyons J (1981) Successful treatment of Candida albicans endophthalmitis with intravitreal amphotericin B. Arch Ophthalmol 99:1565–1567

85. Pflugfelder St C, Flynn HW Jr, Zwickey TA, Forster RK, Tsiligianni A, Culbertson WW, Mandelbaum S (1988) Exogenous fungal endophthalmitis. Ophthalmology 95:19–30

86. Salvanet-Bouccara A, Forestier F, Coscas G, Adenis JP, Denis F (1992) Bacterial endophthalmitis. Ophthalmological results of a national multicenter prospective survey. J Fr Ophtalmol 15:669–678

87. Samad A, Solomon SK, Miller MA, Mendelson J (1995) Anterior chamber contamination after uncomplicated phacoemulsification and intraocular lens implantation. Am J Ophthalmol 120:143–150

88. Sandvig KU, Dannevig L (2003) Postoperative endophthalmitis: establishment and results of a national registry. J Cataract Refract Surg 29:1273–1280

89. Schmitz S, Dick HB, Krummenauer F, Pfeiffer N (1999) Endophthalmitis in cataract surgery. Results of a German survey. Ophthalmology 106:1869–1877

90. Sherwood DR, Rich WJ, Jacobs JS, Hart RJ, Fairchild YL (1989) Bacterial contamination of intraocular and extraocular fluids during extracapsular cataract extraction. Eye 3:308–312

91. Speaker MG, Menikoff JA (1991) Prophylaxis of endophthalmitis with topical povidone-iodine. Ophthalmology 98:1769–1775

92. Sternberg P Jr, Martin DF (2001) Management of endophthalmitis in the Post-Endophthalmitis Vitrectomy Study era. Arch Ophthalmol 119:754–755

93. Ta CN, Egbert PR, Singh K, Shriver EM, Blumenkranz MS, Miño de Kaspar H (2002) Prospective randomized comparison of 3-day versus 1-hour preoperative ofloxacin prophylaxis for cataract surgery. Ophthalmology 109:2036–2040

94. Versteegh MFL, van Rij G (2000) Incidence of endophthalmitis after cataract surgery in the Netherlands. Documenta Ophthalmologica 100:1–6

95. Winward KE, Pflugfelder St C, Flynn HW Jr, Roussel TJ, Davis JL (1993) Postoperative Propionibacterium endophthalmitis. Treatment strategies and long-term results. Ophthalmology 100:447–451

Jacqueline T. Koo, Eric J. Linebarger, Richard L. Lindstrom, David R. Hardten

Core Messages

- Major advances in refractive surgery have driven this field into one of the most exciting in ophthalmology
- Improvements in excimer laser and LASIK technology continue to promise further safety and efficacy
- Lens technology innovations will offer refractive surgeons multiple new options for patients
- Future advances in gene mapping and gene therapy may offer alternative refractive procedures

11.1
Introduction

The subspecialty of refractive surgery is responsible for many of the innovations in the field of ophthalmology. Acceptance of these advancements has come from the incorporation of science and technology to increase the safety, accuracy, and predictability of altering the refractive error of the human eye. These developments offer new tools for the ophthalmologist to improve and enhance vision for our current patients as well as the patients of the future. Eye surgeons are able to correct ametropia by using different surgical techniques in a variety of anatomical locations. This chapter will discuss future trends in refractive surgery that will shape the decisions for refractive surgeons of tomorrow.

The refractive state of the eye is dependent chiefly on three main variables: the cornea, the lens, and the axial length. The refractive power of the eye can be modified by changing the curvature of the principle refractive surfaces (the cornea and lens), altering the index of refraction of different media (cornea, anterior chamber, lens, vitreous) or adjusting the axial length of the eye (sclera).

11.2
Cornea

Historically, the cornea has been the primary interest of the refractive surgeon because of its anatomical accessibility. Corneal refractive surgery, with its multitude of procedures and acronyms, can be simplified into four main mechanisms: (1) corneal tissue removal, (2) addition of tissue volume, (3) compression, and (4) relaxation.

11.2.1
Corneal Tissue Removal

Subtraction techniques use one of a variety of procedures to induce corneal remodelling. Keratomileusis, the removal of a variable amount of corneal stroma, was first proposed by Barraquer [1] in the 1940s and later modified by others. Automated keratomes improved the predictability of keratomileusis, and led to a more popular variation on the technique. Automated lamellar keratoplasty (ALK) became another option for the treatment of myopia and hyperopia in the 1970s and 1980s.

The next advancement in corneal tissue removal would be ushered in by the development of light amplification by stimulated emission of radiation (LASER) technology. By the early 1980s, the precision of the 193-nm excimer laser was seen as a useful tool to reshape the corneal stroma. It has since become the basis for current corneal refractive surgery. The excimer laser has been a major innovation in ophthalmology because of its precise ability to remove tissue with negligible damage to surrounding structures.

Burrato [6] and Pallikaris [33] are credited with combining lamellar surgical techniques developed by Barraquer [1–3], and excimer laser technology in a procedure they termed laser assisted stromal in situ keratomileusis (LASIK). This technique allows for precise sculpting and subtraction of corneal stroma under a protective corneal flap, facilitating broad range correction of hyperopia, myopia and astigmatism while avoiding many of the disadvantages of its forebearer, PRK. LASIK has replaced previous forms of corneal subtraction surgery to become one of the most frequently performed ophthalmic procedures world-wide. The popularity of the LASIK procedure serves as the springboard for even further refinements in refractive surgical technology.

One of the exciting advancements to the current LASIK procedure is wavefront technology. Wavefront technology measures higher order wavefront aberrations of the cornea missed by conventional corneal topography maps. The wavefront aberrometer focuses a measurement beam onto the patient's retina and reflects a wavefront back through the patient's eye. As the wavefront exits, it is distorted by the optics of the eye. Zernike polynomials, mathematical equations formerly developed to understand the optics of space telescopes, convert the wavefront measurements to a waveprint which describes lower order aberrations such as sphere and astigmatism, and higher order aberrations such as spherical aberration, coma and trefoil. The laser is configured to the waveprint to compute a customised corneal ablation to refine refractive treatments.

The commercial applications of wavefront technology in the United States include the VISX CustomVue (VISX, Santa Clara, CA), Alcon LADARVision CustomCornea(Alcon, Orlando, FL), and Bausch and Lomb Zyoptics (Bausch & Lomb, Rochester, NY). FDA trials of these systems have shown excellent results with low to moderate myopes [34]. With this new technology, possible applications of wavefront include myopic and hyperopic enhancements, refractive surgery for hyperopia and mixed astigmatism, presbyopia, and reductions of higher order aberrations and irregular astigmatism. Future advances will develop more mathematical models for the optical distortions of the eye.

Laser technology has also advanced with new gas lasers, solid-state lasers, and intrastromal lasers currently under investigation or awaiting approval for use. Alteration of laser ablation patterns to the cornea will be the first wave of modifications, including the shift from wide beam early generation lasers to faster, more efficient scanning slit, scanning spot, and flying spot lasers. Treatment zones may expand from the current 6- to 7-mm diameter to encompass the entire cornea as well incorporate multi-zone treatments for higher refractive errors and presbyopia. Human clinical trials are underway for patients desiring correction of presbyopia with multifocal laser ablations [8].

The simultaneous correction of astigmatism will become more precise with new laser treatment profiles to adjust the amount of corneal tissue subtraction in various regions of the cornea. Tracking pupillary and iris registration systems may help reduce ablation decentrations and saccadic intrusion artefact. While the current systems are helpful for tracking linear motion in the X, Y and Z axes, newer iris registration methods will use automatic iris registration to track cyclotorsion and the rotational movement of the eye around the Z-axis. Iris location is registered from the diagnostic wavefront unit to the laser. This allows the iris to be in the same position when the laser is treating as it was when the diagnostic unit captured the wavefront information.

New technology is being developed to link tracking systems to instantaneous topographical analysis to provide real-time topographically assisted ablations. This has numerous applications in the treatment of irregular corneal astigmatism. Development of new laser imaging systems may provide more accurate corneal pachymetry than ultrasound instruments and allow for the intraoperative measurements of LASIK flap thickness. The newer systems will possibly use triangulation between a laser and a high-resolution digital camera to create a three-dimensional map of the entire corneal surface, instead of single point measurement as in current ultrasound pachymetry.

Another major area of refinement in LASIK involves changes in microkeratome technology. The possibility of intrastromal ablations, eliminating the need for raising a lamellar flap, is an area of increasing interest. Investigations are also underway for safer, more precise, atraumatic methods of gaining access to the corneal stroma. Super high-velocity water jet technology is being investigated as a plausible alternative to conventional blade systems including the Hydrojet (Medjet, Edison, NJ) [19]. This technology has shown initial promise in creating pristine, atraumatic lamellar flaps, but requires human trials [19]. The Nd:YLF picosecond and 193-nm excimer lasers are also being investigated for use in creating precision lamellar flaps, and expanded work in this area is well underway [23]. Femtosecond laser technology has excited many scientists because of its precise high energy, low heat generating qualities [35]. One current laser, the INTRALASE FS Laser (Intralase, Irvine, CA), uses femtosecond laser technology of 2- to 3-µm spot size to precisely cut tissue by photodisruption. A suction ring holds the eye and the laser disrupts the corneal tissue at the predetermined depth forming plasma bubbles of water and carbon dioxide. These microscopic cavitation bubbles of carbon dioxide and water vapour define the resection plane. The proposed advantages of this laser are the use of lower suction, the greater stability of the flap, uniform flap thickness, and immediate repetition of the flap if loss of suction happens during flap creation. The major disadvantages to this procedure include the increased length of time that the suction ring has to be on the eye because the device takes longer to make a flap than a conventional microkeratome. The flap is more difficult to separate and lift compared to conventional flaps causing some surgeons to require a dull probe to separate the flap from the stromal bed. Given the learning curve involved

in using the INTRALASE and the expense of the laser unit, the system is still developing its appeal to refractive surgeons, yet has great promise.

To avoid the construction of lamellar stromal flaps completely, Atlanta-CIBA Vision Corp. will begin marketing its Centurion SES EpiEdge epikeratome for the Epi-LASIK refractive procedure [19]. The EpiEdge epikeratome is a blunt separator that produces an epithelial sheet, cleaving the epithelium from Bowman's layer, thus eliminating the need for alcohol-based separation, which is toxic to epithelial cells and slows healing. This technology may be useful to improve patient healing and comfort during LASIK.

A biological gel with ablation properties identical to corneal stroma is currently under investigation for use as an adjuvant agent in corneal surface and lamellar surgery. BioMask (Maverick Technologies, Clearwater, FL), is a mouldable, heat-cured synthetic bovine collagen that is applied to the corneal surface prior to ablation [29]. It is initially heated, and then moulded into shape under a contact lens of predetermined base curve. The material has ablation characteristics identical to corneal tissue, which allows irregular corneal surface anomalies to be filled in to a uniform curvature prior to ablation. Initial applications may be in phototherapeutic treatment of corneal scars and dystrophies [41]. Future applications may include the treatment of other types of irregular astigmatism.

The innovation of existing ideas with evolving technology will continue to change the way we approach corneal tissue removal.

Summary for the Clinician

- **Wavefront technology and understanding of higher order aberrations may lead to better LASIK results**
- **Advances in LASIK such as iris-tracking systems, instantaneous corneal topography, and improvements in the microkeratome and laser technology continue to improve the efficacy and safety of this successful procedure**
- **Biological gels may aid in the treatment of irregular astigmatism and corneal surface anomalies**

11.2.2
Corneal Volume Addition

Historically, corneal tissue addition procedures have enjoyed only limited use in a very specific sub-population of patients. The most frequently performed procedure, epikeratophakia, involved the addition of a lenticule of donor corneal tissue added to the host surface after denuding the host epithelium. The donor lenticule was sculpted by a variety of automated techniques to create a corneal lens (hence, the term, "keratophakia") which could be used to treat either hyperopia or myopia in its extreme form [42]. The current and future trends in corneal volume augmentation will centre on synthetic material addition to the corneal surface and stroma, both in the central visual axis and in the periphery.

One of the methods, intrastromal corneal rings, alters corneal shape and refractive error through stromal volume augmentation [7, 14, 36]. This method is based on the principle that arcing corneal collagen lamellae can be flattened centrally by adding tissue volume peripherally. Implantation of peripheral synthetic ring segments will induce central flattening and increased radius of corneal curvature proportional to the thickness of material implanted.

One design, INTACS (Addition Technology, Fremont, CA), involves two arcing 150° segments of approximately 8 mm diameter, ranging in thickness from 0.25 mm to 0.45 mm (Fig. 11.1). These are implanted in the corneal stromal periphery under topical anaesthesia, at approximately 50 % depth. This is accomplished by the creation of a lamellar channel in the peripheral cornea by a stromal separator. This separator is centred on the visual axis under suction, and used to bluntly separated the corneal collagen lamellae. The ring segments are then individually threaded into position. INTACS are currently a viable surgical option for treatment of low to moderate myopia.

This technology has several applicable advantages: it avoids the central visual axis, it is titratable, and it is removable [14, 36]. Ring segments can be removed and replaced with slightly larger or smaller segments to fine tune refrac-

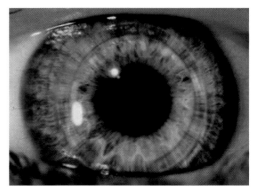

Fig. 11.1. INTACS. (Courtesy of Addition Technology)

tive outcomes, or be removed altogether. While the clinical safety and efficacy data of INTACS inserts appear comparable to older reports of PRK and LASIK, refractive surgeons and patients have not readily embraced this technology. Possible reasons are that the refractive indications are more limited (low degree of essentially spherical myopia), the learning curve required to perform this procedure and the expense of this procedure compared to LASIK or PRK. However, surgeons are looking for applications of this technology for keratoconus and post-LASIK ectasia patients [5].

Research is ongoing to add synthetic material to the cornea to modify the refractive outcome of its central visual axis. Intracorneal lenses have been investigated as a means of correcting myopia, hyperopia and presbyopia [4, 22, 26, 30]. This can be accomplished by implanting an intracorneal lens of like curvature but varying refractive index, thereby changing the effective dioptric power of the cornea. Conversely, implantation of a lens material with similar refractive index, but varying curvature will modify overall corneal curvature and corneal power.

The PermaVision intracorneal lens, (Anamed, Lake Forest, CA) is made of an optically clear, microporous hydrogel (Nutrapore) that mimics the corneal stroma in its water content (78 %), refractive index (1.376), light transmission properties, and permeability characteristics [20]. The material is inert and has been shown in animal studies and early clinical experience to be highly biocompatible. A flap is created in the cornea, the PermaVision lens is centred over the pupil, and the flap is replaced. Early human studies in the United States on intracorneal lenses for the correction of hyperopia are underway [20]. Many future applications are hopeful for this procedure, though questions remain regarding the vision quality achieved, as well as issues with corneal haze and corneal decompensation.

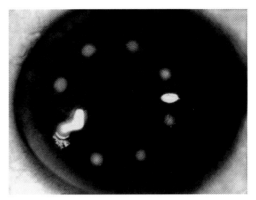

Fig. 11.2. Treatment pattern of conductive keratoplasty

<table>
<tr><td>

Summary for the Clinician

</td></tr>
</table>

- INTACS technology has applications for keratoconus and post-LASIK ectasia patients
- Implantable corneal contact lenses are under research to treat myopia, hyperopia and presbyopia

11.2.3
Corneal Relaxation

Incisional corneal relaxation procedures have been employed to treat myopia, hyperopia and astigmatism dating as far back as the late 1800s. While radial and hexagonal keratotomy have largely been replaced with more precise and efficient methods of altering corneal curvature, astigmatic keratotomy and limbal relaxing incisions continue to be options for neutralising corneal toricity. They can be employed at the time of cataract surgery, or after corneal transplantation and other astigmatism inducing procedures. Future incisional methods may be replaced by pharmacological and biochemical modalities.

11.2.4
Corneal Compression

A variety of peripheral corneal compression techniques have been employed to enhance the central corneal curvature. Much of the current and future technology in corneal compression techniques evolve around controlled administration of energy to the corneal periphery to achieve precise central steepening. Several modalities have been explored to accomplish this goal, including the use of electromagnetic and thermal energy. Although early results were somewhat disappointing, mainly because of surrounding tissue damage and unpredictable outcomes, more recent outcomes using laserless radiofrequency based thermal energy have been encouraging.

Conductive keratoplasty (CK) uses a low-energy, high radiofrequency current which is applied directly to the peripheral corneal stroma through a Keratoplast tip [31]. This procedure causes a homogenous elevation of temperature which shrinks the collagen in the treated area. Each treatment spot produces a cylindrical footprint that extends to approximately 80% of the depth of the mid-peripheral cornea. After a number of treatment spots, the peripheral cornea will flatten and the central cornea will steepen (Fig. 11.2). CK has been used to correct low to moderate hyperopia. Early results show good uncorrected visual acuity, predictability and stability [31]. This procedure eliminates the removal of corneal tissue and the use of a cutting procedure to the cornea. Further studies will be needed to evaluate long-term stability of results, induction of higher order aberrations, and safety for patients with corneal ectasia.

Laser thermokeratoplasty (LTK) describes the controlled application of laser-generated thermal energy to the corneal stroma [13]. LTK incorporates a solid-state holmium:yttrium-aluminum-garnet (Ho:YAG) laser that can be used to create controlled thermal coagulation of corneal stroma with negligible damage to surrounding tissue. The laser is applied in pulsed bursts lasting a couple of seconds and results in focal heating of stromal collagen to approximately 50 °C to achieve central corneal steepening. This procedure has fallen out of favour because of the inconsistent stability and high regression rate of treatments.

Overall, CK holds much promise for the future especially because the technology is reproducible, comparatively inexpensive and easy for the surgeon to master. Newer technology and applications are under research.

Summary for the Clinician

- Conductive keratoplasty remains the most promising of corneal compression techniques because of its safety and surgical ease

11.3
Ciliary Body

Ciliary body research focuses on finding a cure for presbyopia. Alleviating presbyopia remains an important goal for refractive surgery. Computer models and theories on accommodation and lens diaphragm dynamics are leading to new understanding of accommodation and ways to go about rejuvenating its performance.

Two surgical ciliary body techniques are being investigated to reduce presbyopia. One, termed anterior ciliary sclerotomy (ACS), involves creating a series of radial incisions over the ciliary body. This allows circumferential volume expansion of the sclera, increasing the ciliary body to lens distance and rejuvenating accommodation. A second procedure, termed scleral expansion, accomplishes the same goal by implantation of a silastic band near the limbus, which expands potential ciliary body volume. Both procedures are in early development; however, the most promising advancements in presbyopia are in lens implant technology.

Summary for the Clinician

- Ciliary body surgical techniques to reduce presbyopia remain experimental. Further research is needed to find ways to restore accommodative amplitude

11.4
Lens

The arrival of technological advances in lens surgery and replacement has caused this to be one the most exciting areas of refractive surgery. Small incision phacoemulsification and foldable/injectable IOLs have allowed modern cataract surgery to evolve into a refractive surgical procedure. As incisions and lenses are becoming smaller and smaller, refractive surgeons are also offered a wide array of lenses with multiple capabilities including multifocal lenses, accommodating lenses, toric lenses and implantable contact lenses.

Recent advances in refractive lens technology have come in the form of multifocal lens implants, which attempt to provide a functional/compensatory answer to presbyopia while the search for true restoration of accommodation continues.

The Array multifocal lens (Advanced Medical Optics, Irvine, CA) which was FDA approved in 1997 uses a "zonal progressive" design that incorporates five blended aspheric zones of power on the anterior surface of the lens. The lens has had success in clinical trials [40] and is discussed elsewhere in this book. These multifocal lenses offer a pseudo-accommodation effect dependent on the patients' ability to find the appropriate focal point.

Newer technology uses the actual movements of ciliary muscle [11, 12]. Cumming et al. have shown by ultrasound that a posterior capsular intraocular lens will shift by an average of 0.7 mm in the human eye [11]. Based on this research, hinge plate haptics lenses were developed which would move forward with accommodative effort due to the perceived increase in vitreous pressure on the optic. The CrystaLens accommodative IOL (Eyeonics, Aliso Viejo, CA), a silicone lens for surgical implantation into the

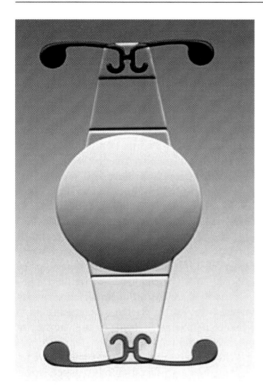

Fig. 11.3. Crystalens. (Courtesy of Eyeonics)

capsular bag, is designed to allow the optic to vault forward on contraction of the ciliary muscle. The lens is a three-piece haptic design made from high index silicone material containing a UV filter (Fig. 11.3). Results of clinical trials of the CrystaLens have demonstrated excellent safety and improved efficacy over multifocal and conventional intraocular lenses with regard to uncorrected distance, intermediate and near vision [12, 16]. The use of this lens in the US is important because it is currently the only accommodating intraocular lens with FDA approval.

Hanna and colleagues also have developed the 1CU (HumanOptics AG, Erlangen, Germany) posterior chamber accommodative intraocular lens. The 1CU is a hydrophobic, acrylic lens with a 5.5-mm optic attached to four hinged haptics which allow anterior movement of the optic during accommodation. Early studies show good efficacy and safety with comparable results to the CrystaLens [24, 28, 32].

In addition, toric IOLs have also become available for use in correcting astigmatism with cataract removal. While some ophthalmologists will use limbal relaxing incisions and astigmatic keratotomy for low levels of astigmatism (<2.00 D) during cataract surgery, these incisions tend to be more unpredictable at higher levels of astigmatism. The FDA approval in 1998 of the STAAR Toric IOL (STAAR Surgical) opened the doors for correction of higher levels of astigmatism to compliment or replace corneal astigmatic incisions. The STAAR Toric IOL is a plate haptic lens design that is currently only available for cylinders of either +2.50 D or +3.50 D. The +2.00 toric lens corrects approximately 1.50 D of keratometric astigmatism, while the +3.50 toric lens corrects approximately 2.25 D. The "TF" model lens has an overall length of 10.8 mm. The longer 11.2-mm "TL" model was later released for spherical powers of <23.5 D. The haptics of the longer lens also have a matte finish to make them less slippery. Results have been promising in correcting astigmatism [37]. However, the major pitfall to these lenses is the close post-operative monitoring for detection of early rotation and misalignment of the lens axis [37].

In contrast to the STAAR Toric IOL, HumanOptics AG (Erlangen, Germany), has worked during the past few years to develop a three-piece, foldable toric IOL. The MicroSil Toric IOL has lens powers ranging between –3.00 and 31.00 D and cylindrical powers ranging from 2.00 to 12.00 D. This MS 6116 TU type lens is a posterior chamber lens which features stable PMMA haptics in a z-design, as well as a 6-mm optic made of silicone. The IOL's overall diameter is 11.6 mm. Implanting the MicroSil Toric lens is somewhat more difficult than inserting a conventional PCIOL because of the shape of its haptics. Early studies show promising results in Europe, but once again, stability of the lens in the capsule is of concern [18].

While many new lenses are being developed to correct for high astigmatism, viable solutions are being offered to correct for high levels of myopia and hyperopia. Clear lens extraction or refractive lens exchange, an extension of cataract surgery for purely refractive goals, is becoming a frequent option for those patients in the extreme levels of myopia and hyperopia.

Summary for the Clinician

- Multifocal intraocular lens offer a pseudo-accommodation effect for patients
- Accommodative intraocular lens implants such as the CrystaLens and the 1CU use the ciliary body to offer accommodation
- Toric lenses are available to correct cataract patients with high levels of astigmatism

11.5
Crystalline Lens Replacement

Since the first implantation of an artificial intraocular lens in 1949, ophthalmologists have envisioned the day when the cataractous human lens would be replaced by a pliable, accommodative lens inside an intact capsular bag [27]. For many years, researchers have investigated this concept through the development of liquid or flexible polymer materials that could be injected into the empty capsular bag. Pfizer Corporation is developing a polymer that surgeons can inject through a 1-mm capsulorhexis to refill the capsular bag, and there are a number of other companies with similar technologies on the horizon. The SmartLens (Medennium, Irvine, CA) is an innovative technology that uses a thermodynamic, hydrophobic acrylic material that is packaged as a 30-mm long, 2-mm wide cylinder rod at room temperature that expands at body temperature to a biconvex, 9.5-mm diameter, 2- to 4-mm thick lens. The transformation from the rod to a biconvex, flexible lens takes about 30 s. The hydrophobic acrylic has a high tackiness that will adhere closely to the capsule to minimise lens epithelial cell migration and reduce mechanical stability and decentration concerns.

Current trends in cataract surgery are to improve cataract removal through generating less heat, improving safety and precision, and increasing efficiency. Conventional phacoemulsification employs ultrasonic vibration to emulsify the cataract. Ophthalmologists around the world have successfully adapted to this technique. Alternatives include the Dodick Laser Photolysis system (A.R.C. Laser, Salt Lake City, UT), which uses a Nd:YAG laser discharging against a titanium target to produce vibrations causing phacolysis of the lens nucleus. Another company, Paradigm Medical, produces the Photon pulsed Nd:YAG laser-driven system, which directly ablates the lens. Outside the United States, at least two companies, both from Germany – Asclepion-Meditec (with its PhacoLase) and WaveLight (with its Adagio System) – have successfully brought erbium:YAG laser-driven phaco systems to the European market. A number of other companies are investigating low-energy approaches to cataract removal, including the SonicWave system from STAAR Surgical, which uses non-thermal sonic energy rather than ultrasonic energy to break up the cataract. Finally, Alcon has licensed a technology called phacogelation or liquefaction, which involves the use of heated saline solution to weaken the chemical bonds of the cataract in preparation for its removal.

With the innovations in crystalline lens replacement, the preservation of an intact capsular bag and protection the corneal epithelium remains of utmost importance. Current cataract surgery is highly dependent on individual surgeon skill. Future cataract surgery technology strives to improve safe and efficient human cataract removal within an intact capsule for every ophthalmologist. "Catarex" (currently licensed to Bausch and Lomb for Atlantic Technology Ventures, New York, NY) involves making a small <1-mm incision in the anterior capsule and inserting a high velocity irrigation port into the lens. The irrigation creates a vortex that emulsifies the cataract and removes it through the same irrigation port to leave behind a fully intact capsular bag. This promising technology remains under investigation [39].

Ametropia following lens replacement has been a challenge for ophthalmologists and will inevitably occur as new refractive techniques alter and complicate lens calculations. The Light Adjustable Lens (Calhoun Vision, Pasadena, CA) offers a non-invasive alternative to adjustment of refractive errors post-implantation following cataract surgery [38]. The LAL is composed of cross-linked silicone polymer matrix, a guest macromer, and a photoinitiator. The

LAL polymerises after application of appropriate wavelength of light onto the selected regions of the implanted lens causing changes in the curvature of the lens and a corresponding increase or decrease in lens power. The process may be repeated until the desired correction is obtained. The surgeon may then irradiate the entire lens causing it to "lock in" the power of the lens. FDA trials are ongoing for this lens [38].

Future genetic and biological research may offer a non-surgical cure for cataracts. Pharmacologic advances to prevent cataracts are being heavily investigated. In the future, for those requiring cataract surgery, lens implants may reduce presbyopia, decrease the exposure of harmful UV rays to the retina, as well as minimise higher order aberrations of glare and halos. Lens extraction and replacement will no longer simply be a way to treat cataracts, but a tool to create visual capabilities above and beyond what currently exists.

Summary for the Clinician

- Research to improve the safety and efficacy of cataract surgery focus on preserving the capsular bag, protecting the cornea and improving the lens implant technology
- The LAL offers a non-invasive technique to change lens power in post-cataract surgery patients
- Pharmacologic methods to prevent and cure cataracts remain under intense research

11.6
Phakic Intraocular Refractive Lenses

The concept of inserting a lens to correct refractive error in a phakic eye dates back several decades. However, many early prototype implant designs were abandoned due to secondary corneal decompensation, glaucoma, and inflammation.

Phakic refractive lens technology was revisited again in the late 1980s by Worst of the Netherlands and Fechner of Germany, who proposed that modifications of existing anterior chamber lens designs could be used to avoid corneal oedema and inflammatory problems associated with previous designs [15, 25]. This was achieved by vaulting the lens design and using the mid-peripheral iris for lens attachment. Baikoff of France then developed another variation on anterior chamber lens design [21]. Consequently, in 1990, a group of Russian ophthalmologists began investigating the concept of a foldable silicone phakic refractive lens that could be fixated in the ciliary sulcus of the posterior chamber [17]. Since then, many phakic intraocular lens designs have emerged. Today, the designs can be classified by the way they are fixated in the eye: (1) anterior chamber angle, (2) iris and (3) posterior chamber.

There are two major anterior chamber angle fixated lenses in production that have published outcomes – the NuVita MA20 and the ZSAL-4. A type of iris-fixated phakic IOL, the Artisan lens (Ophtec, Boca Raton, FL), is a one piece polymethylmethacrylate (PMMA) lens which has iris claws on either side of the optic; the overall length of the implant varies from 7.2 to 8.5 mm, the size of the optic. The haptics are fixed to the mid-periphery of the iris through the mechanism of the claws on either side of the lens. Future designs are working toward a foldable lens. The Implantable Contact Lens (ICL) is a posterior chamber lens developed by Staar Surgical. With the aid of a widely dilated pupil and simple specialised instruments, each footplate of the plate haptic is tucked into the posterior chamber. Another posterior chamber fixated lens is the Phakic Refractive Lens (PRL), manufactured by Medennium, and distributed by CIBA Vision. According to its makers, the lens' distinction is that it is designed to *float* on the crystalline lens – there are no feet to its plate haptics.

In all phakic IOLs, the anterior chamber size is crucial for inclusion or exclusion of patients. Cataract formation, corneal endothelial damage, and glaucoma remain major complications of the surgery. Long-term concerns regarding the implanted phakic IOLs include the increase in size of the natural crystalline with increasing age and cataract formation leading to a decrease in the depth of the anterior chamber and crowding of the posterior chamber, further exaggerating pathologic processes. While the results of phakic IOLs are highly predictable, long-term data are limited.

Current indications for their implantation include extreme refractive errors of both hyperopia and myopia. These lenses have the advantage of correcting extreme refractive errors without loss of accommodation by leaving the natural lens undisturbed. They also avoid any alteration in corneal curvature and asphericity.

Investigation will continue in this particular area of refractive technology and may centre on improved lens designs incorporating accommodative and telescopic capabilities.

Summary for the Clinician

- Phakic intraocular lens implants offer a new refractive solution for high myopes and hyperopes
- Phakic IOL designs are differentiated by their placement in anterior chamber angle, attached to the iris or in the posterior chamber
- Cataract formation, corneal endothelial damage and glaucoma are the main concerns for phakic IOLs

11.7
Conclusion

Refractive surgery remains one of the most exciting aspects of ophthalmology because of the technology and innovations in the field. Future advancements in biotechnology, genetic engineering and neural networks will dramatically further the field of refractive surgery. With the advent of gene mapping, the genes responsible for high myopia, hyperopia and astigmatism may be identified and possible recombinant DNA technology may be able to treat these problems. Gene replacement therapy may solve degenerative eye diseases such as presbyopia and cataracts. Researchers also hope to use implantable chips for retinal diseases which may use this new technology to create in a sense "bionic" eyes and artificial vision. Continued research, experience and testing will bring many solutions and tools for refractive surgeons of the future to provide quality vision to patients.

References

1. Barraquer JI (1949) Refractive keratoplasty. Est Inf Oftal 2:10
2. Barraquer JI (1958) Method of cutting lamellar grafts in frozen cornea. Arch Soc Em Oftalmol Optom 1:271–286
3. Barraquer JI (1964) Keratomileusis for the correction of myopia. Ann Inst Barraquer 5:209–229
4. Barraquer JI (1966) Modification of refraction by means of intracorneal inclusions. Int Ophthalmol Clin 6:53–78
5. Boxer Wachler BS, Chou B, Kessler D (2000) Intacs for keratoconus: early visual results. ISRS Final Program and Abstracts, Summer World Refractive Surgery Symposium, July, p 63
6. Buratto L, Ferrari M, Rama P (1992) Excimer laser intrastromal keratomileusis. Am J Ophthalmol 113:291–295
7. Burris TE, Baker PC, Ayer CT, Loomas BE, Mathis ML, Silvestrini TA (1993) Flattening of central corneal curvature with intrastromal corneal rings of increasing thickness: an eye-bank eye study. J Cataract Refract Surg 19(Suppl):182–187
8. Charters L (2003) LASIK promising for presbyopia using multifocal ablation: multifocal patterns used to improve near vision without compromising distance vision. (Early results). Ophthalmol Times. March 15
9. CIBA (2003) receives FDA approval for first device for Epi-LASIK. Eye World. September
10. Coleman DJ (1986) On the hydraulic suspension theory of accommodation. Trans Am Ophthalmol Soc 84:846–868
11. Cumming JS (2002) CrystaLens Accommodating IOL. Presented at ASCRS conference. Philadelphia, PA
12. Cumming JS, Slade SG, Chayet A (2001) Clinical evaluation of the model AT-45 silicone accommodating intraocular lens: results of feasibility and the initial phase of a Food and Drug Administration clinical trial. Ophthalmology 108:2005–2009; discussion 2010
13. Durrie DS, Schumer DJ, Cavanaugh TB (1994) Holmium:YAG laser thermokeratoplasty for hyperopia. J Refract Corneal Surg 10:S277–280
14. Durrie DS, Asbell PA, Burris TE (1996) Reversible refractive effect: data from Phase 2 study of the 360° ICR in myopic eyes. American Society of Cataract and Refractive Surgery (ASCRS), 1–5 June 1996, Seattle
15. Fechner PU, van der Heijde GL, Worst JGF (1988) Intraokulare Linse zur Myopikorrektion des phaken Auges. Kilin Monatsbl Augenheilkd. 193: 29–34

16. Fine H (2002) Results of Crystalens implantation in 100 eyes. Personal experience. Presented at ASCRS 2002 Conference, Philadelphia

17. Fyodorov SN, Zuev VK, Aznabayev BM (1991) Intraocular correction of high myopia with negative posterior chamber lens. Ophthalmosurgery (Moscow). 3:57–58

18. Gerten G, Schipper I (2003) Toric correction of high astigmatism. Cataract Refract Surg Today. March 2003

19. Gordon E, Parolini B, Abelson M (1998) Principles and microscopic confirmation of surface quality of two new waterjet-based microkeratomes. J Refract Surg 14:338–345

20. Guttman C (2002) Pilot trial encourages further study of intracorneal lens. Ophthalmology Times. June 2002

21. Joly P, Baikoff G, Bonnet P (1989) Mise en place d'un implant negatif de chambre anterieure chex des sujets phaques. Bull Soc Ophtalmol Fr. 89:727–733

22. Keates RH, Martines E, Tennen DG, Reich C (1995) Small-diameter corneal inlay in presbyopic or pseudophakic patients. J Cataract Refract Surg 21:519–521

23. Krueger RR, Juhasz T, Gualano A, Marchi V (1998) The picosecond laser for nonmechanical laser in situ keratomileusis. J Refract Surg 14:467–469

24. Kuchle M, Nguyen NX, Lancgenbucher A et al (2002) Implantation of a new accommodative posterior chamber intraocular lens. J Refract Surg 18:208–216

25. Landesz M, Worst JG, Siertsema JV, van Rij G (1995) Correction of high myopia with the Worst myopia claw intraocular lens. J Refract Surg 11:16–25

26. Lane SS, Lindstrom RL (1991) Polysulfone intracorneal lenses. Int Ophthalmol Clin 31:37–46

27. Leonard P, Rommel J (1982) Lens implantation: 30 years of progress. Junk, The Hague

28. Mastropasqua L, Toto L, Nubile M, Falconio G, Ballone E (2003) Clinical study of the 1CU accommodating intraocular lens. J Cataract Refract Surg 29:1307–1312

29. Stevens SX, Bowyer BL, Sanchez-Thorin JC, Rocha G, Young DA, Rowsy JJ (1999) The BioMask for treatment of corneal surface irregularities with excimer laser photothereapeutic keratectomy.Cornea 18:155–163

30. McCarey BE, Andrews DM (1981) Refractive keratoplasty with intrastromal hydrogel lenticular implants. Invest Ophthalmol Vis Sci 21:107–115

31. McDonald MB, Hersh PS, Manche EE, Maloney RK, Davidorf J, Sabry M (2002) Conductive keratoplasty for the correction of low to moderate hyperopia: U.S. clinical trial 1-year results on 355 eyes. Ophthalmology 109:1978–1989; discussion 1989–1990

32. O'Heineachain R (2002) Two IOL styles prove to be equally accommodating in comparative trial. Eurotimes, Dec 2002

33. Pallikaris IG, Papatzanaki ME, Stathi EZ, Frenschock O, Georgiadis A (1990) Laser in situ keratomileusis. Lasers Surg Med 10:463–468

34. Roach L (2002) Wavefront surges ahead. EyeNet, July 2002

35. Samalonis L (2003) Is it time to make the move to femtosecond-mode lasers? EyeWorld, August 2003

36. Schanzlin D (1996) One year results from Phase 2 clinical trial of the 360° ICR. American Society of Cataract and Refractive Surgery, 1–5 June 1996, Seattle

37. Schneider DM (2003) Toric ICL shows promising initial results for astigmatism: lens features central spherical convex/concave optical zone with cylinder in specified axis location. (Phakic implant).(toric implantable contact lens from STAAR Surgical Co.) Ophthalmol Times, February 1

38. Schwiegerling JT, Schwartz DM et al (2002) Light-adjustable intraocular lenses: finessing the outcome. Rev Refract Surg, February

39. Seibel BS (2002) Endocapsular vortex emulsification technology. Cataract Refract Surg Today, April

40. Steinert RF, Aker BL, Trentacost DJ, Smith PJ, Tarantino N (1999) A prospective comparative study of the AMO ARRAY zonal-progressive multifocal silicone intraocular lens and a monofocal intraocular lens. Ophthalmology 106:1243–1255

41. Stevens SX, Bowyer BL, Sanchez-Thorin JC, Rocha G, Young DA, Rowsey JJ (1999) The Bio-Mask for treatment of corneal surface irregularities with excimer laser phototherapeutic keratectomy. Cornea 18:155–163

42. Werblin TP, Kaufman HE, Friedlander MH, Granet N (1981) Epikeratophakia: the surgical correction of aphakia. 3. Preliminary results of a prospective clinical trial. Arch Ophthalmol 99: 1957–1960

LASIK – Laser In Situ Keratomileusis

Michael C. Knorz

Core Messages

- LASIK provides excellent predictability, stability, visual acuity and quality of vision in low to moderate myopia and hyperopia, but is not recommended for routine use in extreme myopia and high hyperopia
- LASIK has a low incidence of long-term side effects but transient dry-eye syndrome typically occurs, and night vision is somewhat reduced in high corrections
- Retreatments are a normal part of LASIK and occur in about 10% of cases
- Microkeratome-related flap complications are extremely rare today
- The interface after LASIK presents a new space that allows accumulation of cells or fluid, creating new diagnostic entities such as diffuse lamellar keratitis (DLK)
- Severe complications such as corneal ectasia are extremely rare and usually related to preoperatively undiagnosed corneal pathology
- Customised LASIK using wavefront technology induces fewer aberrations and is an evolving technology holding considerable promise

12.1
History

The history of LASIK dates back to 1950 when Jose I. Barraquer was the first to describe adding or removing corneal tissue as an option to changing the refractive status of the eye. He called this procedure keratomileusis [3]. Initially, Barraquer performed a free-hand dissection of the cornea to create a lamellar cut. Later, he developed the mechanical keratome with a suction ring, which has in principle been used until today. Barraquer removed a corneal disc with a thickness of about 350 µm which was deep-frozen and lathed like a contact lens to achieve the desired refractive change. The disc was finally sutured back onto the cornea [4]. Because of the bulky machinery required, the steep learning curve and the high incidence of complications, keratomileusis never gained widespread acceptance. Later on, Luis Ruiz, a student of Barraquer, developed the technique of "keratomileusis in situ". Initially, a corneal disc was removed, and a second cut with a smaller diameter was performed to remove some central corneal tissue, thereby creating flattening of the cornea once the disc was replaced. Later on, this technique was refined by the use of a hinged flap instead of the disc. The diameter and the thickness of the second cut were varied according to an elaborate nomogram to correct different amounts of myopia. This technique, termed "automated lamellar keratoplasty" (ALK), gained considerable popularity especially in the US prior to the approval of excimer lasers by the FDA. The advantages of ALK were the ease of surgery, a fast visual rehabilitation, and limited regression. Disadvantages included lack of precision and a high incidence of irregular astigmatism [26]. While the use of a lamellar cut must be attributed to Barraquer, the combination of a hinged corneal flap with an excimer laser ablation was introduced by Ioannis Pallikaris in 1989. He also coined the term "laser in situ keratomileusis" (LASIK), which became accepted world wide [15]. Back in 1990, Pallikaris' publication attracted little attention. Only when

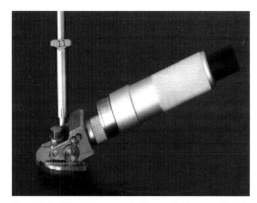

Fig. 12.1. The Automated Corneal Shaper (ACS). This microkeratome accompanied the success story of LASIK and is still in clinical use by some surgeons

Luis Ruiz and others started to combine ALK with excimer laser ablation, called "ALK-Excimer", the procedure to be called LASIK today became popular and attracted the attention of more and more surgeons from all over the world. I still vividly recall listening to the first presentation on "ALK-Excimer" by Luis Ruiz at the annual meeting of the European Society of Cataract and Refractive Surgery (ESCRS) in Innsbruck, Austria, in September 1993. I called him the next day and flew to Bogota to learn this procedure. In those early days, we all performed LASIK for excessive levels of myopia. We felt that, because of the lack of scarring, which was the main issue in PRK at that time, LASIK could be used even in these extreme myopes [12]. We know better today, and more details are given in the section on quality of vision. In the early days, the "Automatic Corneal Shaper" (ACS) (Fig. 12.1), the keratome designed by Luis Ruiz based on the old Barraquer microkeratome, was the instrument of choice. Today, a large variety of microkeratomes is available, and their safety and precision have improved greatly since their first appearance.

As LASIK still uses the same principle as the original keratomileusis technique, it seems justified to assume that long-term complications should be similar. One of the biggest concerns in this regards is the delayed occurrence of corneal ectasia, which has been observed after LASIK in some cases [22]. Although the number

of eyes which underwent keratomileusis is small, a high incidence of ectasia was not observed. It seems likely, therefore, that keratectasia will not develop in a large number of eyes after LASIK but rather be limited to a few cases, most of which are previously undiagnosed forme fruste of keratoconus [22].

Summary for the Clinician

- LASIK has evolved from keratomileusis, introduced by Barraquer, and therefore enjoys a track record of more than 40 years
- Long-term complications such as keratectasia seem rare and are usually caused by preoperatively undiagnosed corneal pathology

12.2
Patient Selection, Technique and Results

12.2.1
Patient Selection

LASIK is a safe and predictable procedure, but it is not indicated for everybody. Based on the published results described above and on the considerations regarding quality of vision (see Sect. 12.4), it can be stated as a general rule that precision and quality of vision are highest in low refractive errors. Excellent results are achieved in low to moderate myopia (up to about –5 D), followed by low hyperopia (up to +3 D), but results are not as good in high myopia (–5 to –10 D) and poor in extreme myopia (over –10 D) and high hyperopia (over +4 D). Obviously, these numbers are not absolute but include some simplification. Besides the amount of correction, other variables such as corneal thickness, diameter of the pupil at various light levels, and the visual demands of the respective patient are extremely important. There has been much controversy regarding the role of pupil size in affecting post-operative quality of vision [19]. Some surgeons will exclude patients whose scotopic pupil size exceeds the diameter of the intended ablation. Others, however, feel that, with ablation zones of 6 mm and larger and well-centred ablations, there may be no relationship between pupil size and the incidence of

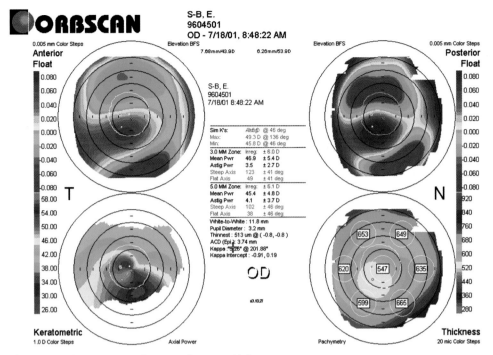

Fig. 12.2. Orbscan topographic map of an eye with keratoconus

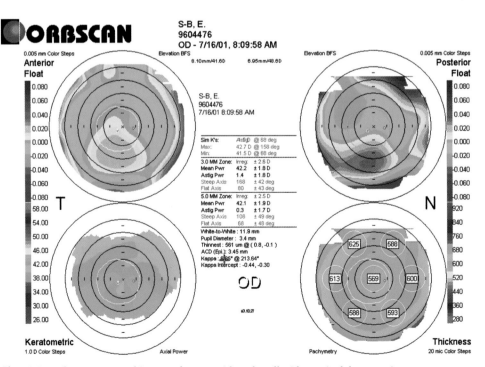

Fig. 12.3. Orbscan topographic map of an eye with early pellucid marginal degeneration

severe halos and other unwanted visual effects. Besides the refractive error, other conditions are also critical. To perform LASIK, the cornea should be normal. It is especially important to rule out any progressive corneal disease such as keratoconus or even forme fruste of keratoconus. Figure 12.2 shows a typical keratoconus, while Fig. 12.3 shows a patient with an early stage of pellucid marginal degeneration. As LASIK weakens the cornea, any pre-existing weakness might be enhanced, resulting in corneal ectasia after LASIK [22]. Besides corneal disease, severe dry-eye syndrome, cataract and advanced glaucoma are contraindications for LASIK. Diabetes seems acceptable, but any stage of diabetic retinopathy presents a contraindication. There should also be no macular degeneration. It is beyond the scope of this chapter to describe the limitations of LASIK in exhaustive detail; however, one useful reference *for patients* is the patient education website established by the American Society of Cataract and Refractive Surgery: www.eyesurgeryeducation.com/Candidate.html.

12.2.2
Technique

LASIK has become a highly standardised procedure which provides excellent and predictable results. It is usually performed as a bilateral simultaneous procedure under topical anaesthesia. Many surgeons also prefer to use some sedation to relax the patient. State of the art is the use of an automated mechanical microkeratome to create a corneal flap with a thickness of between 120–160 µm and a diameter of 8–9.5 mm. The hinge is either placed superiorly or nasally. Once the flap is cut and elevated, excimer laser ablation of the stromal bed is performed. Today's laser systems mostly use some kind of scanning beam or flying spot technology and an active eye tracking to compensate for eye movements. Ablation complications such as central islands, irregular ablations and decentrations are rarely observed today. After the ablation, the corneal flap is replaced. It reattaches without the need for sutures. Post-operatively, a combination of antibiotics and steroids is ad-

ministered for up to 1 week. In addition, lubricating eye drops are used for up to several months, depending on the severity of the postsurgical dry-eye syndrome (see Sect. 12.3).

12.2.3
Results

Looking at the results of LASIK surgery, I will initially report the results of our group of LASIK centres in Germany to demonstrate how LASIK performs outside a clinical study environment. In addition, a few of the most recent clinical studies published will be presented. We evaluated a total of 8,725 non-selected consecutive eyes operated at the FreeVis LASIK Centres in Mannheim, Fuerth, Munich and Hamburg, Germany, in 2001. In all, 7,794 eyes were myopic, while 931 were hyperopic.

Mean preoperative myopia was –4.83±2.39 D (range, –0.5 to –11.0 D). At 1–3 months after LASIK, mean refractive error was –0.04±0.49 D (range, –4 to +2 D). At total of 61% were within ±0.25 D, 84% within ±0.5 D, 95% within ±1 D, and 99% within ±2 D of target refraction. Preoperatively, spectacle-corrected visual acuity was 20/15 or better in 16%, 20/20 or better in 72%, 20/25 or better in 94% and 20/40 or better in 99%. At 1–3 months after LASIK, uncorrected visual acuity was 20/15 or better in 8%, 20/20 or better in 48%, 20/25 or better in 76% and 20/40 or better in 95%. In all, 3% of eyes lost two lines of spectacle-corrected visual acuity.

Results were slightly less accurate in hyperopic LASIK. Mean preoperative hyperopia was 1.12±1.6 D (range, 0–3.75 D). At 1–3 months after LASIK, 50% were within ±0.25 D, 69% within ±0.5 D, 91% within ±1 D and 99% within ±2 D. Preoperatively, spectacle-corrected visual acuity was 20/15 or better in 7%, 20/20 or better in 48%, 20/25 or better in 85% and 20/40 or better in 98%. At 1–3 months after hyperopic LASIK, uncorrected visual acuity was 20/15 or better in 1%, 20/20 or better in 20%, 20/25 or better in 53% and 20/40 or better 87%. A total of 8% lost two lines of spectacle-corrected visual acuity.

Overall, 91.2% of patients were extremely happy, an additional 8.6% were satisfied, and 0.2% were not satisfied with their result.

Looking at LASIK results in the literature, there is a vast number of publications on LASIK, but it is very difficult to find one that reports long-term results on a significant number of patients. Most of those available are no longer up to date, as outdated equipment was used. I will therefore just report two publications. One is by a Canadian group who used a modern flying spot laser (Technolas 217z, Bausch & Lomb, Rochester, NY) on 236 eyes with –0.5 to –7 D of myopia [2]. After 6 months, uncorrected visual acuity was 20/20 or better in 81.9% and 20/40 or better in 94.6%. In all, 73% were within ±0.5 D of target refraction, and 91.2% were within ±1 D. None lost two or more lines of spectacle-corrected visual acuity.

The second publication is by McDonald and coworkers who reported the results of LASIK with the LADARVision excimer laser, another modern flying spot laser, in 177 eyes with myopia of up to –11 D [13]. At 6 months, uncorrected visual acuity was 20/20 or better in 60.5%, 20/25 or better in 80.3%, and 20/40 or better in 93.9%. Refraction was within ±0.5 D in 75.2% and within ±1 D in 94.9%. A loss of two lines of spectacle-corrected visual acuity occurred in 0.6%.

The incidence of retreatments after LASIK varies depending on the level of preoperative myopia, whether or not astigmatism was present, and with age. Overall, an incidence of 10.5% was reported in a representative study which analysed the results of 2485 eyes [9]. A retreatment can therefore not be termed a "complication", but rather a normal part of the procedure. It is caused by a number of factors, the most important one being epithelial healing which tends to counter the shape change induced by the excimer ablation. As retreatments are frequent, and something "normal", patients must be informed accordingly. In addition, surgeons must factor a possible, or likely, retreatment into their calculations when they perform LASIK. This means that the initial LASIK procedure should never be planned to approach the limits of tissue ablation in the respective cornea. There should always be some allowance for a possible retreatment.

Summary for the Clinician

- LASIK is predictable and efficient in myopia and hyperopia. Predictability is highest in low to moderate myopia and somewhat lower in high myopia and hyperopia. LASIK should not be used in extreme myopia and high hyperopia
- Retreatments are a normal part of LASIK and are required in about 10% of cases

12.3
Complications

Dry-eye syndrome is the most important side effect of LASIK. It is caused by the severing of the corneal nerves, which leads to tear film irregularities and also has a neuroparalytical component. Symptoms are dryness and fluctuating vision. Treatment consists of lubricating eye drops or gels and patient counselling. Other options include punctum plugs, permanent punctual occlusion or, lately, the use of cyclosporine eye drops. Symptoms persist for up to several months, rarely years, but ultimately disappear in almost all cases. It is, however, important to inform patients preoperatively about the post-LASIK dry-eye syndrome.

12.3.1
Microkeratome-Related Flap Complications

These complications occur during the microkeratome cut and represent the largest group of flap complications. There is clearly a historical trend that shows improvement of the rate of complications in modern microkeratomes. In a study by Stulting et al. [30], the rate of complications in 1,062 consecutive eyes operated with the Automated Corneal Shaper by 14 surgeons between May 1995 and December 1996 was reported. A total of 27 eyes (2.5%) had flap complications during primary surgery, 17 of which could not be ablated at the time of primary surgery. In a study by Gimbel et al. [7] on the first 1000 consecutive cases operated between April 1995 and February 1997 using the Automated Corneal Shaper by one surgeon, 19 (1.9%) microkeratome-related complications were observed. The incidence of microkeratome-related complications showed a clear learning curve, with 4.5% during the first 100 cases and 0.5% between case 800 and 1000 [7].

In a more recent study of 3826 eyes operated between November 1996 and August 1998, microkeratome-related flap complications occurred in 27 eyes (0.68%) [28]. In 16 eyes, ablation was not possible, and another microkeratome cut was performed after 3 months. Two of the 16 eyes (12.5%) had a microkeratome-related flap complication again, but none of the 16 eyes lost two or more lines of visual acuity. This suggests that making another microkeratome cut after 3 months is generally safe [28]. However, it does not mean that a re-cut should be used in all enhancements. Re-cutting should rather be limited to cases with microkeratome-related flap complications, as presented by Rubinfeld, who reported on several cases with significant visual loss caused by irregular astigmatism due to tissue loss after a re-cut [24].

Pallikaris et al. [16] reported microkeratome-related flap complications in 14.37% (48 of 334 consecutive eyes) operated between September 1997 and November 1998 by one surgeon using the Flapmaker, a disposable microkeratome. Their study is interesting because the authors performed laser ablation in 37 of these eyes despite the flap complication. The ablation resulted in central corneal scars, haze, irregular astigmatism and loss of one line of spectacle-corrected visual acuity in many of the eyes. The author feels that, based on these data, it is strongly recommended not to perform laser ablation at the time a microkeratome-related flap complication occurs. Rather, it should be standard practice to replace the abnormal flap and retreat the eye between 2 and 6 months later by re-cutting it using a thicker flap, if possible, but never a thinner one.

One of the largest and most recent studies reports the incidence of microkeratome-related flap complications in 84,711 eyes operated by 640 surgeons in 28 national open-access laser facilities between November 1998 and May 2000 [11] using both the Automated Corneal Shaper and the Hansatome. Microkeratome-related flap complications occurred in 256 eyes (0.302%).

There were 84 (0.099%) partial flaps, 74 (0.087%) thin or irregular flaps, 59 (0.074%) buttonholes, 29 (0.034%) failures to achieve intraocular pressure and ten (0.012%) free flaps. In a subset of data between December 1999 and May 2000, the authors were also able to compare the Automated Corneal Shaper and the Hansatome. They found a high incidence of 6.38% (21 of 329 eyes) for the Automated Corneal Shaper and a very low incidence of 0.16% (46 of 28,201 eyes) for the Hansatome [11]. The authors state that the low rate of microkeratome-related complications reflects a significant improvement in microkeratome technology.

12.3.2
Other Flap Complications

These include post-operative flap slippage and folds. Flap slippage and folds were reported by Waring et al. [30] using the Automated Corneal Shaper in 13 of 1062 eyes (1.2%). The study by Gimbel et al. [7] reported 18 (1.8%) slipped or folded flaps using the same microkeratome. In a more recent study, Recep et al. [23] reported flap slippage in 21 (1.42%) of 1481 eyes operated between January 1997 and May 1998 using a Moria microkeratome. Flap slippage was detected at 1 h in 15 eyes, at 1 day in two eyes, and at 1 week in three eyes. One eye had a slipped flap both at 1 day and at 1 week. Fine flap striae, so-called microstriae, usually have little or no affect on vision and therefore require no treatment. Large flap folds, or macrostriae, cause loss of vision and require treatment. Figure 12.4 shows macrostriae 1 day after LASIK. In the first few days after surgery, they can usually be managed by refloating and stretching the flap. Macrostriae that are present beyond the first week or two may not respond to simply refloating and stretching, but good results can achieved by suturing the flap [10], or with phototherapeutic keratectomy.

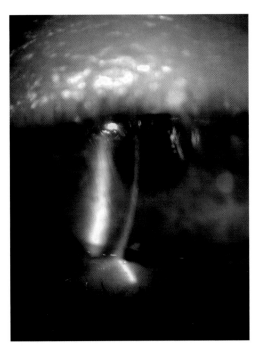

Fig. 12.4. Macrostriae 1 day after LASIK

12.3.3
Interface Complications

There are a variety of complications that can occur at the interface. The most frequent one is diffuse lamellar keratitis (DLK). Epithelial ingrowth, infection and abscess, and fluid accumulation are other complications which are located at the interface.

12.3.3.1
Diffuse Lamellar Keratitis

Diffuse lamellar keratitis is a non-specific response to an insult to the cornea. In rabbits, it was shown that as little as 50 endotoxin units cause grade 2 of diffuse lamellar keratitis [18]. Clinically, diffuse lamellar keratitis presents as a diffuse or multifocal infiltrate defined to the interface, usually 1–6 days after LASIK. It is a diagnostic entity that can be observed after LASIK only as it requires the space within the anterior stroma created by the keratotomy. Within this space, granulocytes and other inflammatory

cells accumulate [5]. Treatment consists of potent topical steroids hourly and daily exams. It is important to intervene early in the post-operative course. In stage 3 (diffuse lamellar infiltrate with snowball-like cell condensate) or deterioration of stage 2 (diffuse mono-layered lamellar infiltrate), re-intervention and irrigation of the interface should be performed immediately. In contrast, should stromal melting or even scarring already be present, it seems advisable not to lift the flap and irrigate as the course cannot be improved [17], and scarring might even be more pronounced due to tissue loss during re-intervention.

Diffuse lamellar keratitis occurs more frequently if epithelial defects are present [25]. It is usually confined to the interface area underlying the epithelial defect. It is extremely important to diagnose it and to use steroids despite the epithelial defects as corneal melting and scarring may develop otherwise. Diffuse lamellar keratitis may also develop without any direct flap manipulation. Harrison and Periman [8] presented a case report of a patient who had a recurrent corneal erosion 3 months after LASIK and developed diffuse lamellar keratitis. Another case of late-onset diffuse lamellar keratitis was reported by Probst and Foley [21]. These cases indicate that diffuse lamellar keratitis has several causes. Most frequently, it seems to be induced by some toxins or allergenic agents introduced during surgery. It can also be caused by trauma to the cornea, e.g. epithelial erosions, even months after LASIK. In these cases the interface seems to provide an empty space where the inflammatory cells can accumulate [8].

12.3.3.2
Epithelial Ingrowth

Epithelial ingrowth requiring surgical removal was reported to occur in 35 (0.92%) of 3786 eyes by Wang and Maloney [29]. In 42 of the 43 eyes, the ingrowth was continuous with the surface epithelium, suggesting a post-operative invasion rather than intraoperative implantation of epithelial cells. A total of 14 of the 43 eyes had a post-operative epithelial defect and six of the 43 eyes had loose epithelium intraoperatively, suggesting a higher incidence of epithelial ingrowth in the presence of an abnormal epithelium. The authors also found a higher incidence of epithelial ingrowth after re-treatments [eight (1.7%) of 480 eyes] [29].

12.3.3.3
Microbial Keratitis

Microbial keratitis is fortunately a rare (1 in 5000 to 10,000 cases) but vision-threatening complication. A review by Alio et al. [1] presents an excellent overview of most of the cases reported, the appropriate therapy and their clinical outcome.

Mycobacterium species recently emerged as a leading pathogen in microbial infections after LASIK [27]. These infections are characterised by a late onset (mean 20 days, range 11 days to 6 weeks) and a prolonged clinical course despite treatment, frequently requiring amputation of the flap [27] or even penetrating keratoplasty.

12.3.3.4
Interface Fluid

The occurrence of interface fluid presents a new diagnostic entity which can be observed only after LASIK. As the collagen fibrils do not appear to heal, the lamellar cut creates a space within the anterior stroma, which can be filled by fluid or other matter. There are some case reports describing interface fluid accumulation [6, 20]. It is caused by steroid-induced glaucoma leading to corneal oedema, and fluid accumulation in the interface. Applanation tonometry on the flap will show low or normal readings, the glaucoma may not be diagnosed and eventually cause optic atrophy [14]. It is important that the rare condition of interface fluid becomes known to all ophthalmologists. It usually follows, or is associated with diffuse lamellar keratitis. The keratitis is treated with steroids, which in turn leads to glaucoma in steroid responders, and the interface fluid accumulates. It is important to diagnose this condition by performing tonometry off the flap or at the limbus, and to initiate proper treatment. Steroids, which are needed to control the diffuse lamellar keratitis, should be tapered off as soon as possible, and anti-glaucoma medication must be added.

Summary for the Clinician

- Post-LASIK dry-eye syndrome is a typical side effect within the first post-operative year and prospective patients should be informed accordingly
- Microkeratome-related flap complications are extremely rare but some microkeratomes, usually disposable ones, exhibit a far above average rate of complications
- The interface after LASIK presents a new space that allows accumulation of cells or fluid, creating new diagnostic entities such as diffuse lamellar keratitis (DLK)
- DLK must be aggressively treated to avoid permanent scarring
- Fluid in the interface suggests steroid-induced glaucoma
- Epithelial ingrowth is rare and caused predominantly by invasion, suggesting that flap quality and apposition are important

12.4
Quality of Vision

All refractive surgical procedures will change the optics of the eye. Part of this change, namely the change in overall refractive power, is the actual purpose of the procedure and therefore welcomed. Another part leads to undesired side effects and should therefore be minimised. When I started to perform LASIK in 1993, the few who performed this procedure corrected refractive errors up to –30 D in some patients. The more we learned about LASIK in the years to follow, the more we became aware of the importance of a new aspect of refractive surgery: the quality of vision we provided to our patients. Our patients and we were excited about an uncorrected vision of 20/25 after we performed a correction of –20 D. However, as time went by, more and more of these patients told us how excited they were, but while they reported good vision in bright light, their next words were "...well, as soon as I am in a room everything gets blurry and foggy. Can you do anything about this?" In the beginning we might not have listened carefully enough, but with increasing experience most of us heard this story over and

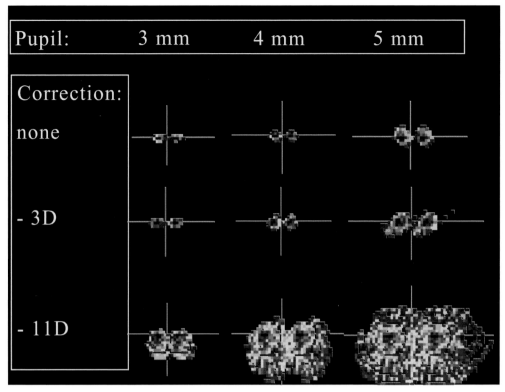

Fig. 12.5. Point images in normal eyes and in eyes after LASIK for myopia at different pupil sizes (images calculated using ray tracing)

over again, and we started to look for possible ways to do better. Our interest focused not only on visual acuity and refraction anymore, but we began to investigate the quality of vision after refractive surgery in great detail.

Here we will look at corneal refractive surgical procedures only, which leaves the change of corneal refraction and the diameter of the pupil to be considered. The change of corneal refraction is defined by the diameter of the part of the cornea that was corrected and by the amount of correction (and, to a lesser extent, by the diameter and the steepness of the transition zone, if any was used).

Retinal images can be calculated using "ray tracing". We used the Technomed C-scan corneal topography system which is no longer commercially available. This system offered a software module called "ray tracing analysis". Simplified, this software will, for a given topographic map, trace rays of light through the re-

spective cornea and pupil and calculate the image on the retina. The effect of the lens will not be included. Any retinal compensation mechanisms (e.g. Stilles-Crawford Effect) will not be considered either. Figure 12.5 shows the simulated retinal images at several pupil sizes and given amounts of correction. Simplified, these two-dimensional graphs can be directly compared with what the patient sees: Two well-defined small blue spots indicate excellent quality of vision, while large halos indicate very poor quality of vision. The halos visible in Fig. 12.5 are similar to the halos a patient will experience around lights at the given pupil size. This, however, does not take into consideration the psychophysical mechanisms of compensation we use unconsciously to compensate for the halos. Fortunately, our brain, much like an image-processing computer, filters the unwanted information (the "halo"), and the halo is not perceived subjectively. This process explains why many of our highly myopic patients who underwent LASIK years ago function reasonably well and do not complain about halos. On the other hand, even if the halos are not perceived, the sheer amount of scattered light will reduce contrast sensitivity and quality of vision in these patients.

In order to compare different myopic corrections, Fig. 12.5 shows a normal eye, an eye which received LASIK for –3 D with a 6-mm planned optical zone, an eye that received LASIK for –5 D with a 6-mm planned optical zone and an eye which had had LASIK for –11 D with a 5-mm planned optical zone. Figure 12.5 demonstrates clearly that the quality of vision decreases with increasing pupil size for a given amount of correction. Comparing a –3 D correction to a normal eye, we see that results are almost identical, and that a faint halo is visible even at large pupil sizes only. This demonstrates a high quality of vision after LASIK in low myopia. Using a 6-mm or larger planned optical zone size, we will therefore provide excellent quality of vision to patients with low myopia.

Results are very different in high myopia. Looking at a –11 D correction with a 5-mm planned optical zone, a significant loss of visual quality becomes obvious even at small pupil sizes. The halos are large and confluent, which will correlate to a clinically significant loss of visual quality. These findings correlate again with our clinical observation, that small optical zones and/or high amounts of correction lead to subjective visual impairment in a certain number of patients. However, a recent clinical study was unable to confirm this correlation [19].

In the correction of myopia we must therefore not only consider the predictability of our treatment but also the quality of vision that can be achieved. We must inform our patients accordingly. We must tell them that quality of vision is likely to be poor in corrections of more than about –10 D, and we should discourage them to undergo LASIK as other procedures, providing better quality of vision, such as phakic IOLs are available in this range of corrections. We must also tell them that some loss of visual quality will occur in corrections of about –5 to –10 D, perhaps more so in patients with large pupils. On the other hand, above results

are very encouraging in low myopia. We can inform our patients that LASIK, in the absence of complications, will not alter their quality of vision significantly. Quality of vision after LASIK is discussed in greater detail in Chap. 19.

Summary for the Clinician

- Quality of vision is an important issue after refractive surgery
- LASIK will not negatively affect quality of vision in low to moderate myopia or hyperopia
- LASIK will reduce quality of vision somewhat in higher myopia (more than –5 D) and high hyperopia (more than +3 D), and patients should be informed about the reduced quality of vision
- The amount of correction that can be performed at the cornea is limited, and extreme myopes as well as high hyperopes will have a poor quality of vision after LASIK and should therefore not be treated

12.5
Customized Ablations

Customized, or wavefront-guided ablations are likely the standard of the future (see also Chap. 14). The technology is available and demonstrates safety and efficacy at least comparable to "standard" LASIK. I had the opportunity to work with the Zyoptix system of Bausch & Lomb, Rochester, NY, from the early days when the system was developed. The Zyoptix system consists of three components: the Zywave aberrometer, the Orbscan IIz corneal tomography system and the Technolas 217z excimer laser. Aberrometer and Orbscan data are linked to the excimer laser via the Zylink software which allows calculation of the treatment which is stored in a file. Before treatment, the file is uploaded into the laser. The treatment itself is just like a standard LASIK procedure. The following section will not focus on the Zyoptix system but describe wavefront-guided treatments from a more general perspective.

12.5.1
Wavefront Measurements

Most aberrometers available today are so-called Hartmann-Shack systems. They measure the overall aberrations of the eye, which include sphere and cylinder, coma, spherical aberration, trefoil and others. Based on these data, the system calculates a refraction which allows a comparison to the manifest refraction and autorefractor data. In a sense, the aberrometer is an advanced autorefractor. It provides accurate refractive data of the optical system of the eye over the whole area of the pupil. The aberrometer-measured refraction represents the mean of the best-fit sphere and cylinder values of the total aberrations measured for a given pupil size. In other words, it gives us an idea what the sphere and the cylinder of the eye measured are. As the aberrometer can only measure the part of the optical system exposed by the pupil, it is mandatory to perform measurements with a dilated pupil. Dilation can be achieved either by performing the exam in a dark room, or by the use of mydriatic agents. The minimum pupil size for a meaningful measurement is 5.5 mm. A smaller pupil will lead to too small an optical zone, and standard LASIK should be used in these cases rather than wavefront-guided LASIK. Another issue to be addressed is the quality of the tear film. As with any optical measurement on the eye, the quality of the result depends heavily on the quality of the optical system. This requires a perfect tear film and an undisturbed eye. Aberrometry must therefore never be performed after a complete eye exam which included applanation tonometry. It is also helpful to administer preservative-free tears in patients with dry-eye syndrome prior to the exam.

12.5.2
Wavefront-Guided Treatments

After measurement, a treatment file is calculated and reviewed by the surgeon. The surgeon must compare the manifest refraction of the eye and the refraction calculated by the aberrometer. In the case of large discrepancies, it is usually recommended to perform a standard ablation. The treatment file is uploaded into the laser and the treatment is performed just like a standard treatment.

12.5.3
What Are the Benefits of Customised LASIK?

Besides a more general benefit that a "custom-tailored" treatment is performed, we must analyse the clinical data to identify other benefits. First and most important is the question whether visual acuity is improved over the preoperative level or not. This so-called eagle vision has caused a lot of public interest. The sad news is that today's data do not support the claim of "eagle vision". We should therefore not claim that "eagle vision" can be achieved. This will rather backfire on us and lead to unhappy patients because of profound misunderstandings and unrealistic expectations.

If supervision cannot be achieved: is customised LASIK better? I strongly believe it is. We must, however, not look at visual acuity alone. As we all know, visual acuity is not the appropriate technique to measure visual function. It rather measures just about 1% of the performance of the visual system. In order to test the full capacity of the visual system, we need contrast sensitivity tests at several pupil sizes or ambient light levels. These tests are currently done by all manufacturers, comparing customised and standard LASIK. Initial results show a better contrast acuity after customised LASIK at low ambient light levels (that is, with large pupils) than after standard LASIK. The reason for this is that customised LASIK does not induce spherical aberration, whereas standard LASIK induced significant amounts of spherical aberration. As of today, the advantage of customised LASIK is therefore not "eagle vision", but "owl vision", a better vision in dim light, a higher quality of vision and less halos than that achieved with standard LASIK.

Summary for the Clinician

- Customised LASIK using wavefront-guided ablations induces fewer optical aberrations and therefore provides a better quality of vision than standard LASIK
- Customised LASIK does not improve visual acuity to supernormal levels (no "eagle vision")
- Customised LASIK is an evolving technique which holds considerable promise

References

1. Alió JL, Pérez-Santonja JJ, Tervo T, Tabbara KF, Vesaluoma M, Smith RJ, Maddox B, Maloney RK (2000) Postoperative inflammation, microbial complications, and wound healing following laser in situ keratomileusis. J Refract Surg 16:523–538
2. Balazsi G, Mullie M, Lasswell L, Lee PA, Duh YJ (2001) Laser in situ keratomileusis with a scanning excimer laser for the correction of low to moderate myopia with and without astigmatism. J Cataract Refract Surg 27:1942–1951
3. Barraquer JI (1949) Queratoplastica refractiva. Estudios Inform. 10:2–21
4. Barraquer JI (1987) Results of myopic keratomileusis. J Refract Surg 3:98–101
5. Bühren J, Baumeister M, Kohnen T (2001) Diffuse lamellar keratitis after laser in situ keratomileusis imaged by confocal microscopy. Ophthalmology 108:1075–1081
6. Fogla R, Rao SK, Padmanabhan P (2001) Interface fluid after laser in situ keratomileusis. J Cataract Refract Surg 27:1526–1528
7. Gimbel HV, Penno EE, van Westenbrugge JA, Ferensowicz M, Furlong MT (1998) Incidence and management of intraoperative and early postoperative complications in 1000 consecutive laser in situ keratomileusis cases. Ophthalmology 105:1839-47; discussion 1847-1848
8. Harrison DA, Periman LM (2001) Diffuse lamellar keratitis associated with recurrent corneal erosions after laser in situ keratomileusis. J Refract Surg 17:463–465
9. Hersh PS, Fry KL, Bishop DS (2003) Incidence and associations of retreatment after LASIK. Ophthalmology 110:748–754
10. Jackson DW, Hamill MB, Koch DD (2003) Laser in situ keratomileusis flap suturing to treat recalcitrant flap striae. J Cataract Refract Surg 29:264–269
11. Jacobs JM, Taravella MJ (2002) Incidence of intraoperative flap complications in laser in situ keratomileusis. J Cataract Refract Surg 28:23–28
12. Knorz MC, Wiesinger B, Liermann A, Seiberth V, Liesenhoff H (1998) Laser in situ keratomileusis for moderate and high myopia and myopic astigmatism. Ophthalmology 105:932–940
13. McDonald MB, Carr JD, Frantz JM, Kozarsky AM, Maguen E, Nesburn AB, Rabinowitz YS, Salz JJ, Stulting RD, Thompson KP, Waring GO (2001) Laser in situ keratomileusis for myopia up to –11 diopters with up to –5 diopters of astigmatism with the summit autonomous LADARVision excimer laser system. Ophthalmology 108:309–316
14. Najman-Vainer J, Smith RJ, Maloney RK (2000) Interface fluid after LASIK: misleading tonometry can lead to end-stage glaucoma. J Cataract Refract Surg 26:471–472
15. Pallikaris IG, Papatzanaki ME, Stathi EZ, Frenschock O, Georgiadis A (1990) Laser in situ keratomileusis. Lasers Surg Med 10:463–468
16. Pallikaris IG, Katsanevaki VJ, Panagopoulou SI (2002) Laser in situ keratomileusis intraoperative complications using one type of microkeratome. Ophthalmology 109:57–63
17. Parolini B, Marcon G, Panozzo GA (2001) Central necrotic lamellar inflammation after laser in situ keratomileusis. J Refract Surg 17:110–112
18. Peters NT, Iskander NG, Anderson Penno EE, Woods DE, Moore RA, Gimbel HV (2001) Diffuse lamellar keratitis: isolation of endotoxin and demonstration of the inflammatory potential in a rabbit laser in situ keratomileusis model. J Cataract Refract Surg 27:917–923
19. Pop M, Payette Y (2004) Risk factors for night vision complaints after LASIK for myopia. Ophthalmology 111:3–10
20. Portellinha W, Kuchenbuk M, Nakano K, Oliveira M (2001) Interface fluid and diffuse corneal edema after laser in situ keratomileusis. J Refract Surg 17:S192–195
21. Probst LE, Foley L (2001) Late-onset interface keratitis after uneventful laser in situ keratomileusis. J Cataract Refract Surg 27:1124–1125
22. Randleman JB, Russell B, Ward MA, Thompson KP, Stulting RD (2003) Risk factors and prognosis for corneal ectasia after LASIK. Ophthalmology 110:267–275
23. Recep OF, Cagil N, Hasiripi H (2000) Outcome of flap subluxation after laser in situ keratomileusis: results of 6 month follow-up. J Cataract Refract Surg 26:1158–1162
24. Rubinfeld RS, Hardten DR, Donnenfeld ED, Stein RM, Koch DD, Speaker MG, Frucht-Pery J, Kameen AJ, Negvesky GJ (2003) To lift or recut: changing trends in LASIK enhancement. J Cataract Refract Surg 29:2306–2317

25. Shah MN, Misra M, Wihelmus KR, Koch DD (2000) Diffuse lamellar keratitis associated with epithelial defects after laser in situ keratomileusis. J Cataract Refract Surg 26:1312–1318
26. Slade SG, Updegraff SA (1995) Complications of automated lamellar keratectomy. Arch Ophthalmol 113:1092–1093
27. Solomon A, Karp CL, Miller D, Dubovy SR, Huang AJ, Culbertson WW (2001) Mycobacterium interface keratitis after laser in situ keratomileusis. Ophthalmology 108:2201–2208
28. Tham VM, Maloney RK (2000) Microkeratome complications of laser in situ keratomileusis. Ophthalmology 107:920–924
29. Wang MY, Maloney RK (2000) Epithelial ingrowth after laser in situ keratomileusis. Am J Ophthalmol 129:746–751
30. Waring GO, Carr JD, Stulting RD, Thompson KP, Wiley W (1999) Prospective randomized comparison of simultaneous and sequential bilateral laser in situ keratomileusis for the correction of myopia. Ophthalmology 106:732–738

LASEK vs PRK

Chun Chen Chen, Dimitri T. Azar

Core Messages

- Photorefractive keratectomy (PRK) has been used widely because of its predictability and safety in treating low to moderate myopia
- Laser subepithelial keratomileusis (LASEK), a modification of PRK, involves the creation of an epithelial flap that is repositioned after laser ablation of Bowman's membrane and the anterior stroma. The epithelial sheet can be generated mechanically or using alcohol
- The viability and integrity of the epithelial flap during the LASEK procedure is crucial for achieving adhesion after flap repositioning and minimising the wound healing process
- Meticulous titration of the dose and exposure time of dilute alcohol solution, and reproducible LASEK technique will be helpful to preserve the viability of the epithelial flap
- Although potential theoretical advantages of LASEK over PRK are decreased post-operative discomfort, faster visual rehabilitation and less haze, several studies have failed to confirm these potential advantages
- LASEK may be a viable alternative for patients with low myopia, thin corneas and life styles that predispose them to flap trauma

13.1
Introduction

Laser subepithelial keratomileusis (LASEK) is a newly developed, modified PRK technique that is based on the detachment of an epithelial flap after the application of dilute alcohol solution, and subsequent repositioning of the flap following laser ablation. The repositioned flap is thought to act as a natural mechanical barrier that diminished post-operative pain and decreases haze formation [27]. LASEK theoretically offers the advantages of avoiding the flap complications of LASIK and, also, addresses the drawbacks of discomfort and delayed recovery associated with conventional PRK.

Laser in situ keratomileusis (LASIK) continues to be the dominant procedure in refractive surgery [15]. It offers more comfort in the early post-operative period, faster visual rehabilitation and minimal haze by maintaining the central corneal epithelium. However, there are increasing reports of LASIK complications, particularly related to flap creation [24, 40, 43]. These include free caps, incomplete pass of the microkeratome, flap wrinkles, epithelial ingrowth, flap melting, diffuse lamellar keratitis, keratectasia and an increase in high-order aberrations [22–24, 33, 40, 43]. Furthermore, LASIK is difficult to perform safely in certain situations, such as very steep or flat corneas, deep-set eyes, anterior scleral buckles and previous glaucoma filtering surgery [4].

Photorefractive keratectomy (PRK) remains an excellent option for mild to moderate corrections, particularly for cases associated with thin corneas, recurrent corneal erosions, or a predisposition to trauma [3]. PRK does not structurally weaken the cornea. Significant post-operative pain, slower visual recovery and haze might happen and be deterrents to the patients.

LASEK has become a viable alternative to PRK and LASIK in selected patients with thin corneas and patients with lifestyles or professions that predispose them to flap trauma, including athletes or military personnel, for example [7]. Early studies suggest that refractive and visual results of LASEK are comparable to those of PRK and LASIK. Lower level of haze formation, relatively fast visual recovery, uniformity of corneal topography and better contrast sensitivity were reported in patients after LASEK surgery [12, 27, 32, 35–37].

13.2
Surgical Technique of LASEK and PRK

By salvaging the central epithelium, LASEK is in essence a hybrid of PRK and LASIK [13]. In the LASEK procedure, the epithelial is partially removed from Bowman's layer after the application of dilute alcohol, connected at the hinge area. Laser ablation is applied directly to Bowman's layer as with traditional PRK. The epithelial flap is repositioned in its original position over the laser ablated stromal surface.

The procedure of LASEK was first performed at the Massachusetts Eye and Ear Infirmary by one of the authors (DTA). The original surgical technique involves preplaced epithelial marked for accurate realignment, a Carones alcohol dispenser to weaken the epithelial sheet by exposure to 18 % alcohol for 25 s, a jeweller's forceps to locate the dissection, a Merocel sponge to peel the epithelial sheet and a 30-gauge Rycroft irrigation cannula to reposition the flap [7]. Camellin and Cimberle described a similar technique that uses a Janach trephine (Janach, Italy) to perform a pre-incision of corneal epithelium, an alcohol solution cone to reserve 20 % alcohol for 30 s, and the short side of an epithelial micro-hoe to detach and fold the epithelium [9]. Epithelial sheet viability and adhesion are the basis for achieving the potential advantages of LASEK [7]. Hence, various techniques are developed in an attempt to preserve epithelial flap viability.

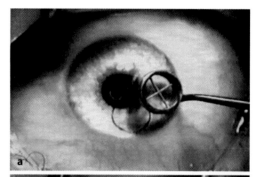

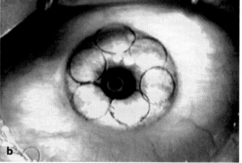

Fig. 13.1 a, b. Marking the paracentral corneal portion (**a**) with an overlapping floral pattern (**b**)

13.2.1
Personal Experience (Azar's Technique)

After anaesthesia and application of a lid speculum, the cornea is marked with overlapping 3.0-mm circles around the corneal periphery (Fig. 13.1). An alcohol dispenser consisting of a customised 7- or 9-mm semi-sharp marker, attached to a hollow metal handle, with a reservoir for the 18 % alcohol (Fig. 13.2), allows irrigation/aspiration of the alcohol after applying firm pressure on the central cornea (ASICO, Westmont, IL) (Fig. 13.3) [7, 11]. After 25–30 s, the solution is absorbed using the suction port (Fig. 13.4) and a dry cellulose sponge (Fig. 13.5). One arm of the Azar LASEK Scissors (ASICO; right and left, Fig. 13.6) is inserted under the epithelium and traced around the delineated margin of the epithelium, leaving 2–3 clock hours of intact margin. The loosened epithelium is peeled as a single sheet using a Merocel sponge, leaving a flap with the hinge still attached (Fig. 13.7). After laser ablation, an anteri-

Fig. 13.2. Azar-Carones LASEK I/A trephine (ASICO AE-2918)

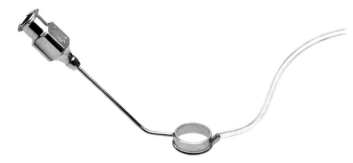

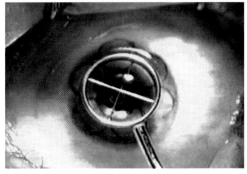

Fig. 13.3. Alcohol circulation

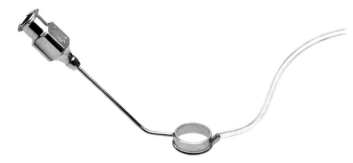

Fig. 13.4. Alcohol absorption

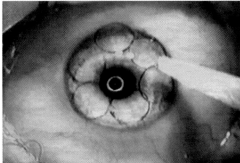

Fig. 13.5. Epithelial flap edge revelation

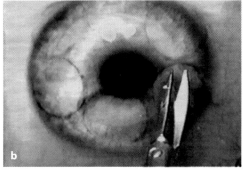

Fig. 13.6 a, b. Flap elevation by the jeweller's forceps (**a**) or the Azar LASEK Scissor (**b**) (ASICO AE-5489, AE-5499)

or-chamber cannula was used to hydrate the stroma and epithelial flap with balanced salt solution. The epithelial flap was replaced on the stroma under intermittent irrigation. Care was taken to realign the epithelial flap using the previous marks and to avoid epithelial defects. The flap then was allowed to dry for 5 min.

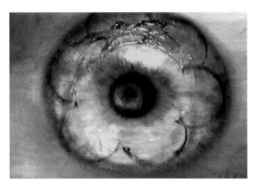

Fig. 13.7. Generation of corneal epithelial flap

13.2.2
Camellin's Technique

The pre-cut incision is performed with a special micro-trephine (Janach, Italy). The depth of micro-trephine is designed to be 70 μm, 80 μm in 8-mm trephines and 90 μm in 9-mm trephine. A blunt portion of the blade at the 12-o'clock position protects the area of the hinge. An alcohol solution cone (Janach, Italy), which is about 0.5 mm or 1 mm larger than the trephine, will be placed on the eye after trephination. Two to three drops of alcoholic solution will be instilled inside the well and left for 25 to 30 s. The pre-cut incision is then dried and thoroughly washed with water. The pre-cut margin is lifted with a hockey spatula to detach the epithelium, and the epithelial flap is gently detached, gathered and folded up at the 12 o'clock position [9, 10, 27].

As the pre-incision is not always perfect, an epithelial micro-hoe is used to complete it. The hoe is pressed firmly downward and pulled about 1 mm toward the pupil centre. Alternatively, the epithelium is detached with the short side of a hockey spatula, making tiny movements almost perpendicular to the margin. The flap is generated and completed along the entire area of trephination up to the hinge.

13.2.3
Vinciguerra's Techinique (Butterfly Technique)

To maintain the viability of epithelial cells, Dr. Vinciguerra proposed a modification of the LASEK technique that preserves the connection between the corneal flap and limbus [42].

The butterfly technique requires the use of the Vinciguerra PRK/LASEK spatula (ASICO, Westmont, IL) to impart a thin abrasion to the paracentral corneal epithelium, from 8 to 11 o'clock in order to spare the optic zone. After positioning the LASEK OZ chamber that is connected to the LASEK pump, apply 20% alcohol for several seconds. The length of time depends on the firmness of the epithelial adhesion noted during the initial abrasion, with a firmer adhesion requiring a slightly longer time. With the Vinciguerra-Carones LASEK spatula, cautiously dissect the epithelium from Bowman's membrane up to the limbus. It is mandatory to keep the cornea well hydrated in order to preserve the obtained loosening effect otherwise the second half of the flap will be dehydrated following completion of dissection of the first half of the flap.

13.2.4
Gel Assisted LASEK

Dr. McDonald used viscous gel (hydroxypropyl cellulose 0.3%) to aid in the separation of the epithelial sheet. The syringe filled with the gel was connected to the cannula. After epithelial trephination, a 2.25 round knife scored down to Bowman's layer for a distance of 1–2 mm. Ten drops of sodium chloride 5% were administered in order to slightly stiffen the cells and were then removed. By sawing back and forth, the epithelial sheet could be lifted. Gel was injected under the epithelium before the cut was made in the middle by scissors. The flap was pushed away after application of gel.

Summary for the Clinician

- LASEK using dilute alcohol is a simple, inexpensive and reproducible technique
- The integrity of the epithelial flap and hinge should be preserved during the LASEK procedure

13.3
Clinical Results of LASEK vs PRK

Azar et al. reported the clinical results of treating 101 myopic patients (131 eyes) with the LASEK procedure [18]. The patients were enrolled between 1996 and 2002. The epithelial defect was complete in 98.8% of eyes by 1 week. Subjective mild pain was reported in 65% of patients. All but one eye had uncorrected visual acuity (UCVA) of 20/40 or better at 6 months. At 1 year, UCVA was 20/40 or better in 94% of eyes. The overall rate of haze formation was 33.1%. No patients had his corneal haze recorded as greater than "mild". The epithelial flap can be consistently created, peeled and returned using the technique previously described (see Sect. 13.2.1).

After treating 249 patients, Camellin reported that intraoperative flap management was easy in 60% of cases, average in 28%, and difficult in 12% [10]. No pain was experienced by 44% of cases in the first 24 h after surgery, and 80% of the post-operative best spectacle corrected visual acuity (BSCVA) was achieved by 90% of patients 10 days post-operatively.

The series of patients treated with LASEK show promising results [5, 7, 12, 18, 26, 27, 31, 32, 34–37]. Scerrati compared the results in two groups of 15 patients treated with LASIK or LASEK. In post-operative corneal topography, BSCVA, and contrast sensitivity, the results of LASEK were superior to those of LASIK [35]. Lohmann et al. and Rouweyha et al. reported the results of treating eyes with high myopia (21 eyes and 32 eyes, respectively) for up to 6 months follow-up [31, 34]. Lohmann et al. presented results whereby all patients were within ±1.0 D of emmetropia. On slit lamp biomicroscopy, all corneas were transparent and no haze was noted at the post-operative points.

Rouweyha et al. also reported UCVA of 20/40 or better in 33 of eyes at day 1; 71% at 2 weeks; and 100% at 3 months.

Lee et al. and Litwak et al. conducted studies comparing LASEK performed in one eye and PRK in the other eye [27, 30]. Lee et al. found that the epithelial defect was healed by the fourth day in eyes that underwent PRK and by the fifth day in eyes that underwent LASEK [27]. The mean epithelial healing time was 3.18±0.50 days and 3.64±0.63 days, respectively, while the difference was not statistically significant (p=0.10). Similarly, Litwak et al. reported that the epithelial defect was completely healed by the fourth day in the PRK and LASEK eyes [30]. The mean epithelial healing time was 3.3±0.5 days and 3.6±0.5 days, respectively (p=0.07).

The subjective pain scores recorded by Lee et al. at 7 days was significantly higher in the PRK eye than the LASEK eye (2.36±0.67 versus 1.63±0.81, p=0.047) [27]. At 1 week, UCVA was 20/25 or better in ten eyes that underwent PRK (37%) and 16 eyes that underwent LASEK (59%). At 3 months, it was 20/25 or better in 15 eyes that underwent PRK (56%) and 17 eyes that underwent LASEK (63%). A total of 17 patients (63%; p>0.05) preferred the LASEK procedure because of faster visual rehabilitation (three eyes), painless recovery (ten eyes), and better visual acuity (four eyes). At 1 month, the mean haze score was 0.86±0.45 in eyes that underwent PRK and 0.46±0.24 eyes that underwent LASEK; this was statistically significant (p=0.02). At 3 months, the difference was not statistically significant (p=0.22).

In the series by Litwak et al., 18 patients (72%) reported more ocular discomfort in the LASEK eye compared to six patients (24%) who complained more about the PRK eye at 1 day [30]. At 3 days, the difference was higher: 80% complained about the LASEK eye and 4% complained about the PRK eye. At 1 week, the UCVA was 20/25 or better in 12 PRK eyes and 12 LASEK eyes (48%). At 1 month the UCVA was 20/25 or better in 19 PRK eyes (76%) and 20 LASEK eyes (80%). No eye had lost one or more lines of best spectacle corrected visual acuity (BSCVA) at the 1-month follow-up examination. At 1 day, patients reported better vision in four LASEK eyes (16%) and 20 PRK eyes (80%). At day 3 patients reported better vision in one LASEK eye (4%) and 24 PRK eyes (96%). There was no development of post-operative corneal haze at 1 month in PRK and LASEK groups.

The comparative studies of LASEK versus PRK showed discrepancies regarding immediate ocular discomfort, subjective UCVA in these two studies. The difference may be inherent in the study population (race and age of the enrolled patient), concentration and duration of dilute alcohol solutions, techniques of epithelial flap elevation and reposition.

Summary for the Clinician

- LASEK is as safe and effective as PRK and LASIK
- It is not clear whether LASEK is associated with substantially less pain and haze or faster visual rehabilitation than PRK

13.4
Electron Microscopy

13.4.1
Preparation of Specimens for Electron Microscopy

The epithelial sheet specimens were obtained from patients undergoing PRK. The epithelial sheets were fixed in half-strength Karnovsky fixative (2% paraformaldehyde and 2.5% glutaraldehyde) in 0.2 M sodium cacodylate buffer (pH 7.4) overnight and post-fixed in 1% osmium tetroxide in 0.2 M sodium cacodylate for 1.5 h. After dehydration in graded alcohol, the eyes were embedded in epoxy resin (Epon-Araldite). Thick sections (1 μm) were stained with toluidine blue, and a suitable area containing basal layers was chosen. The blocks were trimmed accordingly, thin sectioned (80–90 Å), stained with 2% uranyl acetate Reynold's lead nitrate, and examined with a transmission electron microscope (model 410; Philips, Eindhoven, The Netherlands).

13.4.2
Electron Microscopic Analysis of Epithelial Sheets Removed Using 20% Alcohol

Normal corneal epithelia are non-keratinizing, stratified, squamous epithelia five to seven layers thick. Desmosomes are present along all cell membranes abutting other cell membranes. The cells of the basal layer are columnar, and hemidesmosomes are present along their basal plasma membrane adjacent to the basement membrane. Beneath the epithelium is a unilamellar basement membrane that overlies a thick collagen stroma through which anchoring fibres extend from the lamina densa [6, 38].

Azar et al. and Chen et al. studied the electron micrograph of freed epithelial sheets, which were obtained from 20% alcohol exposure for 20 s [7, 11]. The freed epithelial sheet displayed normal stratification. The basal epithelial surface of isolated epithelial sheets showed blebbing of the basal cell membrane and autophagic vacuoles within the cytoplasm of the epithelial basal cells of the freed sheet in two of the four specimens. They also observed variable basement membrane complex configurations beneath the epithelial basal cells: unilamellar basement membrane with focal disruptions (Fig. 13.8a), irregular and discontinuous basement membrane with intact hemidesmosome (Fig. 13.8b), disruptions of basal cell membranes with absent basement membrane (Fig. 13.8c) and duplicated basement membrane containing dense bundles of anchoring fibrils (Fig. 13.8d). The basement membrane layer showed discontinuous and irregular extracellular matrix fragments. The adherence of the basement membrane to the basal layer of the epithelium is vital because it is believed that the basement membrane provides the stability and support that keeps the epithelium intact even with manipulation, thereby preserving the integrity and viability of the entire epithelium. The presence of desmosomes provides anchoring mechanisms for the epithelium to adhere to the ablated stroma. In addition, Gabler et al. also demonstrated that the plane of separation after ethanol exposure in human cadaver eyes was

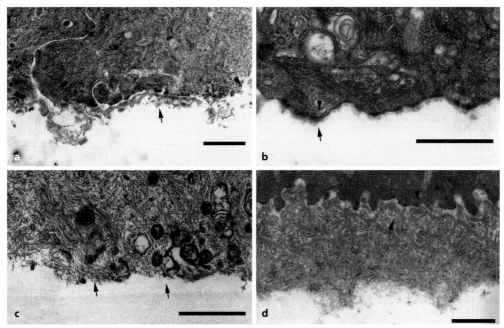

Fig. 13.8 a–d. Transmission electron micrographs of freed epithelial sheets after 20% alcohol application for 25 s (Specimen I, **a**; II, **b**; III, **c**; and IV, **d**). Variable separation of the basement membrane zone was seen. **a** Specimen I showing a localised area of irregular basement membrane zone (*arrow*) and basal cell membrane disruption (*arrowheads*) (original magnification ×17,750). **b** Discontinuous basement membrane zone beneath the basal epithelial cells (*arrows*), evident at higher magnification, was associated with a decreased number of electron-dense hemidesmosomes (*arrowheads*) (original magnification ×30,000).

c The basal cell membranes and the basement membrane (*arrows*) were disrupted in Specimen III. Autographic vacuole formation (*arrowheads*) was extensive in the cytoplasm (original magnification ×1650). **d** Specimen IV: The freed epithelial sheet retained a duplicated basement membrane zone. Pockets of cross-banded anchoring fibrils were arranged in a network between the layers of basal lamina (*arrows*). Electron-dense hemidesmosomes (*arrowheads*) were present along the basal cell membrane (original magnification ×17,750). Bar=1 µm. (Reproduced from [11])

between the lamina densa and the Bowman's layer [20]. By immunofluorescence studies, the cleavage plane of alcohol induced corneal flap was located between the lamina lucida and lamina densa of the basement membrane [16].

Summary for the Clinician

- The electron microscopic and histopathological evaluation indicates that the point of separation during the LASEK procedure was likely to be within the basement membrane or between the basement membrane and the Bowman's layer
- The variation of epithelial-basement membrane configuration after dilute ethanol exposure may be due to variability

between individuals in relation to the adherence of the epithelium to the basement membrane or to the variability of the effect of alcohol on adhesion of epithelial cells

---

13.5
Corneal Wound Healing
After the Refractive Process

While laser refractive surgery offers the promise to correct visual refractive error, biologic variability in the wound healing response is thought to be the major factor limiting the predictability of the outcome of refractive surgery.

The corneal wound healing cascade is complex and involves epithelial mitosis and migration, keratocyte necrosis and apoptosis, myofibroblast transformation, extracellular matrix deposition and remodelling and inflammatory cell infiltration [17, 21 ,25, 29, 44].

13.5.1
Epithelial Wound Healing

During PRK, the central epithelium is completely removed, while in LASEK, the injury to the epithelium is limited to an incision or abrasion through the mid-peripheral epithelium. The epithelial cells immediately adjacent to the damaged areas flatten, shed their microvilli and develop pseudopodial extensions. The epithelial cell starts sliding and migration along the tissue until the epithelial defect is covered [19]. During the process, the epithelium also plays an active role in corneal stromal wound healing. The epithelium can produce both stimulatory and inhibitory cytokines related to plasminogen activation that can affect the release of collagenase and other proteases, as well as inhibitors of collagenase [28]. The epithelial–mesenchymal interaction will maintain a balance between a synthesis of new collagen and proteoglycans with normal assembly and the degradation of the extracellular matrix to allow the restoration of normal structure.

13.5.2
Stromal Wound Healing

As soon as the epithelial barrier is broken by the incision during PRK and LASEK, the stroma begins to imbibe fluid and becomes oedematous adjacent to the wound. After the injury of the corneal epithelium, an underlying keratocyte loss occurs within 1 h. This phenomenon was first recognised by Dohlman et al. [14]. Keratocyte apoptosis, subsequent replenishment with activated keratocytes, is an initiator of the wound healing process that occurs following PRK and LASEK. Animal studies demonstrated that superficial keratocytes undergo programmed cell death mediated by cytokines

released from the injured epithelium, such as interleukin (IL)-1α, Fas/Fas ligand, bone morphogenic protein (BMP) 2, BMP 4 and tumour necrosis factor (TNF)-α [8, 45, 46]. Furthermore, tear fluid also contains a wide range of peptide growth factors and is secreted in increased amount after laser ablation of the stroma [47]. Following PRK, an increased amount of transforming growth factor (TGF)-1 in tear fluid was observed, thus leading to keratocyte proliferation, migration, myofibroblast transformation and synthesis of stromal extracellular matrix components such as fibronectin and collagen [28, 41].

13.6
Epithelial Cell Viability

Corneal epithelial integrity is essential to maintaining balanced epithelial–mesenchymal interactions, which play an active role in the chemokinetics of corneal wound healing, keratocyte apoptosis, myofibroblast transformation and corneal neovascularization [11]. It is hypothesised that the viability of epithelial flap decreases changes in stromal keratocytes and reduces the production of extracellular matrix and collagen. This may result in less post-operative haze formation with LASEK than PRK [4].

The viability of the ethanol-treated epithelial sheet was further studied in tissue culture for cell migration and attachment [11]. One of the three specimens showed outgrowth and attachment of epithelial cells from the epithelial sheet at days 1–15 (Fig. 13.9). These findings were reinforced by the electron microscopic evaluations of the epithelial tissue specimen in vivo.

Concentrations of ethanol ranging from 10 % to 30 % are widely used to remove the corneal epithelium before PRK [2]. Stein et al. reported that using dilute alcohol (25 %) in 91 cases of PRK was a safe, effective and predictive method of removing the epithelium [39]. Abad et al. found that chemical de-epithelialization with dilute ethanol (18 %) appears to be safe and effective and might promote faster rehabilitation [1]. Gabler et al. used 0.1 % trypan blue to test the viability of the epithelial flap of human cadaver eyes after alcohol treatment. They ob-

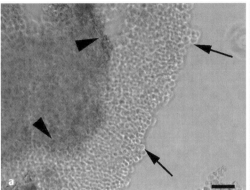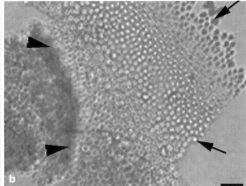

Fig. 13.9 a, b. Inverted phase contrast photographs of the tissue culture from one of the three freed epithelial sheets generated after 20% ethanol treatment for 25 s. **a** Epithelial outgrowth was observed at day 1 extending from the original sheet border (*arrowheads*) to the 1-day outer border (*arrows*). **b** The cell attachment and epithelial outgrowth were persistent until day 15. Bar=50 μm. (Reproduced from [11])

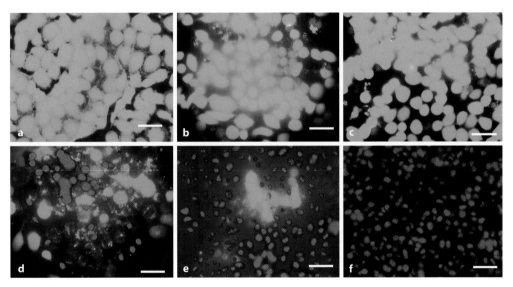

Fig. 13.10 a–g. Fluorescein viability stain with calcein-AM/ethidium homodimer of the cells after 10% (**a**), 20% (**b**), 24% (**c**), 25% (**d**), 26% (**e**), and 40% (**f**) EtOH-H$_2$O treatment for 20 s. Metabolically active cells convert non-fluorescent calcein-AM into green fluorescent polyanionic calcein and exclude ethidium homodimer (**a**). Damaged cell membranes allow permeation of ethidium homodimer and its binding to nucleic acids resulting in red fluorescence (**f**). Bar=50 μm. **g** Cellular survival after different concentrations of alcohol treatment for 20 s. The percentage of viable cells (with exclusive green fluorescence) was calculated by counting cells per ten fields at ×400 magnification. (Reproduced from [11].) Figure 13.10 g see next page

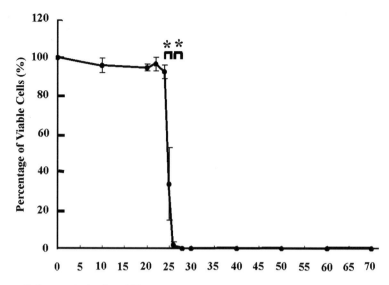

Fig. 13.10 g. Cellular survival after different concentrations of alcohol treatment for 20 s. The percentage of viable cells (with exclusive green fluorescence) was calculated by counting cells per ten fields at ×400 magnification. (Reproduced from [11])

served that the epithelial cells were vital for up to 45 s of 20 % ethanol exposure [20].

Chen et al. detected a dose- and time-dependent effect of dilute alcohol on cultured corneal epithelial cells [11]. The 25 % concentration of dilute alcohol was the inflection point of epithelial survival (Fig. 13.10). A significant increase in cellular death occurred after 35 s of 20 % alcohol exposure (Fig. 13.11). Also, 40 s of exposure further increased apoptosis after 8 h of incubation (Fig. 13.12). These findings are consistent with the clinical observations of varied epithelial attachment to the stromal bed after LASEK surgery.

Summary for the Clinician

- The effect of dilute alcohol on corneal epithelial cell viability is dose- and time-dependent
- Application of the optimal dose and duration of dilute ethanol will facilitate epithelial flap generation, achieve maximal epithelial survival and subsequent adhesion of the repositioned epithelial flap to the stromal bed

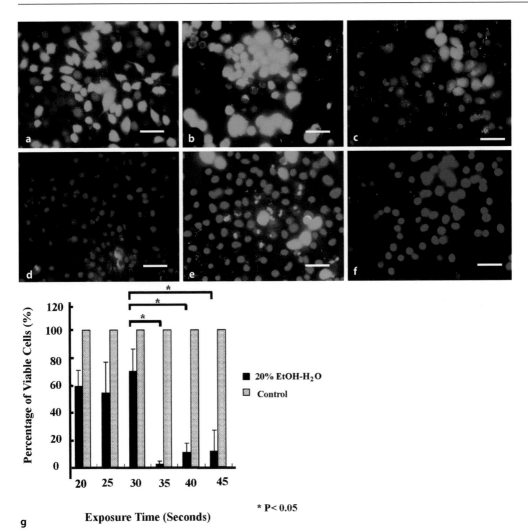

* P< 0.05

Fig. 13.11 a–g. Fluorescein viability stain with calcein-AM/ethidium homodimer of cells exposed to 20% EtOH-H$_2$O for 20 s (**a**), 25 s (**b**), 30 s (**c**), 35 s (**d**), 40 s (**e**), or 45 s (**f**). Calcein-positive green fluorescence indicates metabolically active cells, and ethidium homodimer-positive red fluorescence indicates damage to the cell membrane and binding to nucleic acids. Bar=50 μm. **g** Cellular survival with different exposure times. The percentage of viable cells was calculated from the number of green, red, and bicolored cells counter per ten fields at ×400 magnification. The control group was treated with 100% KSFM (0% ethanol). (Reproduced from [11])

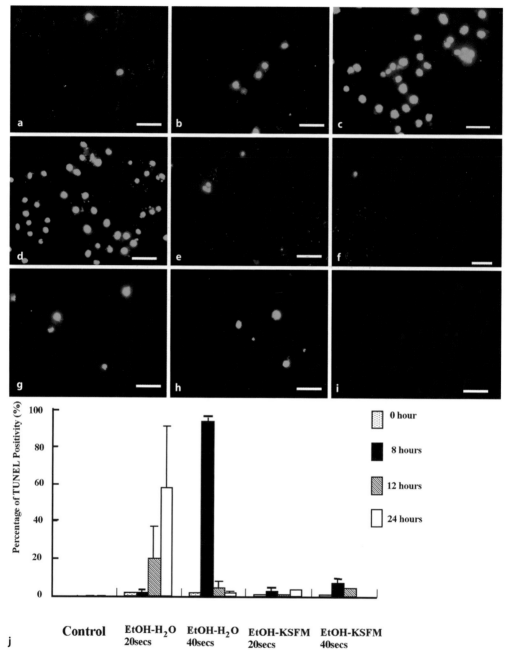

Fig. 13.12 a–j. TUNEL labelling of cultured corneal epithelial cells exposed to 20% EtOH-H$_2$O for 20 s (**a–c**) and 40 s (**d–f**) and to EtOH-KSFM for 40 s (**g–i**). The TUNEL positivity was evaluated after 8 h (**a, d, g**), 12 h (**b, e, h**) and 24 h (**c, f, i**) of incubation. Maximal TUNEL positivity after 20 s of EtOH-H$_2$O exposure was detected at 24 h of incubation (**c**, 58.05±33.10) and after 40 s of EtOH-H$_2$O exposure at 8 h of incubation (**d**, 94.12±1.21%). Substantially lower TUNEL positivity was seen after 8, 12, and 24 h of incubation with EtOH-KSFM for 40 s (**g**, 0.65± 0.02%; **h**, 7.11±1.49%; **i**, 4.52±1.05%). **j** TUNEL positivity after 8, 12, and 24 h of incubation of 20% EtOH-H$_2$O for 20 and 40 s and 2% EtOH-KSFM for 20 and 40 s compared to controls. Control groups were treated with 100% KSFM for 20 s. (Reproduced from [11])

References

1. Abad JC, Bonnie A, Talamo JH et al. (1996) Dilute alcohol versus mechanical debridement before photorefractive keratectomy. J Cataract Refract Surg 22:1427–1433
2. Abad JC, Bonnie A, Power WJ et al. (1997) A prospective evaluation of Alcohol-assisted versus mechanical epithelial removal before photorefractive keratectomy. Ophthalmology 104:1566–1574
3. Ambrosio R JR, Wilson S (2003) LASIK vs LASEK vs PEK: advantages and indications. Semin Ophthalmol 18:2–10
4. Anderson NJ, Beran RF, Schneider TL (2002) Epi-LASEK for the correction of myopia and myopic astigmatism. J Cataract Refract Surg 28:1343–1347
5. Autrata R, Rehurek J (2003) Laser-assisted subepithelial keratectomy for myopia: two- year follow-up. J Cataract Refract Surg 29:661–668
6. Azar DT, Spurr-Michaud SJ, Tisdale AS et al. (1992). Altered epithelial-basement membrane interactions in diabetic corneas. Arch Ophthalmol 110:537–540
7. Azar DT, Ang RT, Lee JB et al. (2001) Laser subepithelial keratomileusis: electron microscopy and visual outcomes of flap photorefractive keratectomy. Curr Opin Ophthalmol 12:323–329
8. Baldwin HC, Marshall J (2002) Growth factors in corneal wound healing following refractive surgery: a review. Acta Ophthalmol Scand 80:238–247
9. Camellin M, Cimberle M (1999) LASEK may offer the advantages of both LASIK and PRK. Ocular Surg News 28–29
10. Camellin M, Cimberle M (2000) LASEK has more than 1 year of successful experience. Ocular Surg News 18:14–17
11. Chen CC, Chang JH, Lee JB et al (2002) Human corneal epithelial cell viability and morphology after dilute alcohol exposure. Invest Ophthalmol Vis Sci 43:2593–2602
12. Claringbold TV II (2002) Laser- assisted subepithelial keratectomy for the correction of myopia. J Cataract Refract Surg 28:18–22
13. Dastjerdi MH, Soong HK (2002) LASEK (laser subepithelial keratomileusis). Curr Opin Ophthalmol 13:261–263
14. Dohlman CH, Gasset AR, Rose J (1968) The effect of the absence of corneal epithelium or endothelium on the stromal keratocytes. Invest Ophthalmol Vis Sci 7:520–534
15. Duffey RJ, Leaming D (2003) US trends in refractive surgery: 2002 ISRS survey. J Refract Surg 19:357–363
16. Espana EM, Grueterich M, Mateo A et al (2003) Cleavage of corneal basement membrane components by ethanol exposure in laser-assisted subepithelial keratectomy. J Cataract Refract Surg 29:1192–1197
17. Fantes FE, Hanna KD, Waring GO et al. (1990) Wound healing after excimer laser keratomileusis (photorefractive keratectomy) in monkeys. Arch Ophthalmol 108:665–675
18. Feit R, Taneri S, Azar DT et al. (2003) LASEK results. Ophthalmol Clin North Am 16:127–135
19. Fountain TR, de la Cruz Z, Green WR (1994) Reassembly of corneal epithelial adhesion structures after excimer laser keratectomy in humans. Arch Ophthalmol 112:967–972
20. Gabler B, Von Monhrenfels CW, Lohmann CP (2001) LASEK: a histological study to investigate the vitality of corneal epithelial cells after alcohol exposure. Invest Ophthalmol Vis Sci 42:S680
21. Gao J, Gelber-Schwalb TA, Addeo JV et al. (1997) Apoptosis in the rabbit cornea after photorefractive keratectomy. Cornea 16:200–208
22. Gimbel HV, Anderson Penne EE, Van Westenbrugge JA et al. (1998) Incidence and management of intraoperative and early postoperative complications in 1000 consecutive laser in situ keratomileusis cases. Ophthalmology 105:1839–1847
23. Hersh PS, Brint SF, Maloney RK et al. (1998) Photorefractive keratectomy versus laser in situ keratomileusis for moderate to high myopia: a randomized prospective study. Ophthalmology 105:1512–1522
24. Holland SP, Srivannaboon S, Reinstein DZ (2000) Avoiding serious corneal complications of laser assisted in situ keratomileusis and photorefractive keratectomy. Ophthalmology 107:640–652
25. Jester JV, Petroll WM, Cavanagh HD (1999) Corneal stromal wound healing in refractive surgery: the role of myofibroblasts. Prog Retin Eye Res 18:311–356
26. Kornilovsky IM (2001) Clinical results after subepithelial photorefractive keratectomy (LASEK). J Refract Surg 17:S222–223
27. Lee JB, Seong GJ, Lee JH et al. (2001) Comparison of laser epithelial keratomileusis and photorefractive keratectomy for low and moderate myopia. J Cataract Refract Surg 27:565–570
28. Li DQ, Tseng SCG (1995) Three patterns of cytokine expression potentially involved in epithelial-fibroblast interactions of human ocular surface. J Cell Physiol 163:61–79

29. Li DQ, Tseng SCG (1996) Differential regulation of cytokine and receptor transcript expression in human corneal and limbal fibroblasts by epidermal growth factor, transforming growth factor-α, platelet-derived growth factor B, and interleukin-1β. Invest Ophthalmol Vis Sci 37:2068–2080

30. Litwak S, Zadok D, Garcia-de Quevedo V et al. (2002) Laser-assisted subepithelial keratectomy versus photorefractive keratectomy for the correction of myopia. A prospective comparative study. J Cataract Refract Surg 28:1330–1333

31. Lohmann CP, von Mohrenfels CW, Gablet B et al. (2001) LASEK: a new surgical procedure to treat myopia. Invest Ophthalmol Vis Sci 42:S599

32. Lohmann CP, von Mohrenfels WC, Gablet B et al. (2002) Laser epithelial keratomileusis (ELISA). Laser epithelial keratomileusis (LASEK). Klin Monatsbl Augenheilkd 219:26–32

33. Moreno-Barriuso E, Lloves JM, Marcos S et al. (2001) Ocular aberrations before and after myopic corneal refractive surgery: LASIK-induced changes measured with laser ray tracing. Invest Ophthalmol Vis Sci 42:1396–1403

34. Rouweyha RM, Chung AZ, Yee RW (2001) Laser-assisted epithelial in situ keratomileusis (LASEK) outcomes in high myopia. Invest Ophthalmol Vis Sci 42:S599

35. Scerrati E (2001) Laser in situ keratomileusis vs. laser epithelial keratomileusis (LASIK vs. LASEK). J Refract Surg 17[Suppl]:S219–S221

36. Shah S, Sebai Sarhan AR, Doyle SJ et al. (2001) The epithelial flap for photorefractive keratectomy. Br J Ophthalmol 85:393–396

37. Shahinian L Jr (2002) Laser- assisted subepithelial keratectomy for low to high myopia and astigmatism. J Cataract Refract Surg 1334–1342

38. Spurr SJ, Gipson IK (1985) Isolation of corneal epithelium with Dispase II or EDTA: effects on the basement membrane zone. Invest Ophthalmol Vis Sci 26:818–827

39. Stein HA, Stein RM, Price C et al. (1997) Alcohol removal of the epithelium for excimer laser ablation: outcome analysis. J Cataract Refract Surg 23:1160–1163

40. Tham VM-B, Maloney RK (2000) Microkeratome complications of laser in situ keratomileusis. Ophthalmology 107:920–924

41. Vesaluoma M, Teppo AM, Gronhagen-Riska C et al. (1996) Release of TGF]1 and VEGF in tears following photorefractive keratectomy. Curr Eye Res 16:19–25

42. Vinciguerra P, Camesasca FI (2002) Butterfly laser epithelial keratomileusis for myopia. J Refract Surg 18[Suppl]:S371–S373

43. Wang Z, Chen J, Yang B (1999) Posterior corneal surface topographic changes after laser in situ keratomileuesis are related to residual corneal bed thickness. Ophthalmology 106:406–409

44. Wilson SE, He YG, Weng J et al. (1996) Epithelial injury induces keratocyte apoptosis: hypothesized role for the interleukin-1 system in the modulation of corneal tissue organization and wound healing. Exp Eye Res 62:325–327

45. Wilson SE, Mohan RR, Ambrosio R Jr et al. (2001) The corneal wound healing response: cytokine-mediated interaction of the epithelium, stroma, and inflammatory cells. Prig Retin Eye Res 20:625–637

46. Wilson SE, Mohan RR, Hong JW et al. (2001) The wound healing response after laser in situ keratomileusis and photorefractive keratectomy: elusive control of biological variability and effect on custom laser vision correction. Arch Ophthalmol 119:889–896

47. Zhao J, Nagasaki T, Maurice DM (2001) Role of tears in keratocyte loss after epithelial removal in mouse cornea. Invest Ophthalmol Vis Sci 42:1743–1749

Refractive Keratotomy: Does It Have a Future Role in Refractive Surgery?

Mitchell P. Weikert, Douglas D. Koch

Core Messages

- Corneal incisions increase the radius of curvature perpendicular to the incision. Radial incisions flatten the central cornea, while arcuate incisions flatten the corneal meridian on which they are centred
- The effect of radial and arcuate keratotomy increases with age, as well as length and number of incisions
- Post-operative hyperopic shift and diurnal fluctuation are seen in some patients following radial keratotomy
- The largest role for refractive keratotomy lies in the management of astigmatism
- Peripheral corneal relaxing incisions can reduce astigmatism alone, combined with cataract surgery, or following PRK, LASIK and penetrating keratoplasty, but are limited in their treatment range

14.1
Introduction

Myopia affects approximately 25% of adults in the United States [24, 43], while 15%–40% of the normal population have significant astigmatism [3, 14]. These conditions can usually be corrected with eyeglasses and contact lenses; however, many patients pursue refractive surgery to decrease their dependence upon these devices. Although refractive surgery has its roots in radial (RK) and astigmatic keratotomy, the advent of excimer laser surgery has led to a tremendous decrease in their use as the primary methods for the surgical correction of refractive error [9]. As technological advances continue in

photorefractive keratectomy (PRK), LASER in situ keratomileusis (LASIK), phakic/pseudophakic intraocular lens (IOL) design and crystalline lens removal, the question arises: "Is there a future role for refractive keratotomy in modern refractive surgery?" In an effort to address this question, this chapter will review the history [5, 26] and principles behind refractive keratotomy, as well as its evolution through multiple clinical trials, subsequent complications and current applications.

14.2
History of Refractive Keratotomy

The use of keratotomy to correct refractive error originated in the mid-nineteenth century when Snellen [42] suggested that a corneal incision placed perpendicular to the steep corneal meridian might induce flattening along that meridian. The first procedure was not performed until 16 years later when, in 1885, Schiötz used a penetrating limbal incision to decrease astigmatism following cataract surgery [41]. Lucciola reported the first cases of non-penetrating corneal incisions in 1886, where he also attempted to reduce astigmatism by flattening the steep corneal meridian in ten patients [28]. The earliest, systematic studies were performed by Jan Lans, when he studied the effect of corneal incisions on the refractive status of rabbits [20]. He defined the basic principles of refractive keratotomy and was the first to identify coupling.

The next major advances came from Japan in the mid-twentieth century with the work of Tsutomu Sato [37, 38]. Sato placed incisions through the corneal endothelium to reduce myopia after observing corneal flattening in keratoconus patients following rupture of Descemet's membrane. He employed posterior, radial corneal incisions for low levels of myopia (2 D) and combined them with anterior, radial incisions to treat higher levels. Though initially successful, his posterior incisions eventually resulted in corneal decompensation, which appeared approximately 20 years after the surgery.

Fyodorov, Durnev, Yenaliev and other physicians in the Soviet Union were the next major group to advance the techniques of incisional refractive surgery with their work in the 1970s [5]. Expanding on the foundation built by Sato, they refined his technique by creating nomograms that incorporated multiple surgical variables to produce more predictable results. Their initial attempts to introduce RK to the United States in the early 1970s were unsuccessful. However, after observing their success in the USSR, Bores performed the first RK procedures in the US in 1978.

Though the procedure was initially quite controversial, interest grew and the National Eye Institute (NEI) was motivated to step in and fund the Prospective Evaluation of Radial Keratotomy (PERK) Study [49]. The PERK Study began in 1980 as a 5-year, multi-centre, self-controlled clinical trial to evaluate the safety and efficacy of radial keratotomy in the treatment of physiologic myopia. Though limited by its narrow range of surgical variables, the PERK Study's high rate of retention and well-controlled data collection provided valuable information on the natural history of incisional refractive surgery.

The 1980s and early 1990s found many investigators refining different aspects of the procedure. Salz [36], Jester [15], Lindstrom [22], Duffey [10] and others developed human cadaver eye models to study the effects of incisional zone diameter, length, depth and pattern on the reduction of myopia and astigmatism. Deitz [7] first incorporated the patient's age into the list of variables that determined the surgical incision pattern. Lindstrom [1, 21] continued to investigate the correction of astigmatism with arcuate, transverse, and trapezoidal incisions. Casebeer [5], in addition to using age as a variable in his nomograms, expanded the range of optical zones, incorporated astigmatic correc-

tion, embraced the concept of surgical enhancement, and developed a bidirectional blade to safely incorporate the benefits of Russian and American techniques. These advances helped to increase the accuracy, safety and predictability of refractive keratotomy, but as experience grew, several problems inherent in the surgical procedure became apparent.

By the mid-1990s, the complications of hyperopic drift, diurnal variation, glare, and variability of response were well known. At this same time, excimer laser refractive surgery emerged from the earlier technique of automated lamellar keratoplasty. Though initially much more expensive, PRK and LASIK saw rapid technological advances and soon their advantages became readily apparent. By the late 1990s, they had replaced refractive keratotomy as the dominant technique for the surgical correction of refractive error. Though currently in limited use, incisional corneal surgery remains a useful tool in the surgeon's repertoire of refractive procedures.

14.3
Principles of Refractive Keratotomy

Corneal incisions behave as if tissue was added, increasing the radius of curvature perpendicular to the incision. Radial incisions increase corneal circumference in the mid-periphery and, since the cornea is otherwise fixed at the limbus, cause a compensatory flattening of the central cornea (Fig. 14.1a, b). Since this central flattening decreases the corneal refractive power, the technique has been used to reduce myopia. The relative reduction in corneal power increases with the length, depth and number of incisions (Fig. 14.2a, b). Radial cuts that extend more toward the anterior cornea produce a smaller central clear zone (also called the optical zone), but have a greater flattening effect. Increasing the number of incisions causes a proportional decrease in the corneal refractive power, although this relationship is not linear.

Arcuate and transverse incisions (Fig. 14.3) increase the radius of curvature along the meridian perpendicular to their location, resulting in flattening of the meridian and a reduction in its refractive power. In addition to flattening along the

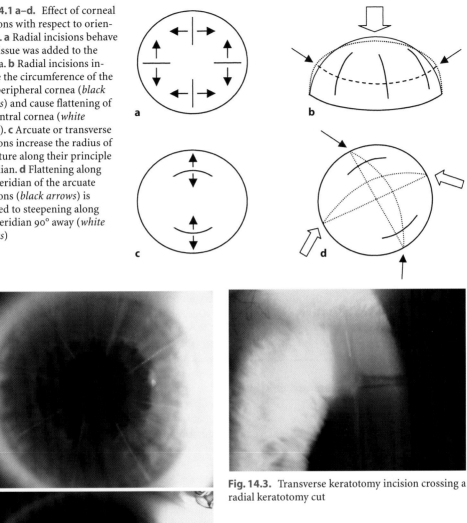

Fig. 14.1 a–d. Effect of corneal incisions with respect to orientation. **a** Radial incisions behave as if tissue was added to the cornea. **b** Radial incisions increase the circumference of the mid-peripheral cornea (*black arrows*) and cause flattening of the central cornea (*white arrow*). **c** Arcuate or transverse incisions increase the radius of curvature along their principle meridian. **d** Flattening along the meridian of the arcuate incisions (*black arrows*) is coupled to steepening along the meridian 90° away (*white arrows*)

Fig. 14.3. Transverse keratotomy incision crossing a radial keratotomy cut

Fig. 14.2 a, b. Radial keratotomy. **a** Eight-incision RK with a single transverse incision crossing the 12:30 cut. Note that the 1:30 incision contains several epithelial cysts which appear as *white dots* along the line of the cut. **b** Four-incision RC with slightly decentered optical zone

principle meridian, the cornea steepens along the meridian 90° away (Fig. 14.1 c,d). This concept has been called coupling and was described by Thornton in his restatement of Gauss's law of elastic domes. Thornton's "law of modified living elastic domes" states that the change in the perpendicular meridian is proportional to the change in the primary meridian reduced by the increase in circumference [44]. Such behaviour is analogous to a cross cylinder change in the corneal refractive power and is usually described as the ratio of flattening in the primary meridian to steepening in the orthogonal meridian. A coupling ratio of 1:1 produces equal and opposite changes along the perpendicular meridians and thus has no effect on the spherical equivalent.

The flattening effect of arcuate and transverse keratotomy (AK and TK) increases with incision number, length and depth. Arcuate incisions have a slightly greater effect than transverse incisions because their actual length is about 10 % greater along the curve [4]. In addition, anterior incisions will also have more effect than peripheral incisions for a given arc length. The coupling ratio can be highly variable, but generally increases with the distance from the limbus (i.e. more anterior incisions produce more flattening relative to steepening). The coupling effect is reduced in the presence of radial incisions, which limit the transmission of coupling forces through the corneal tissue.

Summary for the Clinician

- Corneal incisions increase the radius of curvature perpendicular to the incision
- Coupling is the ratio of flattening in the primary meridian to steepening in the orthogonal meridian

14.4
Techniques of Refractive Keratotomy [5]

Current techniques of refractive keratotomy utilise precision diamond blades to achieve predictable and reproducible incision profiles. Diamond blades may be of fixed or adjustable length and generally have a protective guide that slides along the corneal surface with little resistance. Adjustable knives have built-in micrometers that determine the length of blade exposed beyond the protective foot plates. Initially calibrated with pre-set coin-shaped gauge blocks, blades were later adjusted under specially designed microscopes for increased accuracy. Corneal markers are used to delineate the location and length of the radial, arcuate and transverse incisions. They are centred on the visual axis or pupil, depending on the chosen technique. The horizontal or vertical axis of the cornea is marked with the patient sitting up to account for the ocular torsion that may occur when the patient lies down. This helps to minimise error in the placement of AK and TK incisions.

Historically, radial keratotomy has evolved through three basic styles. The first was the "Russian" technique where incisions began at the limbus and were directed toward the central cornea in a centripetal manner. The Russian blade (Fig. 14.4a) cuts with its vertical edge, creating a uniformly deep incision with a nearly perpendicular profile at its anterior termination. Though it produces good results, the Russian style carries the risk of inadvertent extension into the visual axis. The "American" or centrifugal technique uses a slanted blade (Fig. 14.4b) and cuts from the edge of the central optical zone toward the limbus. While it carries less risk of cutting through the visual axis, the American style tends to compress the central corneal tissue, producing non-uniform incision profiles that are rounded near the central cornea. The "double-pass" technique was later developed to combine the advantages of the Russian and American styles. The double-pass blade (Fig. 14.4c) has a fully cutting slanted edge and an opposite vertical edge that is only sharp near the tip. The first half of the double-pass cut is of the American style in a centrifugal direction. After reaching the limbus, the blade is directed back toward the corneal centre (Russian style) within the same incision. The sharp vertical tip refines the incision profile, while the dull vertical portion protects against extension into the visual axis. Blade depth is usually set to 100 % of the ultrasonic pachymetry measurement at the edge of the optical zone for all three techniques.

Blades used for AK or TK (Fig. 14.4d) often have a rectangular shape and are trifaceted, with sharpened edges on the end and each side. The flat blade profile creates a "rudder-like" effect, which facilitates the arcuate movement of the knife. When the blade is introduced into the cornea, this flat profile creates significant tissue compression causing the incision depth to be less than the blade setting. For this reason, blade depth is often set to levels greater than the ultrasonic pachymetry measurements taken at the incision location.

Summary for the Clinician

- Russian style or centrifugal incisions produce a more uniform profile, while American style or centripetal incisions are safer
- The cornea should be marked with the patient sitting up to minimise the error in astigmatic keratotomy secondary to ocular rotation

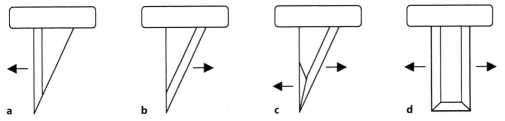

Fig. 14.4 a–d. Refractive keratotomy blade styles. **a** Russian, vertical cutting edge. **b** American, slanted cutting edge. **c** Dual pass, slanted, full cutting and partial, vertical cutting edge. **d** Arcuate blade with rectangular profile

Table 14.1. Data from the 5-year follow-up of the PERK Study

Patients (*n*)		Eyes		Follow-up	Patient age
Total	@ 5-Year follow-up (%)	Total	@ 5-Year follow-up (%)	Years (mean ±SD)	Years (mean ±SD)
435	413 (95%)	793	757 (95%)	5.2±0.6 (range 3–6.3)	33±7.3 (range 21–58)

Table 14.2. Summary of the results for the PERK Study at the 5-year follow-up evaluation

Pre-operative SE range (diopters)		Lower (−2.00 to −3.12)	Middle (−3.25 to −4.37)	Higher (−4.50 to −8.00)	Total (−2.00 to −8.00)
Number of patients @ 5 years		124	140	149	413
Number of eyes @ 5 years		234	271	252	757
UCVA (% eyes)	≥20/20	75%	63%	43%	60%
	≥20/40	95%	89%	79%	88%
	≥20/160	99%	98%	94%	97%
SE (dioptres, mean ±SD)		+0.34±1.08	+0.06±1.30	−0.55±1.75	
Δ SE (dioptres, mean ±SD)		+2.92±1.10	+3.84±1.35	+5.11±1.79	+3.98±1.69
SE (% eyes)	−1.00 to +1.00	75%	67%	49%	64%
	>+1.00	18%	20%	14%	17%
	<−1.00	7%	13%	37%	19%
Bilateral RK	Number of patients	98	115	119	332
	No correction Worn	85 (87%)	70 (61%)	60 (50%)	215 (65%)
BCVA (number of eyes)	Lost ≥2 lines	25 (3%)	–	–	–
	Lost 1 line	106 (14%)	–	–	–
	No change	348 (46%)	–	–	–
	Gained 1 line	241 (32%)	–	–	–
	Gained ≥2 lines	32 (4%)	–	–	–

Table 14.3. Results of five clinical studies in radial keratotomy. The studies differ in technique, blade style, incision pattern, and astigmatism correction, but illustrate the range of results found in the literature. In general, lower levels of preoperative myopia had better refractive and visual outcomes

		Studies [50]	[2]	[39]	[7]	[54]
Patients (n)		427	101	107	458	128
Eyes (n)		793	156	198	972	241
Percentage of eyes reported		87	67	79	68	78
Age (years)	Mean ±SD	33±7.3	NR	33±9.6	34.2	39
	Range	21–58	NR	19–75	18–62	22–62
Follow-up (years)	Mean ±SD	10.1±1.0	5.2	4.85	1.2	3.0
	Range	4.9–11.8	4.7–6.4	3.0–6.3	0.75–1.25	2.5–3.7
Surgical data						
Protocol		PERK	Fyodorov	Fyodorov	Kansas City	Casebeer
Dates		1982–88	1980–81	1980–81	1982–85	1990–92
Incisions	Primary (n)	8	8 or 16	8 or 16	8	4–8
	Maximum (n)	16	16	16	10–16	16
Blade style	Style	American Diamond	Russian Metal	Russian Metal	American Metal	Russian Diamond
Clear zone diameter (mm)		3.0–4.5	3.0–5.0	3.0–5.0	2.7–6.0	2.5–5.0
Age in nomogram		No	No	No	Yes	Yes
Astigmatism correction		No	Yes	Yes	No	Yes
Bilateral (%)		78	54	85	NR	88
Enhancement (%)		12	58	NR	0.6	37
Pre-operative myopia						
CR SE (D)	Mean ±SD	−3.47±NR	−5.00±2.90	−4.40±1.90	−4.40±1.90	−4.07±1.89
	Range	−2.00 to −8.00	−16.00 to −1.50	−10.38 to −1.50	−11.88 to −0.62	+0.25 to −9.62
Treatment groups (D)	Lower	−2.00 to −3.12	−1.50 to −16.00	−1.50 to −2.88	−0.62 to −3.00	+0.25 to −3.12
	Middle	−3.25 to −4.38		−3.00 to −5.88	−3.12 to −6.00	−3.25 to −4.38
	Higher	−4.50 to −8.00		−6.00 to −10.38	−6.00 to −10.25	−4.50 to −9.62
Post-operative results						
CR SE	Mean ±SD	+0.51±1.64	+0.30±2.12	−0.50±2.00	+0.09±1.20	+0.45±0.76
	Range	−4.88 to +6.25	−9.50 to +6.75	−7.62 to +5.00	−5.62 to +9.00	−1.00 to +4.13
CE SE (%)	−0.50 to +0.50 D	38	NR	NR	NR	66
	−1.00 to +1.00 D	60	53	56	76	84
	>+1.00 D	23	33	15	12	NR
	<−1.00 D	17	14	29	12	NR

Table 14.3. Continued

		Studies [50]	[2]	[39]	[7]	[54]
UCVA 20/20 (%)	Total	53	37	7	47	55
	Lower	66	NR	11	65	60
	Middle	50	NR	7	44	64
	Higher	43	NR	0	30	46
UCVA 20/40 (%)	Total	85	76	62	88	96
	Lower	92	NR	75	96	98
	Middle	86	NR	65	89	100
	Higher	77	NR	36	77	93
BCVA Loss (%)	1 Line	15	8	19	NR	1
	2 Lines	3	6	10	2	3

NR, not reported.

14.5 Major Clinical Trials in Refractive Keratotomy

The PERK Study [50] was the first large clinical investigation into the safety and efficacy of incisional refractive surgery. The nine-centre, self-controlled study was funded by the NEI in 1980 and enrolled 435 patients with physiologic myopia ranging from –2.00 to –8.00 dioptres (D). Astigmatic correction was not attempted and re-operations were discouraged during the first year after the procedure. The study adhered to a strict surgical technique of eight-incision radial keratotomy. Patients were divided into three groups by their baseline cycloplegic refractive error: "lower" with –2.00 to –3.12 D, "middle" with –3.25 to –4.37 D, and "higher" with –4.50 to –8.00 D of myopia. The central optical or clear zone was the only surgical variable adjusted for each patient group and was 4.0 mm for the lower group, 3.5 mm for the middle group, and 3.0 for the higher group. A diamond knife was used to create the RK incisions, which were centred on the line of sight. Blade depth was set to 100 % of the thinnest of four ultrasonic pachymetry measurements made at the edge of the central clear zone at 3, 6, 9, and 12 o'clock. The blade setting was verified with a calibration block and incisions were centrifugal or American in style. Topical anaesthesia was used and post-operative medications consisted of a topical antibiotic and cycloplegic, but no steroids. Surgery on the second eye was delayed for at least 1 year and re-operations consisted of eight more RK incisions placed between the original eight cuts.

The 5-year results for the PERK Study [51] are summarised in Tables 14.1 and 14.2. The study achieved high retention rates, with 95 % of eyes available for follow-up during the 5-year post-operative period. Uncorrected visual acuities (UCVA) of 20/40 or greater were achieved in 88 % of eyes. A total of 64 % had spherical equivalent (SE) cycloplegic refractions within 1 D of emmetropia. In general, results improved as the level of preoperative myopia decreased. In all, 76 % of patients elected to have surgery on their second eye and 65 % of these patients wore no spectacle or contact lens correction at 5 years.

The procedure proved to be safe with only 3% (25 patients) losing two lines or more in best-corrected visual acuity (BCVA). Of these patients, 18 still had BCVAs of at least 20/20 and 24 were correctable to 20/40 or better. The remaining patient developed a cataract and lost seven lines of BCVA.

The PERK Study provided a reliable database for the outcomes of a single, well-defined technique of radial keratotomy. It also established a standard for the future evaluation of newer refractive surgical procedures and techniques. Several fundamental principles came to light early in the PERK Study, the most significant of which was the effect of age on the refractive response to surgery. Although not factored into the study's surgical plan, age was the only patient variable that predictably affected the outcome of RK. The results from PERK and other studies showed that older patients received 0.70–1.00 D of greater effect per decade of life for a given optical zone and incision number. Eyes with 5 D of myopia or less achieved better UCVA and lower residual refractive error. The ideal post-operative refraction was found to be −0.50 to −1.00 D. This residual myopia allowed good UCVA, delayed the onset of symptomatic presbyopia, offset hyperopic drift and maintained the refractive state to which the patient was accustomed. Though praised for its methodology, quality of data acquisition and retention rate, the study had several weaknesses, such as lack of age consideration, limited optical zone selection, lack of astigmatism correction, use of the American incision style and discouragement of enhancements.

The technique of RK continued to evolve during and after the PERK Study, as the procedure became more popular. In the mid-to-late 1980s, the range of myopic correction was reduced (typically −1.50 to −6.00 D) and age became a major component in surgical planning. Diamond blade depth was set under a microscope, as incisions became deeper (90%–95%) and were centred on the undilated pupil. The Russian technique increased in popularity, after it was found to produce incisions of more uniform depth and profile. Fewer cuts were used in the initial correction of low-to-moderate myopia, with under-correction as the target and future enhancement anticipated.

Several studies ran concurrently with the PERK Study or followed in the literature, though none equalled its scale and control. Some incorporated the concepts learned from the PERK protocol and included astigmatism correction via radial, arcuate or transverse keratotomy. The results of five studies [2, 7, 39, 52, 54] with large enrolments and/or long follow-up are shown in Table 14.3. Although they differ in RK technique, surgical instrument choice, and treatment range, some important points can be seen with their comparison. All of these studies reduced myopia, as illustrated by the difference in the mean pre- and post-operative spherical equivalents (SE). However, the standard deviation for the post-operative mean SE was wide, indicating that it was often difficult to reach emmetropia on an individual basis. The proportion of patients within 1 D of emmetropia ranged from 53% to 84%, while 62%–96% obtained uncorrected visual acuities of 20/40 or better (20/20 vision was achieved in seven to 55%). In general, patients with lower levels of preoperative myopia achieved better uncorrected visual acuities with less residual refractive error.

Using the Casebeer technique, the Werblin study [54] achieved the best results. The Casebeer technique employed many of the principles learned through the evolution of RK. Age and refractive error were used to determine the size of the optical zone and number of incisions. Fewer incisions were made during the initial procedure, with a target of mild myopia. Arcuate incisions were used for the correction of astigmatism. Surgical enhancement was embraced as a means of titrating incision length and number to achieve higher rates of emmetropia. Diamond blades were calibrated under a microscope and the Russian (and later, double-pass) incision style resulted in predictable depths with smoother profiles.

Summary for the Clinician

- Older patients received 0.70–1.00 D of greater effect per decade of life for a given optical zone and incision number

14.6
Complications of Refractive Keratotomy

Although multiple studies have demonstrated the safety and efficacy of RK, long-term follow-up has revealed several complications inherent to the procedure. The most significant of these result from the biomechanical changes induced in the cornea. They include hyperopic drift and diurnal fluctuation in visual acuity.

14.6.1
Hyperopic Drift

A gradual shift toward hyperopia occurs in 20%–50% of eyes following RK. The 10-year results from the PERK Study showed that 43% of eyes underwent a spontaneous hyperopic shift by ≥1.00 D between the 6-month and 10-year post-operative evaluations. Deitz [8] and Arrowsmith [2] found similar shifts in 54% and 22% of their patients, respectively. The PERK study's mean post-operative refractive error increased from −0.36±1.09 D at 6 months to +0.51±1.64 D after 10 years, reflecting a mean change of +0.87 D. The rate of hyperopic drift decreased after 2 years from 0.21±0.02 D/year to 0.06±0.004 D/year (Fig. 14.5). This lower average rate of change agreed with the rate found by Deitz between follow-up examinations at 3.7 and 8.5 years.

Though the hyperopic shift progressed slowly, the PERK data showed no evidence of a plateau and Deitz documented continued progression as far as 12 years after surgery. The maximum refractive change in the PERK study at 10 years was +6.37 D, while the Deitz study had a peak change of +3.75 D from the 1-year to the 8.5-year evaluation. PERK patients with higher levels of myopia who received longer incisions (smaller central clear zone) displayed larger post-operative shifts in refractive error. No correlation was found with other variables, such as age and intraocular pressure. Werblin [53] found higher rates of late hyperopic shift (1–3 years after surgery) in patients with higher levels of preoperative myopia (>6.0 D). While his patients with lower preoperative myopia

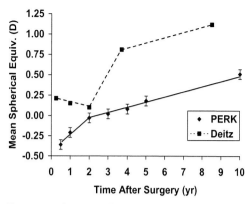

Fig. 14.5. Change in the mean spherical equivalent of the cycloplegic refraction over time for the PERK Study [52] from 6 months to 10 years and for the Deitz Study [8] from 3 months to 8.5 years. Both studies show a progressive shift toward hyperopia that does not plateau. The rate of the hyperopic shift (0.06 D/year) is similar in both studies after approximately 4 years

tended toward a plateau in their rate of refractive change, the higher myopes demonstrated no such levelling. For patients under-corrected following their initial surgery, some hyperopic drift may be advantageous, as it brings them closer to emmetropia. However, patients with little post-operative refractive error or early presbyopia may experience increasing difficulty and dissatisfaction as they progress beyond emmetropia into hyperopia.

14.6.2
Diurnal Fluctuation

Diurnal fluctuation in visual acuity, cycloplegic refraction, keratometry and corneal topography has been well documented following RK. Published rates have ranged from 2% to 60% [40]. In a subset of patients available for examination 11 years after surgery in the PERK Study [31], the mean change in the SE of the CR was found to be −0.31±0.58 D from morning to evening. The diurnal shift was myopic in 97% of eyes, with a magnitude greater than 0.50 D in 51% and a peak change of −1.62 D. The refractive cylinder increased by more than 0.50 D in 31% of patients. Central corneal steepening of 0.50–1.94 D, as measured by keratometry, was seen in 35%. A total of 13% experienced a 2–7 Snellen line decrease in their uncorrected visual acuity. In the patients with bilateral RK, these changes were found to be highly symmetrical. It should be noted that this set of patients was somewhat biased.

Corneal topography was examined in another set of PERK patients 10 years after RK [16]. This group showed a mean increase in myopia of 0.36±0.58 D from the morning to the evening. The average corneal power calculated from the topographic data increased by 0.52±0.45 D, reflecting a steepening in the corneal shape. These changes correlated with the change in manifest SE, as well as the best spectacle-corrected visual acuity. It should be noted that the patient populations included in the above studies were biased toward those with a functional complaint. Depending on their baseline refractive error, patients may note worsening or improvement in their uncorrected vision. For example, hyperopes may note better distance vision as they shift toward emmetropia, while patients with residual myopia may describe worsening acuity as the day progresses. Early presbyopes may complain of reading difficulty in the morning, which resolves in the afternoon or evening. This fluctuation is often frustrating to patients and can be difficult to manage if they rely on spectacle correction.

14.6.3
Other Complications

Other complications seen with RK include loss of contrast sensitivity (CS) and glare. Some studies have shown significant decreases in contrast sensitivity [30, 46], especially in the early post-operative period, while others have shown no significant change. Ginsburg published CS results for a subset of PERK patients approximately 1 year after surgery. Under photopic conditions, they found no clinically meaningful loss of CS in operated versus unoperated eyes of the same patient. However, they did show a statistically significant decrease in CS for higher spatial frequencies (12 and 18 cycles per degree),

though the measurements were still within the normal range. Eyes with RK tended toward lower CS when the pupil size equalled or exceeded the size of the central clear zone, but this was not statistically significant. Patients with smaller clear zones had more subjective complaints and also trended toward a decrease in CS.

Patients who complained of glare on psychometric testing showed significant losses in CS at middle and higher spatial frequencies. However, no correlation was found between the psychometric glare index and the CS function. Glare complaints did not correlate with the level of preoperative myopia and were attributed to a loss in visual quality from the RK. It should be noted that this testing was performed under photopic conditions. Many post-RK patients note symptoms of glare under conditions of dim illumination, such as night driving. Contrast sensitivity may decrease under these conditions as the pupil dilates beyond the clear zone and the RK incisions play a greater role in scattering light.

The introduction of excimer laser refractive surgery in the mid-1990s led to a precipitous decline in the use of RK as the primary means of surgically correcting myopia. However, Damiano and associates [6] used RK to treat residual myopia following LASIK in patients whose corneal pachymetry was too thin to permit laser-based enhancement. Their series of 60 eyes in 41 patients had a mean reduction in spherical equivalent from –8.09 D to –0.43 D, following both procedures. A total of 41% achieved an UCVA ≥20/20, while 94% were greater than or equal to 20/40. No eye lost more than two lines in BCVA. In this study, RK improved the refractive results in a patient population that could not be managed with LASIK alone.

The efficacy of both PRK and LASIK is superior to that of RK, with improved visual outcomes, higher predictability and increased patient satisfaction. Unfortunately, even with their excellent safety profiles, these procedures are not risk-free. Well-documented complications of LASIK include infection, diffuse lamellar keratitis, poorly cut flaps, flap striae, post-operative ectasia and the need for corneal transplantation. In addition, PRK may induce subepithelial haze and both procedures are subject to under- and overcorrection, as well as mild myopic regression with time.

In certain applications, refractive keratotomy can provide a low-cost and low-risk alternative to excimer laser surgery for the management of refractive error. Perhaps the most common use of incisional corneal surgery today lies in the reduction of astigmatism.

Summary for the Clinician

- A gradual shift toward hyperopia occurs in 20 %–50 % of eyes following radial keratotomy
- A morning-to-evening shift toward myopia, with associated corneal steepening, is seen in a subset of RK patients

14.7
Refractive Keratotomy for the Management of Astigmatism

Although regular astigmatism can be corrected with spectacles or contact lenses, even with optimal correction, patients may continue to experience asthenopia, meridional magnification, off-axis blur and visual field restriction [4, 44]. Irregular astigmatism can be improved with rigid gas permeable contact lenses; however, many patients are contact lens-intolerant or lack the manual dexterity required for their use. For these reasons, surgical methods are often sought for the reduction of astigmatism.

The ideal candidate for the surgical management of astigmatism was characterised by Lindstrom and coauthors [27]. They described a patient with astigmatism in excess of 2.0 D, whose fellow eye has less than 1.5 D of astigmatism, astigmatism at a different meridian or a similar level and meridian of astigmatism, but is also scheduled for cataract surgery. If the fellow eye is similar in astigmatic power and location, surgical correction may be unnecessary. The surgeon's primary goal should be to preserve the preoperative corneal asphericity, reduce small amounts of preoperative astigmatism or reduce large amounts of astigmatism without shifting the meridian [18].

Since PRK and LASIK can treat myopic, hyperopic, and mixed astigmatism, they are typically the procedures of choice for healthy eyes, without contraindication, that fall within their treatment ranges. However, in eyes with cataracts, corneal transplants, or other issues that could reduce the efficacy and safety of laser treatment, refractive keratotomy can be an effective and low-cost option for surgically reducing astigmatism. Procedures that fall under the umbrella of astigmatic refractive keratotomy include adjusting the cataract incision placement, opposite clear corneal incisions (CCI), arcuate keratotomy (AK), transverse keratotomy (TK) and limbal or peripheral corneal relaxing incisions (LRI/PCRIs).

14.7.1
Cataract Incision Placement

Clear corneal incisions (CCIs) made during cataract surgery have been known to induce astigmatism by flattening the meridian on which the incision is centred. The amount of this surgically induced astigmatism (SIA) varies with incision length and placement. Pfleger [32] examined 103 consecutive eyes following temporal CCI cataract surgery with incision sizes of 3.2 mm (Group A), 4.0 mm (Group B), and 5.2 mm (Group C). The mean SIA at 1 year following surgery was found to be 0.09 D, 0.26 D and 0.54 D in Groups A through C, respectively. A shift in the meridian of astigmatism greater than 30° was seen in 14 % of Group A patients, 24 % of Group B, and 27 % of Group C. Kohnen and colleagues [19] also compared the SIA created by temporal, two-step CCIs of varying size. They studied 60 eyes of 60 patients with incision sizes of 3.5 mm (Group A, self-sealing), 4.0 mm (Group B, self-sealing), and 5.0 mm (Group C, single radial suture). At 6 months after surgery, the mean SIA was found to be 0.37±0.14 D in Group A, 0.56±0.34 D in Group B, and 0.70±0.50 D in Group C.

Masket [29] compared 45 eyes following phacoemulsification cataract extraction performed through a 3.0×2.5-mm temporal CCI, without enlargement. Vector analysis of corneal topography and simulated keratotomy showed approximately 0.5 D of SIA, with less than 0.25 D observed in the surgical meridian. Corneal topography was stable by 2 weeks following surgery. Vass and Menapace [47] measured 0.28–0.53 D of temporal flattening in 20 patients with 3.0 mm temporal CCIs. When compared with normal controls, the cataract surgery patients showed no associated nasal flattening or vertical steepening. He and colleagues [13] found no significant change in astigmatism at 3 months following cataract surgery through a 2.8-mm CCI.

Based on these and other studies, approximately 0.0–0.5 D of SIA can be expected from temporal CCIs less than or equal to 3.2 mm. If available, corneal topography is recommended as part of the standard pre-cataract surgery evaluation. If the topographic and keratometric astigmatism are against-the-rule (ATR), consider centring the temporal CCI along the steep meridian. In right eyes, this can easily be accomplished for steep meridians falling between 150 and 30°. Left eyes are more difficult, with a comfortable range of 0–30°.

Summary for the Clinician

- Temporal clear corneal incisions less than 3.2 mm produce 0.0–0.50 D of flattening along the meridian of the wound

14.7.2
Opposite Clear Corneal Incisions

Given the flattening effect of CCIs described above, Lever and Dahan [25] proposed that a similar incision placed opposite to the temporal CCI might enhance the flattening effect along the steep meridian. Opposite CCIs were placed in 33 eyes of 26 patients with pre-existing astigmatism greater than 1.75 D (mean 2.81±0.74 D, range 2.00–5.00 D). The steepest meridian was identified and two straight stab incisions were made parallel to the iris plane with a diamond keratome. In patients with ATR astigmatism, the incisions were placed at 3:00 and 9:00. The temporal incision was used for cataract surgery, while the nasal incision was not used. CCIs were located at 6:00 and 12:00 in patients who had with-the-rule (WTR) astigmatism. Cataract

surgery was performed through the superior wound and the inferior wound was left alone. Oblique astigmatism was treated in a similar manner, with the surgeon choosing the most comfortable location. Incision length varied from 2.8 to 3.5 mm, depending on the level of pre-operative astigmatism (no nomogram was provided). The mean post-operative astigmatism was reduced to 0.75±0.60 D (range plano to +1.75 D) at a mean follow-up of 5.4 months (range 1–12 months). Vector analysis showed a mean astigmatism correction of 2.25 D. The opposite CCI wounds were well sealed on postoperative day 1 and no complications were noted, although the follow-up was limited.

The procedure effectively reduces astigmatism; however, it carries additional risk associated with the extra penetrating corneal wound. Careful early postoperative management is essential. Given the age-dependent results of refractive keratotomy, one might expect similar behaviour with this technique, but this was not addressed. Although CCIs can reduce astigmatism, their range is limited. Partial thickness, arcuate or transverse corneal incisions provide a means for correcting higher levels of astigmatism.

14.7.3
Arcuate and Transverse Keratotomy

Arcuate and transverse relaxing incisions have been used to treat astigmatism since the earliest days of refractive surgery. Multiple studies have documented the effect of various optical zones and incision lengths on astigmatism reduction and coupling ratio.

The ARC-T Study [33, 34] was a multi-centre, prospective evaluation of single-stage AK for the management of 1–6 D of naturally occurring astigmatism. A total of 160 eyes of 95 patients received standardised AK at a 7-mm optical zone according to a modification of the Lindstrom surgical nomogram [26] (Table 14.4). After 1 month, RK for myopia and second stage AK for residual astigmatism was performed on eyes that needed further correction. The mean refractive cylinder decreased from 2.82 to 0.50 D at 1 month. Of the eyes, 61% had at least

1.0 D of residual astigmatism, while 17% had at least 2.00 D. Eyes that underwent a second surgery averaged 1.60 D of astigmatic reduction for the additional procedure and 2.90 D total.

The coupling ratio, defined as the ratio of flattening in the incised meridian to steepening in the opposite meridian, was 0.95±0.10 for the refractive change and 0.84±0.05 for the keratometric change at 1 month following single-stage AK [11]. Of the patients, 18% lost one line of best spectacle-corrected visual acuity and only 1% (two eyes) lost two lines. Under-correction and over-correction were common. The number of incisions, incision length, age and gender were the factors that predicted increased astigmatic response.

To decrease the risk of overcorrection, Buzard [4] employed a nomogram using shorter and shallower arcuate incisions (Table 14.5). In all, 46 eyes of 29 patients received two arcuate incisions at an optical zone of 7.0 mm with

Table 14.4. ARC-T modification [33] of the Lindstrom nomogram for arcuate keratotomy with a 7.0-mm optical zone. Blade depth is set to 50 μm greater than the ultrasonic pachymetry measured 1.5 mm temporal to the visual axis

Incision		Predicted refractive cylinder change (D)
Number	Length	
1	45	0.02 × age (years) + 0.40
2	30	0.02 × age (years) + 0.40
1	60	0.03 × age (years) + 0.60
1	90	0.04 × age (years) + 0.80
2	45	0.04 × age (years) + 0.80
2	60	0.06 × age (years) + 1.20
2	90	0.08 × age (years) + 1.60

lengths of 45, 60, or 90°. Blade depth was set to 80% of the pachymetry measurement at the incision location. Of the eyes 50% received enhancement for under-correction by deepening and lengthening the incisions. The mean preoperative refractive astigmatism of 3.41±1.44 D (range 1.25–7.75 D) was reduced to 1.30±1.00 D (range 0.00–5.50 D) at 6 months following surgery. The mean changes in keratometric astigmatism for the 45-, 60-, and 90-degree incisions were 1.66±0.64 D, 2.69±1.24 D, and 2.83±1.04 D, respectively. Two patients (4%) were overcorrected with axis shifts of 51 and 105°. All patients had a reduction in their astigmatism; however, the large standard deviations illustrate the variable response that can be seen with AK, even with conservative nomograms and planned enhancements.

Arcuate incisions have been combined with cataract surgery to reduce pre-existing astigmatism. Titiyal and colleagues [45] prospectively evaluated the effect of paired, intraoperative AK incisions placed at a 7-mm optical zone during phacoemulsification cataract surgery through a 3.5-mm CCI at the steep meridian. A total of 17 eyes of 14 patients received AK incisions combined with cataract surgery, while 17 eyes of 14 other patients formed a control group receiving cataract surgery alone. The AK group showed a mean reduction in astigmatism of 1.26±0.54 D as compared to the control group, which showed a decrease of 0.48±0.60 D. The coupling ratio was 1.10±0.43 in the AK group versus 0.82±0.38 in the controls. Thus, AK combined with cataract surgery proved more effective than cataract surgery alone in reducing pre-existing astigmatism.

Arcuate corneal incisions have also been used following penetrating keratoplasty (PKP) [35]. They are typically placed anterior to the

Table 14.5. Buzard nomogram for arcuate keratotomy with a 7.0-mm optical zone. Blade depth is set to 80% of the ultrasonic pachymetry measured at the incision location

Length	20	25	30	35	40	45	50	55	60	65	70	75	80
45	1.70	1.85	2.00	2.15	2.30	2.45	2.60	2.75	2.90	3.05	3.20	3.35	3.50
60	2.78	2.78	3.00	3.23	3.45	3.68	3.90	4.13	4.35	4.58	4.80	5.03	5.25
90	3.70	3.70	4.00	4.30	4.60	4.90	5.20	5.50	5.80	6.10	6.40	6.70	7.00

graft–host junction at optical zones of 5–7 mm, and can range in length from 45° to 90°. Published nomograms (for example, Table 14.4) for AK incisions should be applied conservatively, as corneal forces can behave unpredictably when influenced by the annular scar of the graft–host junction. While the astigmatic response to AK incisions is variable in normal eyes, it can be highly unpredictable in eyes with corneal transplants. Corneal topography can be helpful in directing incision placement and relative length. Incisions should be centred on the visual axis, even if the graft is decentred. Optical zones less than 5 mm should be avoided because the incisions may induce irregular astigmatism. In cases of high post-PKP astigmatism, the effect of AK incisions can be augmented by compression sutures placed 90° away from the steep meridian.

Finally, AK has been used as an adjunct procedure for the management of residual astigmatism following PRK and LASIK. Kapadia analysed the effect of paired AK incisions performed before PRK in 37 eyes with astigmatism 1.50 D and after PRK in 86 eyes with +0.75 D. In the AK-before-PRK group, mean astigmatism decreased from 2.40±0.6 D (range 1.00–4.00 D) to 0.60±0.60 D (range 0.0–2.25 D) following the incisional surgery. The AK-after-PRK group showed a reduction from 1.50±0.60 D to 0.40±0.40 D, with a vector change in the axis of 65±68°. AK enhancement was performed in 16% of eyes that had AK before PRK and in 21% of eyes that had AK after PRK. Coupling was less predictable at high levels of astigmatism. In either case, stability of the first procedure should be documented before performing the second procedure.

Though AK can effectively reduce astigmatism, several disadvantages have limited its use. Response to the procedure can be unpredictable and over-correction may result in a shift of the astigmatic axis, which can be poorly tolerated. As the optical zone decreases, incisions placed closer to the visual axis may induce glare and/or irregular astigmatism. These factors have led to the placement of arcuate incisions in the peripheral cornea, thereby decreasing the risk of complications.

Summary for the Clinician

- Arcuate keratotomy effectively reduces astigmatism alone, combined with cataract surgery, or following penetrating keratoplasty
- Arcuate keratotomy may be unpredictable, with creation of irregular astigmatism, a shift in the astigmatic axis, and induction of glare

14.7.4
Peripheral Corneal Relaxing Incisions

Limbal relaxing incisions (LRIs) form a subset of AK where incisions are made in the peripheral cornea. Some advocate the term "peripheral corneal relaxing incisions" (PCRIs), since they are placed slightly anterior to the corneal limbus. Because they have several advantages when compared to AK and TK, Gills and other authors have championed the use of PCRIs to correct astigmatism during cataract surgery. These advantages include preservation of the optical quality of the cornea, decreased risk of glare induction, reduced postoperative discomfort, a more consistent 1:1 coupling ratio, less potential for overcorrection, a lower risk of axis shift and a decreased likelihood of irregular astigmatism.

Wang, Misra and Koch [48] retrospectively analysed the efficacy of PCRIs placed at the end of cataract surgery in 115 eyes of 94 patients. Blade depth was fixed at 600 μm and incisions were centred on the steep corneal meridian, just anterior to the limbal vessels. Patients with pre-existing, keratometric WTR astigmatism of 0.75 D or ATR astigmatism 1.0 D were included in the study. The Koch nomogram used age and preoperative keratometric astigmatism to titrate the PCRI length and number. When paired incisions were placed along the horizontal meridian, the CCI was incorporated into the PCRI. Limbal landmarks were noted and the cornea was marked with the patient sitting upright to permit accurate, intra-operative location of the steep meridian. Eyes receiving PCRIs were compared to a control group undergoing CCI phacoemulsification cataract surgery alone. Astigmatism changes were computed along the meridian of the PCRI(s) (with-the-wound, WTW) and the meridian 90° away (against-the-wound, ATW) using the Holladay-Cravy-Koch formula.

The control group showed an overall mean reduction in astigmatism relative to the CCI of -0.17 ± 0.48 D (-0.31 ± 0.39 D for right eyes and -0.07 ± 0.65 D for left eyes). The mean age of patients receiving PCRIs was 69 ± 12 years. At 4 months following surgery, patients with preoperative WTR astigmatism and a single 6.0-mm PCRI showed a reduction in WTW-ATW astigmatism of -0.55 ± 0.67 D. Paired 6.0-mm incisions induced a larger mean astigmatic reduction of -1.18 ± 0.91 D in the WTR group. Eyes with preoperative ATR astigmatism had mean WTW-ATW changes of -2.18 ± 0.91 D, -2.02 ± 0.60 D, and -2.72 ± 0.61 D for single 4.5-mm, single 6.0-mm, and paired 6.0-mm PCRIs, respectively. All astigmatic changes were statistically significant when compared to the changes in the control group. WTW-ATW values decreased with increasing age and with increasing magnitude of preoperative WTR astigmatism. No such correlation was found in the group with preoperative ATR astigmatism. The overall percentage of eyes with keratometric astigmatism ≤1.0 D increased from 33% to 75%. Incisions along the horizontal meridian had a greater effect than those along the vertical. Overcorrection occurred in all treatment groups, but increased with the length and number of PCRIs.

In this study, PCRIs effectively reduced astigmatism when combined with cataract surgery. Although they had an acceptable safety profile, the mean treatment benefit was limited to less than 1.2 D in patients who had WTR astigmatism and less than 2.75 D in patients who were ATR. The results of the study were used to modify their PCRI nomogram, which is shown in Table 14.6.

Toric intraocular lenses provide an alternative method for reducing astigmatism in cataract surgery. However, there is only one FDA-approved model available and the range of astigmatism correction is very limited. Gills [12] combined LRIs with toric IOL implantation to reduce higher levels of preoperative astigmatism. Thirteen eyes of 10 patients with astigmatism >2.50 D (mean 5.54 D, range 2.62–7.75 D) received a Staar toric IOL in combination with a single LRI, paired LRIs or an LRI combined with a corneal relaxing incision. All patients had post-operative refractive cylinder ≤0.75D. The mean induced keratometric cylinder was -2.34 ± 0.56 D, while the mean induced refractive cylinder was -3.61 ± 0.48 D. Post-operative uncorrected and best-corrected visual acuities were $\geq20/40$ in 69% and 92% of patients, respectively. BCVA improved by four or more Snellen lines in 38%. While outcomes of the study were good, the mean follow-up was limited to 4 months.

Table 14.6. Koch nomogram for 600-μm deep peripheral corneal relaxing incisions placed at the end of temporal CCI phacoemulsification cataract surgery

	Preoperative astigmatism (D)	Age (years)	PCRIs (n)	Length
WTR	0.75–1.00	<65	2	45°
		≥65	1	45°
	1.01–1.50	<65	2	60°
		≥65	2	45°
	>1.50	<65	2	80°
		≥65	2	60°
ATR/Obl	1.00–1.25	–	1	35°
	1.26–2.00	–	1	45°
	>2.00	–	2	45°

WTR, "with-the-rule" astigmatism; ATR/Obl, "against-the-rule" or oblique astigmatism.

Koch and Sanan [17] used PCRIs to treat residual astigmatism following PRK in four eyes and LASIK in two eyes. Two patients received single relaxing incisions with a reduction in the refractive cylinder from 1.40–0.50 D at 1 month. Topographic astigmatism decreased from 1.30–1.10 D over this same interval. In the four patients that received paired incisions, refractive astigmatism was reduced from 1.40 to 0.50 D and the topographic astigmatism from 1.60 to 0.70 D at 1 month. Mean UCVA improved to 20/20 from the preoperative level of 20/40. Although this was a small series with limited follow-up, it showed that post-PRK and post-LASIK astigmatism can be effectively managed with PCRIs. Relatively low levels of correction were achieved, however no patients were overcorrected.

Relaxing incisions can also be used to treat post-keratoplasty astigmatism [35]. They are typically placed in, or just anterior to the graft–host junction, with a target depth of 70%–80%. As with AK, incision lengths range from 45° to 90°. The response can be highly variable, with published astigmatic reductions ranging from 0 to 15 D. Intraoperative qualitative keratometry can help guide incision length and location, but may not be predictive of the final results. As mentioned above, compression sutures along the flat meridian can enhance the PCRI effect. Selective suture removal is usually delayed for 4–8 weeks. Reductions in astigmatism of 2.8–14.9 D have been reported with various combinations of relaxing incisions, compression sutures and enhancement procedures.

Summary for the Clinician

- Peripheral corneal relaxing incisions effectively reduce astigmatism when combined with cataract surgery. Larger reductions were seen in patients with ATR astigmatism than in those who had WTR astigmatism
- PCRIs can be combined with toric intraocular lens implantation to reduce higher levels of astigmatism
- PCRIs can reduce astigmatism following PRK, LASIK and penetrating keratoplasty, but are limited in their treatment range

---

14.8 Conclusion

Refractive keratotomy laid the foundation for modern refractive surgery and was the dominant procedure for the correction of myopia and myopic astigmatism during the 1980s and early 1990s. The mid-1990s saw the introduction of excimer laser refractive surgery, with its improved efficacy, safety and predictability. The use of RK and AK decreased steadily through the end of the decade and now represents less than 1% of refractive procedures performed by members of the American Society of Cataract and Refractive Surgery [23].

The current role for refractive keratotomy lies primarily in the management of astigmatism. Though usually combined with cataract surgery, arcuate corneal incisions may be used alone or in conjunction with penetrating keratoplasty, PRK and LASIK to reduce astigmatism. PCRIs have been shown to be effective and carry less risk of glare induction, overcorrection, axis shift and creation of irregular astigmatism. As advances continue in the areas of intraocular lens design, crystalline lens removal and excimer laser refractive surgery, we are likely to see further decline in the use of refractive keratotomy. However, at this time, refractive keratotomy remains a low-cost and low-risk alternative for the management of astigmatism.

References

1. Agapitos PJ, Lindstrom RL, Williams PA, Sanders DR (1989) Analysis of astigmatic keratotomy. J Cataract Refract Surg 15:13–18
2. Arrowsmith PN, Marks RG (1989) Visual, refractive, and keratometric results of radial keratotomy. Five-year follow-up. Arch Ophthalmol 107: 506–511
3. Bear J, Richler A (1983) Cylindrical refractive error: a population study in western Newfoundland. Am J Optom Physiol Opt 60:39–45
4. Buzard KA, Laranjeira E, Fundingsland BR (1996) Clinical results of arcuate incisions to correct astigmatism. J Cataract Refract Surg 22:1062–1069
5. Casebeer JC (1995) Casebeer Incisional Keratotomy. Slack Inc., Thorofare, NJ

6. Damiano RE, Kouyoumdjian GA, Forstot SL, Kasen WB, Moore CR (2003) Combined laser in situ keratomileusis and radial keratotomy for the treatment of moderate to high myopia. J Cataract Refract Surg 29:908–911

7. Deitz MR, Sanders DR, Raanan MG (1987) A consecutive series (1982–1985) of radial keratotomies performed with the diamond blade. Am J Ophthalmol 103:417–422

8. Deitz MR, Sanders DR, Raanan MG, DeLuca M (1994) Long-term (5- to 12-year) follow-up of metal-blade radial keratotomy procedures. Arch Ophthalmol 112:614–620

9. Duffey RJ, Leaming D (2003) US trends in refractive surgery: 2002 ISRS survey. J Refract Surg 19:357–363

10. Duffey RJ, Tchah H, Lindstrom RL (1988) Spoke keratotomy in the human cadaver eye. J Refract Surg 4:9–11

11. Faktorovich EG, Maloney RK, Price FW, Jr (1999) Effect of astigmatic keratotomy on spherical equivalent: results of the Astigmatism Reduction Clinical Trial. Am J Ophthalmol 127:260–269

12. Gills J, Van der Karr M, Cherchio M (2002) Combined toric intraocular lens implantation and relaxing incisions to reduce high preexisting astigmatism. J Cataract Refract Surg 28:1585–1588

13. He W, Lu P, Zhang X, Li J, Xu J, He X (2000) A clinical investigation on cataract surgery with 2.8 mm incision. Zhonghua Yan Ke Za Zhi 36:282–284

14. Hirsch M (1965) Changes in astigmatism during the first eight years of school: an interim report from OJAI Longitudinal Study. Am J Optom 40:127–131

15. Jester JV, Venet T, Lee J, Schanzlin DJ, Smith RE (1981) A statistical analysis of radial keratotomy in human cadaver eyes. Am J Ophthalmol 92:172–177

16. Kemp JR, Martinez CE, Klyce SD et al. (1999) Diurnal fluctuations in corneal topography 10 years after radial keratotomy in the Prospective Evaluation of Radial Keratotomy Study. J Cataract Refract Surg 25:904–910

17. Koch DD, Sanan A (1999) Peripheral corneal relaxing incisions for residual astigmatism after photoastigmatic keratectomy and laser in situ keratomileusis. J Refract Surg 15:S238–239

18. Kohnen T, Koch DD (1996) Methods to control astigmatism in cataract surgery. Curr Opin Ophthalmol 7:75–80

19. Kohnen T, Dick B, Jacobi KW (1995) Comparison of the induced astigmatism after temporal clear corneal tunnel incisions of different sizes. J Cataract Refract Surg 21:417–424

20. Lans LJ (1898) Experimentelle Untersuchungen uber Entsehung von Astigmatismus durch nichperforirende Corneawunden. Arch fur Ophthalmologie 45:117–152

21. Lavery GW, Lindstrom RL (1985) Clinical results of trapezoidal astigmatic keratotomy. J Refract Surg 1:70–74

22. Lavery GW, Lindstrom RL (1985) Trapezoidal astigmatic keratotomy in human cadaver eyes. J Refract Surg 1:18–24

23. Leaming DV (2003) Practice styles and preferences of ASCRS members-2002 survey. J Cataract Refract Surg 29:1412–1420

24. Leibowitz HM, Krueger DE, Maunder LR et al. (1980) The Framingham Eye Study monograph: an ophthalmological and epidemiological study of cataract, glaucoma, diabetic retinopathy, macular degeneration, and visual acuity in a general population of 2631 adults, 1973–1975. Surv Ophthalmol 24:335–610

25. Lever J, Dahan E (2000) Opposite clear corneal incisions to correct pre-existing astigmatism in cataract surgery. J Cataract Refract Surg 26:803–805

26. Lindstrom RL (1990) The surgical correction of astigmatism: a clinician's perspective. Refract Corneal Surg 6:441–454

27. Lindstrom RL, Agapitos PJ, Koch DD (1994) Cataract surgery and astigmatic keratotomy. Int Ophthalmol Clin 34:145–164

28. Lucciola J (1886) Traitement chirugical de l'astigmatisme. Arch d'Ophthalmol 16:630

29. Masket S, Tennen DG (1996) Astigmatic stabilization of 3.0 mm temporal clear corneal cataract incisions. J Cataract Refract Surg 22:1451–1455

30. McDonald MB, Haik M, Kaufman HE (1987) Color vision and contrast sensitivity testing after radial keratotomy. Am J Ophthalmol 103:468

31. McDonnell PJ, Nizam A, Lynn MJ, Waring GO, 3rd (1996) Morning-to-evening change in refraction, corneal curvature, and visual acuity 11 years after radial keratotomy in the prospective evaluation of radial keratotomy study. The PERK Study Group. Ophthalmology 103:233–239

32. Pfleger T, Skorpik C, Menapace R, Scholz U, Weghaupt H, Zehetmayer M (1996) Long-term course of induced astigmatism after clear corneal incision cataract surgery. J Cataract Refract Surg 22:72–77

33. Price FW, Grene RB, Marks RG, Gonzales JS (1995) Astigmatism reduction clinical trial: a multicenter prospective evaluation of the predictability of arcuate keratotomy. Evaluation of surgical nomogram predictability. ARC-T Study Group. Arch Ophthalmol 113:277–282

34. Price FW, Jr., Grene RB, Marks RG, Gonzales JS (1996) Arcuate transverse keratotomy for astigmatism followed by subsequent radial or transverse keratotomy. ARC-T Study Group. Astigmatism Reduction Clinical Trial. J Refract Surg 12:68–76

35. Riddle HK, Jr., Parker DA, Price FW, Jr (1998) Management of postkeratoplasty astigmatism. Curr Opin Ophthalmol 9:15–28

36. Salz J, Lee JS, Jester JV et al. (1981) Radial keratotomy in fresh human cadaver eyes. Ophthalmology 88:742–746

37. Sato T (1939) Treatment of conical cornea by incision of Descemet's membrane. Acta Societica Ophthalmological Japonica 43:541

38. Sato T (1953) A new surgical approach to myopia. Am J Ophthalmol 36:823–829

39. Sawelson H, Marks RG (1989) Five-year results of radial keratotomy. Refract Corneal Surg 5:8–20

40. Schanzlin DJ, Santos VR, Waring GO 3rd et al. (1986) Diurnal change in refraction, corneal curvature, visual acuity, and intraocular pressure after radial keratotomy in the PERK Study. Ophthalmology 93:167–175

41. Schiötz H (1885) Ein Fall von hochgradigem Hornhautastigmatismus nach Starextraction Besserung auf operativem Wege. Arch fur Augenheilk 15:178–181

42. Snellen H (1869) Die Richtunge des Hauptmeridiane des Astigmatischen Auges. Albrecht von Graefes Arch Klin Ophthalmol 15:199–207

43. Sperduto RD, Seigel D, Roberts J, Rowland M (1983) Prevalence of myopia in the United States. Arch Ophthalmol 101:405–407

44. Thornton SP (1990) Astigmatic keratotomy: a review of basic concepts with case reports. J Cataract Refract Surg 16:430–435

45. Titiyal JS, Baidya KP, Sinha R et al. (2002) Intraoperative arcuate transverse keratotomy with phacoemulsification. J Refract Surg 18:725–730

46. Tomlinson A, Caroline P (1988) Effect of radial keratotomy on the contrast sensitivity function. Am j Optom Phys Sci 103:468

47. Vass C, Menapace R (1994) Computerized statistical analysis of corneal topography for the evaluation of changes in corneal shape after surgery. Am J Ophthalmol 118:177–184

48. Wang L, Misra M, Koch DD (2003) Peripheral corneal relaxing incisions combined with cataract surgery. J Cataract Refract Surg 29:712–722

49. Waring GO 3rd, Moffitt SD, Gelender H et al. (1983) Rationale for and design of the National Eye Institute Prospective Evaluation of Radial Keratotomy (PERK) Study. Ophthalmology 90: 40–58

50. Waring GO 3rd, Lynn MJ, Gelender H et al. (1985) Results of the prospective evaluation of radial keratotomy (PERK) study one year after surgery. Ophthalmology 92:177–198, 307

51. Waring GO 3rd, Lynn MJ, Nizam A et al.(1991) Results of the Prospective Evaluation of Radial Keratotomy (PERK) Study five years after surgery. The Perk Study Group. Ophthalmology 98:1164–1176

52. Waring GO 3rd, Lynn MJ, McDonnell PJ (1994) Results of the prospective evaluation of radial keratotomy (PERK) study 10 years after surgery. Arch Ophthalmol 112:1298–1308

53. Werblin TP, Stafford GM (1996) Hyperopic shift after refractive keratotomy using the Casebeer System. J Cataract Refract Surg 22:1030–1036

54. Werblin TP, Stafford GM (1996) Three year results of refractive keratotomy using the Casebeer System. J Cataract Refract Surg 22:1023–1029

Phakic Intraocular Lenses

Dennis C. Lu, David R. Hardten, Richard L. Lindstrom

Core Messages

- Phakic IOLs may be appropriate for some potential refractive surgery patients in whom keratorefractive surgery is unsuitable
- Patients to consider include those with higher ametropia or those with thin corneas
- Phakic IOLs are classified into three categories: anterior chamber angle fixated, anterior chamber iris fixated and posterior chamber lenses
- The main potential complication of anterior chamber lenses is contact with the endothelium whereas the main complication of posterior chamber lenses is iatrogenic cataract formation
- Assessment of key anatomic factors, such as anterior chamber depth and endothelial cell count, is critical in evaluating a patient

15.1
Introduction

The latter part of the 20th century has been a revolutionary age for refractive surgery. There has been an explosive growth in the number of technologies that have developed for refractive surgery. Most of the focus has been placed on the corneal component of the optical system, such as with the current wavefront technologies. Although the corneal refractive surgeries have been effective for low to moderate degrees of myopia and hyperopia, their efficacy and predictability has been more limited for higher degrees of refractive error. Recently there has been a revival in interest on the lenticular component of the optical system – leading to advances in phakic intraocular lenses, refractive lens exchange and accommodative and multifocal intraocular lenses. The lenticular refractive procedures have provided an effective alternative solution for the correction of higher degrees of ametropia and for eyes that are otherwise unsuitable for keratorefractive procedures.

15.1.1
Limitations of Keratorefractive Procedures

Conductive keratoplasty has been limited to low degrees of hyperopia. Likewise, Intacs is confined to the correction of low degrees of myopia without astigmatism. The excimer laser procedures such as photorefractive keratectomy (PRK), laser subepithelial keratomileusis (LASEK) and laser in situ keratomileusis (LASIK) are more versatile with regards to the range of refractive errors that they are able correct. However, even LASIK, which is the most versatile, has less predictable results and optical quality at the higher ranges of ametropia as a result of larger alterations in corneal biomechanics and wound healing. Larger degrees of tissue ablation in turn may lead to the induction of increasing amounts of higher order aberrations [41]. The emergence of wavefront guided ablation, however, promises to reduce higher order aberrations when compared to traditional excimer laser ablation. Yet, the corneal thickness imposes a significant limit on the degree of ametropia that may be corrected as deep ablations may increase the risk of induced corneal ectasia [45,

48]. In addition, with PRK or LASEK, higher degrees of correction can lead to increased risk of subepithelial haze and regression [6, 17, 40].

15.1.2
Role of Lenticular Refractive Procedures

Because lenticular refractive procedures need not contend with the variables of corneal wound healing and altered corneal geometry, refractive outcomes are more predictable and stable when compared to LASIK at higher degrees of correction. In fact, barring surgical related issues such as incisional astigmatism and IOL centration, the wavefront remains largely unchanged in phakic IOLs compared to corneal refractive procedures [27]. As with cataract surgery, the predictability in refractive outcome depends in large part on the selection of the IOL power. An additional advantage of lenticular refractive surgeries is that removal or exchange of the IOL is possible.

Several types of lenticular refractive procedures are currently being performed today: phakic IOL implantation, refractive lens exchange (RLE) and cataract extraction with a monofocal, multifocal or accommodative IOL. Accommodative IOLs currently represent a relatively new technology but may prove to be a promising refractive device in the future. While RLE has provided a viable solution for the highly ametropic patient in the presbyopic age group, phakic IOL implantation provides a distinct advantage for the younger age group in that this technique preserves accommodation. Implantation of phakic IOLs is a versatile procedure in its ability to correct myopia and hyperopia. Furthermore toric IOLs are currently being developed for the concurrent correction of astigmatism. However, phakic IOLs currently lack the accuracy of excimer laser procedures at the lower degrees of ametropia. Because patients who have undergone phakic IOL implantation may have residual spherical and cylindrical error, they may undergo additional LASIK enhancement procedures to achieve better uncorrected visual acuity (UCVA) [60]. The stepwise approach of phakic IOL implantation followed by an excimer laser enhancement to correct the residual refractive error has been termed "bioptics" by Zaldivar [60].

15.2
Evolution and Classification of Phakic IOLs

The concept of using an anterior chamber lens implant in a phakic eye to correct high myopia was originally explored by Strampelli in the 1950s [54] and later by Barraquer in 1959 [13]. However, the phakic anterior chamber lenses of this generation suffered from unacceptably high complication rates related to endothelial cell loss, iridocyclitis and hyphema. Consequently, implantation of phakic anterior chamber was abandoned but later revived in the 1980s. During this decade, three competing designs arose: Fechner and Worst et al. proposed use of an iris fixated lens [21], Baikoff et al. used an angle-supported lens modified from the Kelman multiflex lens [11] and Fydorov designed a phakic posterior chamber intraocular lens [24]. Currently, phakic IOLs are classified according to the way in which they are fixated: (1) anterior chamber angle fixated, (2) anterior chamber iris fixated and (3) posterior chamber. Each of these designs has inherent advantages as well as unique potential complications.

15.2.1
Anterior Chamber Angle-Fixated Lenses

The main advantage of the anterior chamber angle-fixated lens is the ease of insertion and the familiarity that most ophthalmologists have with insertion of anterior chamber intraocular lenses (ACIOL). Current designs incorporate a foldable or non-foldable IOL that requires an incision between 3.0 and 6 mm, depending on the size of the IOL.

15.2.1.1
Design Considerations

The unique complications of phakic IOLs are primarily mechanical in nature and result from the anatomic relationships between the IOL and its neighbouring ocular structures. With the an-

Table 15.1. Complications arising from phakic IOL contact with ocular structures

Contact with:	Complication:
Endothelium	Endothelial loss, corneal oedema
Iris	Pigment dispersion, chronic uveitis
Pupil	Pupillary block, angle closure glaucoma
Irido-corneo-scleral angle	Pupil ovalisation, peripheral anterior synechiae
Crystalline lens	Cataract formation

terior chamber lenses, the main complications arise from: (1) Contact with the endothelium resulting in endothelial cell loss and corneal oedema; (2) contact with the iris leading to pigment dispersion and chronic uveitis; (3) pupillary block leading to acute angle closure glaucoma; (4) deformation of the irido-corneo-scleral angle structures by the haptics, resulting in pupil ovalisation, peripheral anterior synechiae, glaucoma and occasionally (5) contact with the natural crystalline lens leading to cataract formation. In addition, IOL decentration, tilt, pupil ovalisation, and the smaller IOL optic required by anterior chamber lenses can all contribute to the symptoms of glare and halos for which these IOLs are notorious (Table 15.1).

In order to minimise contact between the IOL and the ocular structures, the following design parameters must be considered: (1) vaulting angle of the IOL, (2) diameter of the optic, (3) thickness and profile of the optic, both centrally and peripherally and (4) geometry of the haptics, including the number of haptic contact points and distribution of compressive forces in the irido-corneo-scleral angle. Clearly, the anterior chamber depth, white-to-white distance, pupil size, corneal pachymetry, and specular microscopy must be measured prior to surgery. Excessive vaulting of the IOL results in endothelial contact while inadequate vaulting leads to pigmentary dispersion and/or acute pupillary block glaucoma. A peripheral iridectomy or iridotomy is therefore recommended for all phakic IOLs. The profile of the optic must be designed to minimise contact with the endothelium and iris, which can be achieved by decreasing either or both the thickness and diameter of the optic. However, altering the geometry of the IOL will affect the optics: thickness influences

the dioptric power of the IOL, and a smaller optic diameter can lead to glare and halos. Finally the geometry of the haptics must be designed to provide an even distribution of forces while minimising excessive contact with angle structures. An even distribution of haptic forces is necessary in order to provide correct centration while preventing IOL rotation and pupil ovalisation.

15.2.1.2
Non-foldable Anterior Chamber Angle Fixated Lenses

Baikoff's original ZB implant (Domilens, Lyons, France), which was a modification of the Kelman Multiflex lens, incorporated a biconcave negative-powered angle-fixated lens (Fig. 15.1). This design suffered from unacceptably high rates of endothelial cell loss, with reported rates of 16%–19% at 1 year and 20%–28% at 2 years [12, 39, 43, 42]. The lens employed a 4.5-mm optic angulated at 25° and consisted of four haptic contact points. This geometry resulted in exces-

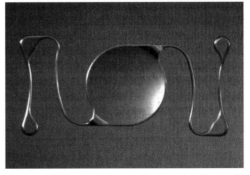

Fig. 15.1. First generation ZB anterior chamber angle fixated implant. (Reprinted with permission from [10])

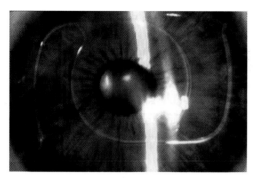

Fig. 15.2. NuVita anterior chamber angle fixated implant. (Reprinted with permission from [10])

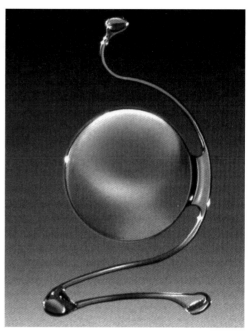

Fig. 15.3. Vivarte foldable anterior chamber angle fixated implant. (Reprinted with permission from [10])

sive contact between the optic edge and the endothelium when patients rubbed their eyes [43]. Subsequently, Baikoff minimised endothelial contact in his second generation design, the ZB5 M lens, by decreasing the angulation to 20° and by reducing the optical edge thickness at the expense of reduced effective optical diameter. The ZB5 M significantly reduced the rate of endothelial cell loss and provided reasonable optical quality [2, 12, 43]. Thus the lens enjoyed reasonable longevity between 1990 and 1997. Several studies reported reduction of endothelial cell loss to ranges of 4.5%–5.5% at 1 year and 5.6%–6.8% at 2 years [2, 12]. The main complications of this lens were related to the haptic design and the reduced optical zone: pupil ovalisation in 22.6% and night time halos in 27.8% [2, 12].

The successor to the ZB5 M is the NuVita MA20 (Bausch & Lomb Surgical/Chiron Vision, Irvine, CA), which is currently available in Europe but not yet approved for use in the United States (Fig. 15.2). Modifications to the z-shaped haptic profile and redistribution of compressive forces have reduced the incidence of iris ovalisation [12]. In addition the geometry of the optic was altered to an anterior convex/posterior concave profile. This profile minimises endothelial contact while increasing the effective optical zone (4.5 mm) within the same overall optic diameter (5.0 mm). According to the manufacturer, the increased effective optical zone and use of an antireflective process applied to the optic edges, termed Peripheral Design Technology, combine to reduce the incidence of glare and halos [9].

Various other manufacturers have produced angle-fixated IOLs that are modifications of Baikoff's original designs: the ZSAL 4 (Morcher, Stuttgart, Germany) and the Phakic 6 (Ophthalmic Innovations International, Ontario, CA). The ZSAL 4 was developed by Pérez-Santonja et al. and became commercially available in Europe in 1995. The design is similar to the NuVita but implements a larger 5.0 effective optical zone within a 5.5 mm plano-concave optic at an angulation of 19°. Though this design provided reasonable optical quality and reduced the incidence of night time halos, it did not reduce the incidence of complications related to haptic design: pupil ovalisation, IOL rotation and chronic low-grade uveitis. However, the rate of endothelial cell loss was lower: 3.50% at 12 months and 4.18% at 24 months [43]. The ZSAL 4 is supplied in powers ranging from –6 to –20 D in increments of 1.00 D, and is available in lens lengths of 12.5 or 13.0 mm.

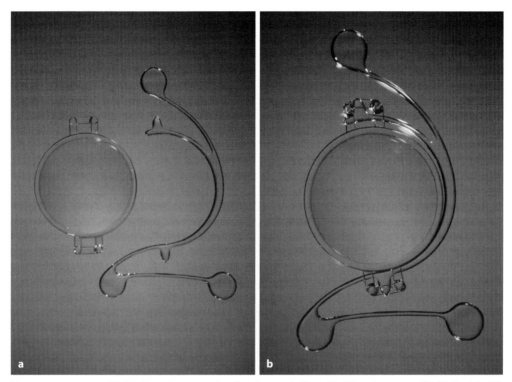

Fig. 15.4. a Unassembled Kelman Duet anterior chamber angle fixated implant (courtesy of Tekia Inc.) **b** Kelman Duet implant assembled (courtesy of Tekia Inc.)

The Phakic 6 implant shares similarities to the ZSAL 4 but features a larger 6-mm optic in efforts to reduce the incidence of halos. However, the larger optic poses the increased risk of endothelial contact. Long term studies are not yet available. Furthermore, the implant is available with heparin-surface modification, which aims to reduce the formation of synechiae. The Phakic 6 is available in myopic ranges of –2 to –25 D and hyperopic ranges of +2 to +10 D. The lens lengths range from 12.0 to 14.0 mm [47].

15.2.1.3
Foldable Anterior Chamber Angle Fixated Lenses

Innovative designs and novel materials have led to the development of foldable angle-fixated lenses that can be inserted through small incisions. The Vivarte (manufactured by Ioltech, La Rochelle, France and distributed by Ciba Vision) is a single piece IOL composed of hy-drophilic acrylic (Fig. 15.3). A unique manufacturing process allows for the selective polymerisation of each IOL component and thereby produces a soft optic and footplate while creating a rigid haptic. Thus, the soft optic allows the IOL to be folded while the rigid haptic provides support within the angle at three contact points. The optic diameter is 5.5 mm and is available in lengths of 12.0, 12.5, 13.0 and 13.5 mm. The power ranges from –7 to –25 D in 0.5 D increments.

Using a different approach to the design of a "foldable" angle-fixated lens, the Kelman Duet employs a two piece IOL wherein the components are sequentially inserted through a small incision and assembled in the anterior chamber (Fig. 15.4 a,b). At present, the PMMA haptic is manufactured in lengths of 12.0, 12.5, 13.0 and 13.5 mm, and the silicone optic is produced at a diameter of 5.5 mm. Power of the lens ranges from –8 to –20 D [57]. The device is currently undergoing clinical trials in Europe and is not yet approved for use in the United States.

15.2.2
Anterior Chamber Iris-Fixated Lenses

In order to move the IOL further away from the endothelium and to avoid damage to angle structures, Worst proposed an alternative design for the anterior chamber intraocular lens in 1977 termed the "iris claw" lens. In this design, the lens is fixated anterior to the iris plane by two diametrically opposing haptic claws that incarcerate a portion of mid-peripheral iris (Fig. 15.5 a,b). This process has been termed "enclavation". Originally used to correct aphakia following cataract surgery, Worst later modified the iris claw lens into a negative powered biconcave design to correct myopia in phakic patients in 1986. In 1991, the lens adopted a convex-concave profile with a larger optical zone of 5.0 mm and a total length of 8.5 mm [37]. Since then, this model has been employed and was renamed the Artisan myopia lens in 1998 by the manufacturer (Ophtec, Groningen, The Netherlands) without a change in the design. An additional model with a 6.0-mm optical zone was added for patients with larger pupils. Advanced Medical Optics (AMO, Santa Ana, CA) is planning to market the lens in the United States upon approval under the name Verisyse.

In order to allow for unimpeded constriction and dilation of the pupil, the lens is fixated at the immobile midperipheral iris. Because enclavation is the most challenging part of the procedure, centration of the lens over the pupil can sometimes be difficult [35]. However, the lens may be fixated at any angle – horizontally, vertically, or obliquely – depending on surgeon preference.

Currently, the Artisan is a non-foldable PMMA lens capable of ultraviolet filtration and has different models available for the correction of myopia and hyperopia. Foldable designs are currently under investigation. In addition, a toric design has recently become available for the concurrent correction of astigmatism. The two models for myopia have differing optic diameters but the same overall length of 8.5 mm. Model 206 has a 5.0-mm optic with power ranging from –3 to –23.5 D in 0.5 D increments. Model 204 has a larger 6.0 mm optic and is conse-

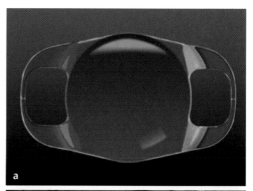

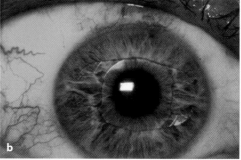

Fig. 15.5. a Artisan lens (courtesy of Ophtec BV). **b** Artisan lens properly positioned in a myopic eye (courtesy of Ophtec BV)

quently limited to a smaller range of powers because of its proximity to the endothelium: –3 to –15.5 D in 0.5 D increments. According to the manufacturer, the distance from the optic edge to the endothelium ranges from 1.5 to 2.0 mm depending on the dioptric power and the anterior chamber depth, as well as the diameter of the optic. For the correction of hyperopia, the model 203 incorporates a 5-mm optic with an overall length of 8.5 mm and is available in dioptric powers ranging from +1 to +12 D in 0.5 D increments.

Ophtec has introduced two different toric models. In model A, the torus axis is oriented parallel to the axis of the claw whereas in model B the torus axis is perpendicular. Most surgeons prefer horizontal insertion of the IOL and would therefore use model A for with-the-rule astigmatism and model B for against-the-rule astigmatism. The toric IOL is available in myopic powers ranging from –3 to –23.5 D in 0.5 D increments, hyperopic powers of +2 to +12 D in

0.5 D increments, and cylindrical correction from 1.0 to 7.0 D. It is comprised of a spherical anterior surface and a spherocylindrical posterior surface. Because the lens requires an incision of approximately 5.5 mm, the amount of induced astigmatism created by the incision and sutures must be taken into account when choosing the appropriate lens.

The Artisan lenses for myopia and hyperopia are currently in phase III of the FDA clinical trials in the United States, and the results have been encouraging. In Europe, the Artisan lens has already obtained the CE mark for myopia and hyperopia after having undergone a large multicentre trial. The toric and foldable lens designs are still in the investigational stages in Europe.

15.2.3
Posterior Chamber Lenses

While the most daunting risk in anterior chamber lenses is endothelial damage, the major concern in posterior chamber lenses is iatrogenic cataract formation. Thus, optimising the clearance of the IOL between the crystalline lens and the iris has been the primary focus in their design. Contact with the crystalline lens would provoke iatrogenic cataract formation, while contact with the iris may result in iris chafing and attendant chronic uveitis. Furthermore, an anteriorly positioned IOL may result in pupillary block and resultant angle closure glaucoma. Thus, a preoperative peripheral iridotomy is recommended. Two approaches have evolved in maintaining the optimal IOL position between the iris and lens: (1) sulcus fixation with appropriate vaulting and, more recently, (2) harnessing the aqueous flux dynamics to float the hydrophobic IOL away from the crystalline lens in such a way that any type of fixation is avoided. Staar Surgical AG (Nidau, Switzerland) manufactures the Implantable Contact Lens (ICL), which employs the sulcus fixated design. By contrast, Medennium Inc. (Irvine, CA) incorporates the floatation approach in their Phakic Refractive Lens (PRL).

15.2.3.1
Sulcus-Fixated Posterior Chamber Lenses

As with anterior chamber angle fixated lenses, the concept of vaulting is critical in determining the success of a posterior chamber sulcus fixated lens. In turn, the vaulting angle is influenced by the length of the IOL and the sulcus-to-sulcus distance. Choosing an IOL that is too short relative to the sulcus-to-sulcus distance will result in inadequate vaulting and resultant cataract formation [22]. Furthermore, a short IOL may result in decentration. By contrast, a long IOL length will lead to excessive vaulting, which in turn can lead to pigmentary dispersion or acute pupillary block glaucoma. Thus correct sizing of the IOL is critical in preoperative planning. The ideal vaulting is thought to be 500 µm over the crystalline lens (Fig. 15.6). Currently, no accurate method exists to measure the sulcus-to-sulcus distance, and therefore it is extrapolated from white-to-white measurements.

The ICL evolved from Fyodorov's original design, which was first used to correct high myopia in 1986. In order to avoid the endothelial contact that was associated with anterior chamber lenses, Fyodorov pioneered the design of the first posterior chamber phakic intraocular

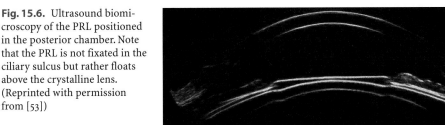

Fig. 15.6. Ultrasound biomicroscopy of the PRL positioned in the posterior chamber. Note that the PRL is not fixated in the ciliary sulcus but rather floats above the crystalline lens. (Reprinted with permission from [53])

lens. Staar Surgical made further modifications to the design, and the first implantations were accomplished in 1993 [8, 58]. After several refinements, Staar Surgical now offers the current model of the ICL: the ICH V4 (Fig. 15.7). The ICL is a single piece plate-haptic foldable lens that may be inserted through an incision of less than 3 mm. The lens is composed of a proprietary material termed Collamer (Staar Surgical AG, Nidau, Switzerland), a hydrophilic collagen polymer (34% water and <0.1% collagen), that appears to be highly biocompatible and allows the crystalline lens to maintain a normal metabolism. Both myopic and hyperopic models are available. Toric models are currently undergoing clinical trials and will correct up to 6 D of astigmatism. The myopic lens is concave-concave in design and is available in powers ranging from −3 to −20 D. The hyperopic model is convex-concave and is available in powers from +1.50 to +20.00 D. Depending on the power of the lens, the optical zone varies between 4.5 and 5.5 mm. While the thickness is only 50 µm at the optical zone, the thickness increases to 100 µm at the footplates and up to 500–600 µm at the haptic zone. Although the width is fixed at 7.0 mm, the lengths range from 11.0 to 13.0 mm in 0.5-mm increments. Choice of lengths is critical in determining the appropriate position and vaulting above the crystalline lens.

Short term results of the ICL have been encouraging and quality of vision has been excellent. Clinical trials are still evaluating the long term results and safety. The ICL gained the European CE mark of approval in 1997. In the United States, the ICL began FDA trials in 1997 and the spherical models have been recommended for approval by the FDA Ophthalmic Devices Advisory Panel and are awaiting final approval [52]. Toric models are in the early phases of the FDA trials.

15.2.3.2
Non-fixated Posterior Chamber Lenses

The posterior chamber lens manufactured by Medennium Inc., named the Phakic Refractive Lens (PRL), requires no fixation (Figs. 15.8, 15.9). This lens floats on the crystalline lens by nature of its hydrophobic material in conjunction with the aqueous flux dynamics. This lens is composed of a highly purified, optically clear silicone. Because of its lack of fixation, stability of centration and rotation are concerns. For these reasons, this particular design may not be suitable for a toric lens. According to the manufacturer, centration is achieved by the self-centering design of the optic body.

The PRL is a one-piece foldable plate haptic lens that may be inserted through a 3.2-mm incision. Because it does not require sulcus fixation, sizing is not as critical with the PRL as it is with the lenses that require fixation and vaulting. Thus the manufacturer offers one length of 11.3 mm for the myopic model and one length of 10.6 mm for the hyperopic model. A 10.8 mm

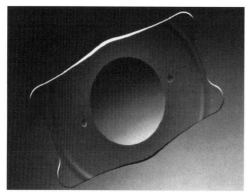

Fig. 15.7. STAAR implantable contact lens. (Reprinted with permission from [59])

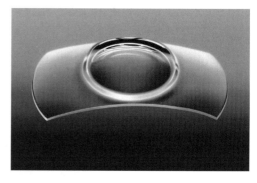

Fig. 15.8. Phakic refractive lens. (Reprinted with permission from [56])

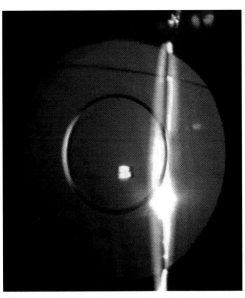

Fig. 15.9. Slit lamp photograph of the PRL properly positioned. (Reprinted with permission from [53])

- Geometry of the haptics, including the number of haptic contact points and distribution of compressive forces in the irido-corneo-scleral angle for angle fixated implants

15.3 Evaluation of the Phakic IOL Patient

Because implantation of a phakic IOL is an elective procedure for the correction of ametropia, patient selection and education is imperative. The surgeon must have a clear understanding of the surgical options available, as well as the contraindications and indications of each. A thorough discussion of the risks, benefits and alternatives must then be undertaken in order to allow the patient to make an informed decision. Realistic patient expectations are essential to a successful outcome.

myopic model was previously offered but was discontinued because of decentration issues [28]. In both the hyperopic and myopic models, the width of the lens is 6.0 mm. Thickness varies according to the dioptric power, with a maximum thickness of 0.6 mm. The myopic model is offered in powers ranging from –3 D to –20 D in half diopter increments, which allows for correction of myopia up to –23.0 D. For the hyperopic model, power ranges from +3 D to +15 D in half diopter steps and corrects a maximum of +11 D. Whereas the diameter of the optical zone for the myopic model varies between 4.5 and 5.0 mm depending on the power, the diameter for the hyperopic model is fixed at 4.5 mm.

The PRL has gained the CE mark of approval in the European Union and is currently undergoing Phase III FDA trials in the United States.

Summary for the clinician:

Important considerations when choosing a phakic IOL:
- Vaulting angle of the IOL
- Diameter of the optic
- Thickness and profile of the optic, both centrally and peripherally

15.3.1 General Patient Factors

In general, patients less than age 18 should not have any refractive surgery, as their refractive error has not stabilised. Refractive stability may occur at an older age for patients with higher levels of myopia. Patients with unrealistic expectations of "perfect vision" after surgery should also be identified. These patients will generally be unhappy with the outcome.

15.3.2 Refraction

Phakic IOLs are suitable for myopia in the range of –8 D to –22 D and hyperopia in the range of +3 D to +10 D. The Artisan toric iris-fixated lens is able to correct from 1 to 7 D of astigmatism, while the toric Staar ICL may correct up to 6 D of astigmatism. Lower refractive errors are better suited for corneal refractive procedures, unless the patients' corneas are unsuitable with regards to thickness or topography. For best results, the refractive error should be stable prior to the surgery. Both cycloplegic and non-cycloplegic refractions should be performed to determine the contribution of accommodation.

15.3.3
Anatomic Factors

In anterior chamber lenses, the depth required to avoid endothelial contact depends in part on the power of the IOL, but in general requires at least 3.2 mm as measured from the epithelium [26]. Posterior chamber phakic IOLs also require a sufficient anterior chamber depth of at least 3.2 mm in order to allow for atraumatic insertion and manipulation of the IOL. The anterior chamber depth may be determined via A-scan ultrasound or by the Orbscan II. A large pupil may result in postoperative glare and haloes, and yet many patients still find this acceptable.

15.3.4
Pre-existing Ocular Pathology

Implantation of phakic IOLs should be performed on healthy eyes without pre-existing ocular pathology. Thus a thorough slit lamp examination should be performed. Of particular concern, patients with pre-existing cataract may fare better with natural lens replacement or cataract surgery. Phakic IOLs, particularly anterior chamber lenses, may be associated with endothelial cell loss. Eyes with iris abnormalities, such as iridocorneal endothelial syndrome, may not have adequate angle support for anterior chamber lenses [26]. A history of anterior uveitis is also a relative contraindication, as intraocular surgery may reactivate quiescent disease. Any history of peripheral retinal pathology warrants a thorough dilated fundus exam and preoperative prophylactic laser treatment may be helpful [23]. Ancillary tests should include specular microscopy and pachymetry. Furthermore, corneal topography should be obtained to identify keratoconus.

15.3.5
IOL Sizing for Fixated Lenses

Correct sizing of the IOL is critical in determining the proper vaulting angles for the anterior chamber angle-fixated and posterior chamber sulcus-fixated lenses. For the anterior chamber lenses, the white-to-white (W-to-W) measurement is used to estimate the diameter of the iridocorneal angle and the appropriate lens size is subsequently chosen. As for the ICL posterior chamber lens, the ciliary sulcus distance is extrapolated from the white-to-white measurements. For myopic patients, 0.5 mm is added to the W-to-W length. With hyperopic correction, the ICL length is the same as the W-to-W. By contrast, sizing of the IOL is less of an issue for the iris-fixated Artisan Lens and the Phakic Refractive Lens, both of which do not require vaulting or angle fixation.

15.3.6
IOL Calculations

The calculation of power in phakic IOLs is different from that in cataract surgery. For phakic IOLs, the lens manufacturers typically provide nomograms with which to determine the appropriate power. These nomograms are based upon standard vertex conversion formulas. With cataract surgery, a refracting element – namely the crystalline lens – is removed, and thus the preoperative refraction does not directly affect IOL calculations. By contrast, no refracting element is removed in phakic IOL implantation. Hence, the power of the phakic IOL is simply determined from the patient's refraction and adjusted according to vertex conversion formulas. Consequently, axial length is not a variable in phakic IOL calculations. For anterior chamber phakic lenses, the calculation of power is based upon the Van der Heijde nomogram. For the ICL posterior chamber lens, software supplied by the manufacturer will compute the IOL power at the ciliary sulcus plane.

15.3.7
Peripheral Iridectomy or Iridotomy

Because of the potential to cause pupillary block and resultant angle closure, all phakic IOLs require preoperative peripheral iridotomies or intraoperative iridectomies. Surgical iridectomy carries the risk of traumatic cataract or zonular dialysis in the phakic patient. The manufacturers recommend that two iridotomies be placed superiorly 90° apart in the event that part of the IOL occludes one of the iridotomies.

> #### Summary for the Clinician
>
> Considerations in the evaluation
> and planning:
> - Assessment of the anterior chamber depth is critical for both anterior and posterior chamber lenses
> - IOL sizing is critical for angle or sulcus fixated lenses and may be estimated from white-to-white measurements
> - Nomograms for IOL power are determined from the patient's refraction and adjusted for vertex distance
> - Peripheral iridotomies are required for all types of phakic IOLs

15.4
Surgical Technique

Depending upon the surgeon's familiarity with the technique, general, retrobulbar, peribulbar or topical anaesthesia may be used. The anterior chamber lenses require preoperative miosis, while the posterior chamber lenses require preoperative dilation. A viscoelastic is injected through a paracentesis port prior to the insertion of the lens in order to form the anterior chamber and to protect the endothelium and lens during manipulation of the IOL.

15.4.1
Anterior Chamber Angle Fixated

The size and location of the incision depends upon whether the lens is foldable or non-foldable. The meridian of the incision is chosen so as to minimise astigmatism. In repositioning these lenses, care must be taken to minimise pupil ovalisation.

15.4.1.1
Non-foldable Angle Fixated Lenses

With non-foldable lenses, the incision may be created via a corneal or corneoscleral approach and the size of the incision ranges from 5.5 to 6.0 mm depending upon the size of the IOL optic. Though a glide may facilitate insertion of the IOL into the angle, the glide itself may pose a potential hazard to the crystalline lens. The lens is inserted into the anterior chamber with forceps and repositioned with a Sinskey hook. The corneoscleral incision is then sutured and the viscoelastic is removed.

15.4.1.2
Foldable Angle Fixated Lenses

The two types of "foldable" lenses, both of which have tripod haptics, require vastly different techniques. The Vivarte lens may be folded and inserted with forceps through a 3.2-mm incision. Because of its smaller size, the self-sealing incision may be created in clear cornea or via a corneoscleral approach. The knee of the tripod haptic is inserted first and the trailing haptic is positioned with a Sinskey hook. The lens is then repositioned with hooks via two paracentesis ports situated perpendicular to the main wound.

The Kelman Duet lens is not actually foldable but consists of two separate components – the optic and the haptic – that are sequentially inserted through a small incision and assembled in the anterior chamber. Two 1-mm clear corneal incisions are created at 3 and 9 o'clock and facilitate manipulation of the components. The haptic is first inserted with forceps through one of the incisions and repositioned in the angle. The optic is then injected into the anterior chamber. Two diametrically opposed tabs on the optic are then fastened to corresponding "snaps" on the haptic.

15.4.2
Anterior Chamber Iris Fixated

Two opposing paracentesis ports are created on either side of the main incision and serve as entry sites for enclavation of the iris to the lens. The angle of these incisions is therefore directed downward towards the mid-peripheral iris rather than parallel to the iris as in cataract surgery. The main incision may be corneal or corneoscleral and varies between 5 and 6.5 mm depending on the size of the lens chosen. Using long-angled forceps, the lens is then inserted into the anterior chamber, taking care to avoid the natural lens. With a Sinskey hook, the implant is then rotated into the horizontal position for superior incisions or the vertical position for horizontal incisions. While stabilising the lens with the Artisan implantation forceps (Ophtec), a specifically designed enclavation needle (Operaid) is then inserted through one paracentesis site and used to draw a portion of mid-peripheral iris into one claw of the lens. A similar process is performed for the opposing claw while taking care to centre the optic over the iris. If centration is poor or the pupil ovalisation is excessive, the iris may be released with the enclavation needle and the lens may be repositioned. The main incision is then closed with sutures. Unlike the angle or sulcus fixated lenses, the iris-fixated lens may be centred over the pupil even if the pupil is not centred in relation to the limbus [26].

15.4.3
Posterior Chamber Angle Fixated

Proper loading of the lens into the injection cartridge is a critical step in the implantation of the ICL. Because the ICL is manufactured with a predetermined vault, correct orientation within the cartridge is necessary and may be verified by positioning markers on the lens. Two oppos-

ing paracentesis ports are created on either side of the main incision and allow for manipulation of the ICL. The ICL is injected through a clear cornea incision, which is approximately 3.0–3.2 mm. Once inside the anterior chamber, each footplate of the plate haptic is gently tucked under the pupil using specially designed spatulas that are inserted through the paracentesis ports. Care must be taken not to touch the surface of the crystalline lens. When proper positioning is verified, the pupil is pharmacologically constricted with miotics.

15.4.4
Posterior Chamber Phakic Refractive Lens

Although the design of the PRL differs from that of the ICL, the implantation procedure is practically identical. Two opposing paracentesis ports are created on either side of a 3.2-mm clear cornea incision. The lens may be inserted with either specially designed forceps or with an injector. Like the ICL, the four corners of the plate haptic style lens are then gently tucked underneath the pupil with specially designed spatulas. Unlike the ICL, the PRL does not require fixation within the ciliary sulcus.

15.5
Post-operative Course and Enhancements

The visual recovery with phakic IOL implantation is rapid. Intraocular inflammation is minimal compared to cataract extraction with phacoemulsification because no ultrasound energy is transmitted to the ocular structures. Unlike the excimer laser procedures, there is no regression effect with phakic IOLs because corneal healing is not required. Patients with phakic IOL implantation may desire a subsequent excimer laser enhancement procedure for residual spherical or astigmatic refractive error.

15.6
Results

There are several ways to evaluate the effectiveness and quality of vision following refractive surgery. The most common method is to evaluate the percentage of patients achieving 20/40 and 20/20 and the percentage that fall within 0.50 D and 1.00 D of emmetropia. Another method is to compare the mean preoperative spherical equivalent to the mean postoperative spherical equivalent. In addition, the efficacy index is defined as the ratio of the post-operative UCVA to the pre-operative BCVA. Larger ratios are the desired outcome. Loss of BCVA is a measure of safety and may be reflected in the safety index, which is the ratio of post-operative BCVA to pre-operative BCVA. More recently, the emergence of aberrometers now allows for the evaluation of the wavefront and quality of vision.

The results of the major clinical studies are summarised in the following tables. Table 15.2 summarises the myopic results for the ICL, PRL, Artisan, NuVita, and the ZSAL-4. Likewise, Table 15.3 summarises the hyperopic results.

15.6.1
Myopic Results

Few long-term studies exist for phakic IOLs and a direct comparison of each different type is difficult because of rapid changes in the lens designs. Furthermore, the range of refractive errors corrected varies from study to study, with some studies enrolling the more extreme refractive errors. This context must be considered when evaluating the outcomes. In general, the results have been encouraging with regards to refractive outcomes, efficacy, and safety. As a whole, the latest generation of phakic IOLs appears to be quite safe with regards to loss of BCVA. On average, 5% of eyes lost one line of visual acuity, while <1% of eyes lost two or more lines of vision. About one-third of patients gained two or more lines of vision.

The Artisan lens has remained unchanged since 1991 and thus has the largest series of patients available for evaluation. As demonstrated by Table 15.2, both the Artisan lens and the ICL lens have demonstrated remarkable results, with 20%–30% achieving an UCVA of 20/20 or better and 70%–80% achieving an UCVA of 20/40 of better.

Recently, Vukich compared data of 559 LASIK eyes with 210 ICL eyes for the treatment of myopia in the range of 8–12 D [46, 56]. At 1 year, the LASIK eyes achieved 20/20 UCVA in 36% and 20/20 BCVA in 82% compared to 52% and 90% of the ICL eyes, respectively. Predictability was within 0.5 D at 1 year in 57% of LASIK eyes and 69% of the ICL eyes. Furthermore, the LASIK eyes showed an average regression from –0.06 D at 1 week to –0.51 D at 1 year while the ICL group had no regression. Wavefront analysis of ten eyes in each group at least 6 months post-operatively revealed coma of 0.46 µm and spherical aberration of 0.39 µm in the LASIK eyes compared to 0.22 and 0.13 µm, respectively, for ICL eyes.

15.6.2
Hyperopic Results

As demonstrated by Table 15.3, correction of high hyperopia with phakic IOLs appears to be a relatively safe procedure with regards to loss of BCVA. An average of 7% of eyes lost one line of BCVA, and 1.8% lost two or more lines of BCVA. An average of 17% gained two or more lines of BCVA. All the reported safety indices were greater than one. Moreover the hyperopic phakic IOLs demonstrated very good predictability, with 70% of eyes falling within 0.5 D of the targeted refraction and 93% of eyes falling 1 D. In addition, the phakic IOLs produced relatively good results with respect to UCVA.

Table 15.2. Major case series involving implantation of a phakic intraocular lens to correct myopia. (Table courtesy of Anthony J. Lombardo, MD, from [32])

Lens	First author [reference]	Eyes (n)	Mean follow-up (months)	Mean pre-op S.E. (D)	Range of re-fraction (D)	Efficacy Mean post-op S.E. (D)	Post-op ±0.5 D (%)	Post-op ±1.0 D [%]	UCVA 20/20 (%)	UCVA 20/40 (%)	Efficacy index	Safety BCVA loss of 1 line (%)	BCVA loss 2 or more lines (%)	BCVA gain 2 or more lines (%)	Safety index
ICL	Bloomenstein [15]	65	24	−8.47	−3.00 to −16.25	−0.31	75	92	52	92	N.R.	8	0	1.5	N.R.
	Arne [7]	58	6	−13.85	−8.00 to −19.25	−1.22	N.R.	57	N.R.	N.R.	0.84	5	0	40	1.46
	Uusitalo [55]	38	13	−15.10	−7.75 to −29.00	−2.00	71	82	5.3	53	N.R.	6.3	0	41	N.R.
	Gonvers[a] [25]	22	7	−11.5	−6.87 to −15.50	−1.19	32	45	18	68	N.R.	0	0	N.R.	N.R.
	Menezo[b] [38]	12	18	−16.00	−11.50 to −28.00	−0.73	33	43	0	75	1.04	0	0	75	1.59
	Bleckmann[c] [14]	7	7	−8.14	N.R.	−0.13	N.R.	N.R.	N.R.	N.R.	1.01	N.R.	N.R.	N.R.	1.43
PRL	Hoyos [28]	17	12	−18.46	−11.85 to −26.00	−0.22	53	82	N.R.	N.R.	1.04	0	0	18	1.14
Artisan	Budo [16]	249	36	−12.95	−5.0 to −20.0	−0.6	57	79	34	77	1.03	2.0	1.2	43	1.31
	Maloney [34]	155	6	−12.69	−5.50 to −22.50	−0.54	55	90	26	83	N.R.	9.5	0	12	N.R.
	Alexander [1]	135	6	−12.66	−4.88 to −22.75	−0.35	63	90	N.R.	83	N.R.	3.0	0.74	22	N.R.
	Menezo[d] [36]	94	49	−14.73	−7 to −28	−0.84	49	80	13	62	1.00	0	0	82	1.52

S.E., spherical equivalent; UCVA, uncorrected visual acuity; BCVA, best-corrected visual acuity; N.R., not recorded.
[a]ICM V3 and V4; [b]ICM V2–V4; [c]Concurrent limbal relaxing incisions to reduce corneal astigmatism; [d]Worst-Fechner and Worst.

Table 15.2. Continued

Lens	First author [reference]	Eyes (n)	Mean follow-up (months)	Mean pre-op S.E. (D)	Range of refraction (D)	Efficacy Mean post-op S.E. (D)	Post-op ±0.5 D (%)	Post-op ±1.0 D [%]	UCVA 20/20 (%)	UCVA 20/40 (%)	Efficacy index	Safety BCVA loss of 1 line (%)	BCVA loss 2 or more lines (%)	BCVA gain 2 or more lines (%)	Safety index
	Landesz [30]	78	11	– 17	–6.25 to –28.00	–2	50	68	30	73	1.00	6.4	2.6	28	1.21
	Dick[e] [19]	45	6	– 8.90	–1.25 to –21.25	–0.50	83	100	6.3	85	1.03	0	0	33	1.25
	El Danasoury [20]	43	12	–13.93	–9.50 to –19.38	–0.64	42	65	21	88	N.R.	5	0	16	N.R.
	Malecaze [33]	25	12	–10.19	–8.00 to –12.00	–0.95	24	60	N.R.	60	0.71	12	0	24	1.12
ZSAL-4	Pérez-Santonja [43]	23	24	–19.56	–16.75 to –23.25	–0.65	56	83	0	61	1.12	N.R.	0	N.R.	1.45
NuVita	Allemann [5]	20	24	–18.95	–14.75 to –22.75	–1.93	10	10	5	N.R.	0.68	0	0	65	1.67

S.E., spherical equivalent; UCVA, uncorrected visual acuity; BCVA, best-corrected visual acuity; N.R., not recorded.
[a]ICM V3 and V4; [b]ICM V2–V4; [c]Concurrent limbal relaxing incisions to reduce corneal astigmatism; [d]Worst-Fechner and Worst; [e]Toric model.

Table 15.3. Major case series involving implantation of a phakic intraocular lens to correct hyperopia. (Table courtesy of Anthony J. Lombardo, MD, from [32])

Lens	First author [reference]	Eyes (n)	Mean follow-up (months)	Mean pre-op S.E. (D)	Range of refraction (D)	Efficacy Mean post-op S.E. (D)	Post-op ±0.5 D (%)	Post-op ±1.0 D [%]	UCVA 20/20 (%)	UCVA 20/40 (%)	Safety Efficacy index	BCVA loss of 1 line (%)	BCVA loss 2 or more lines (%)	BCVA gain 2 or more lines (%)	Safety index
ICL	Bloomenstein [15]	20	24	+5.55	+3.00 to +7.75	+0.06	80	95	40	80	N.R.	25	5	10	N.R.
	Pesando [44]	15	12	+7.77	+4.75 to +11.75	+0.02	69	92	0	46	N.R.	0	7.7	N.R.	N.R.
	Sanders [51]	10	6	+6.63	+2.50 to +10.88	+0.20	80	90	70	100	N.R.	0	0	20	1.13
	Rosen [49]	9	3	+4.26	+2.25 to +5.62	+0.26	89	89	44	89	0.98	11	0	22	1.16
	Bleckmann[a] [14]	7	8	+2.65	N.R.	+0.30	N.R.	N.R.	N.R.	N.R.	0.96	N.R.	N.R.	N.R.	1.05
PRL	Hoyos [28]	14	12	+7.77	+5.25 to +11.00	-0.38	50	79	N.R.	N.R.	0.60	7.1	0	0	1.00
Artisan	Alió [4]	29	14	+6.06	+3 to +9	+0.10	79	97	7	66	0.83	3.4	0	28	1.11
	Dick[b] [19]	22	6	+3.25	0 to +6.5	-0.24	50	100	18	96	1.03	0	0	14	1.25

S.E., spherical equivalent; UCVA, uncorrected visual acuity; BCVA, best-corrected visual acuity; N.R., not recorded.
[a]Concurrent limbal relaxing incisions to reduce corneal astigmatism; [b]Toric model.

15.6.3
Toric Results

One study describing the surgical outcomes of a toric phakic IOL was recently published [19]. A total of 48 myopic eyes with a mean preoperative spherical equivalent of –8.90 ±4.52 and 22 hyperopic eyes with a mean preoperative spherical equivalent of +3.25 ±1.98 D were implanted with the Artisan toric IOL. There was a significant reduction in spherical and cylindrical errors after surgery. The average magnitude of the refractive astigmatism was reduced from 3.7 D pre-operatively to 0.7 D post-operatively. Predictability was excellent: all eyes were within 1.00 D of the targeted refraction and 72.9 % were within 0.5 D.

15.7
Complications

The complications that are unique to each type of phakic IOL have been detailed in a previous section. While the major concern in anterior chamber lenses is endothelial cell loss, the critical concern in posterior chamber lenses is cataract formation. Table 15.4 summarises the complications for each type of lens as reported by the major studies. In general, the complication rates have shown continued improvement with each successive generation of lenses.

Endothelial cell loss rates have been acceptably low with the latest generation of anterior chamber lenses. It is important to distinguish endothelial cell loss from the initial surgical in-sult versus the gradual decline that results from intermittent IOL contact and chronic low grade inflammation. Most studies have concluded that the majority of endothelial cell loss has occurred at the time of surgery with only minimal loss thereafter. The studies with the longest follow-up of each of the lenses show a 12 % loss at 4 years with the ICL [18], a 13 % loss at 4 years with the Artisan [37], and a 9 % loss at 7 years with the ZSAL-4 [2].

The risk of cataract formation is greatest in the posterior chamber lenses. Because of improvements in vaulting, the latest generation of ICLs have been shown to have a reduced rate of cataract formation [50]. The Artisan lens also carries a risk of anterior subcapsular cataracts as well as anterior nuclear vacuoles associated with the trauma of insertion.

Pupil ovalisation is primarily a risk of anterior chamber phakic IOLs, with reported rates between 16 % and 40 %. They are generally progressive in nature and may be due to chronic irritation of the phakic IOL footplates in the anterior chamber angle. A small percentage of eyes have ovalisation that is non-progressive in nature and related to improper insertion.

Because anterior chamber lenses require smaller optic sizes that minimise the risk of endothelial contact, they are associated with the risk of glare and halos. In order to minimise these symptoms, the ZSAL-4 and NuVita lenses have optic edge modifications. The 5-mm model of the Artisan lens has a higher risk of symptoms, but Ophtec has offered a larger 6-mm optic to reduce glare and halos. However, this model is only available in powers up to 15.5 D.

Table 15.4. Reported complications in major case series involving implantation of a phakic intraocular lens. (Table courtesy of Anthony J. Lombardo, MD, from [32])

Lens	First author [reference]	Eyes (n)	Mean follow-up (months)	Endothelial cell loss	Pupil irregularity (%)	Pigment dispersion or lens deposits (%)	IOL decentration or rotation (%)	Chronic glaucoma (%)	Pupillary block glaucoma (%)	Cataract (%)	Glare or halos (%)
ICL	Sanders [50]	523	17	N.R.	N.R.	N.R.	N.R.	N.R	N.R.	2.9	N.R.
	Bloomenstein [15]	85	24	N.R.	0	0	0	N.R.	1.2	21	0
	Arne [7]	58	6	-2.0% at 2 years	0	100	N.R.	3.4	N.R.	3.4	54
	Uusitalo [55]	38	22	N.R.	N.R.	N.R.	5.3	0	7.9	7.9	N.R.
	Dejaco-Ruhswurm[a] [18]	34	>24	-12.3% at 4 years	N.R.	N.R.	N.R.	N.R.	N.R.	N.R.	N.R.
	Gonvers[b] [25]	32	7	N.R.	N.R.	88	N.R.	62	0	12.5	N.R.
	Menezo [38]	12	18	N.R.	0	42	17	0	0	25	8.3
	Sanders [51]	10	6	N.R.	0	0	N.R.	0	0	0	N.R.
	Rosen [49]	9	3	N.R.	N.R.	22	N.R.	N.R.	22	N.R.	N.R.
PRL	Hoyos [28]	31	12	N.R.	N.R.	3.2	18	N.R.	6.4	3.2	13
Artisan	Budo[c] [16]	249	36	-9.4% at 3 years	0.4	N.R.	8.8	N.R.	0.8	0.4	8.8
	Maloney[d] [34]	155	6	+0.23% at 6 mo.	1.2	N.R.	N.R.	0	0	2.4	2.4
	Alexander[e] [1]	135	6	+0.3% at 6 mo.	1.5	0	0.74	0	0	1.5	3
	Menezo[f] [37]	111	38	-13.42% at 4 years	0.9	N.R.	13.4	4.5	0	0	1.8
	Landesz [31]	78	24	+6.1% at 2 years	0	N.R.	N.R.	N.R.	0	2.6	13

aICM V2-V4 and ICH V2-3; bICM V3 and ICM V4; c5 mm optic only; d5 and 6 mm optic; e5 and 6 mm optic; fWorst-Fechner and Worst.

Table 15.4. Continued

Lens	First author [reference]	Eyes (n)	Mean follow-up (months)	Endothelial cell loss	Pupil irregularity (%)	Pigment dispersion or lens deposits (%)	IOL decentration or rotation (%)	Chronic glaucoma (%)	Pupillary block glaucoma (%)	Cataract (%)	Glare or halos (%)
	Dick [19]	70	6	-4.5% at 6 months	0	1.4	1.4	0	0	0	5.7
	El Danasoury [20]	43	12	-0.7% at 1 year	0	N.R.	2.2	N.R.	N.R.	N.R.	2.2
	Pérez-Santonja [42]	30	24	-17.6% at 2 years	N.R.	N.R.	N.R.	N.R.	N.R.	N.R.	N.R.
	Alió [4]	29	12	-9.4% at 1 year	5.3	15.8	3.4	N.R.	0	N.R.	6.8
	Malecaze [33]	25	12	-1.8% at 1 year	N.R.	N.R.	N.R.	0	N.R.	N.R.	52
ZSAL-4	Alió [2], Alió^g [3]	263	59,72	-9.3% at 7 years	16	N.R.	N.R.	7.2	0	3.4	10
	Pérez-Santonja [43]	18	24	-4.2% at 2 years	17	13	48	0	0	0	26
NuVita	Allemann [5]	20	24	-14% at 2 years	40	N.R.	80% with >15° rotation	4.8	0	0	20

N.R., not recorded. ^g ZB5 M and ZSAL-4.

15.8
Conclusions

The results of phakic IOL technology thus far have been encouraging. Although they may not achieve the same level of accuracy as excimer lasers at the lower ranges of ametropia, phakic IOLs are able to provide more predictable results at the higher ranges. Furthermore, the refractive outcomes of phakic IOLs offer more long term stability as compared to corneal refractive procedures, which must contend with the variability of corneal healing. In fact, phakic IOLs offer superior quality of vision with fewer induced higher order aberrations because they lack the variability of tissue healing. Consequently, there has been some speculation as to whether the future of "custom" refractive surgery lies with lenticular refractive surgery versus corneal refractive surgery. With custom cornea treatments, precision technology is being used to ablate an imprecise surface, namely the cornea. On the other hand, the smooth and precise refracting surface of phakic IOLs, as demonstrated by scanning electron microscopy studies [29], lack the micro-aberrations of ablated cornea and hence induce fewer aberrations. Furthermore, phakic IOLs may soon be designed to incorporate wavefront correction. Clearly, both technologies – the phakic IOLs and excimer laser technology – each have their own shortcomings as well as their own unique strengths. Thus at present, they will continue to exist in a symbiotic relationship that will allow us to further advance the results of refractive technology.

References

1. Alexander L, John M, Cobb L et al (2000) U. S. clinical investigation of the Artisan myopia lens for the correction of high myopia in phakic eyes. Report of the results of phases 1 and 2, and interim phase 3. Optometry 71:630–642
2. Alió JL, de la Hoz F, Pérez-Santonja JJ et al (1999) Phakic anterior chamber lenses for the correction of myopia: a 7-year cumulative analysis of complications in 263 cases. Ophthalmology 106:458–466
3. Alió JL, de la Hoz F, Ruiz-Moreno JM, Salem TF (2000) Cataract surgery in highly myopic eyes corrected by phakic anterior chamber angle-supported lenses(1). J Cataract Refract Surg 26:1303–1311
4. Alió JL, Mulet ME, Shalaby AM (2002) Artisan phakic iris claw intraocular lens for high primary and secondary hyperopia. J Refract Surg 18:697–707
5. Allemann N, Chamon W, Tanaka HM et al (2000) Myopic angle-supported intraocular lenses: two-year follow-up. Ophthalmology 107:1549–1554
6. Anderson Penno E, Braun DA, Kamal A, Hamilton WK, Gimbel HV (2003) Topical thiotepa treatment for recurrent corneal haze after photorefractive keratectomy. J Cataract Refract Surg 29:1537–1542
7. Arne JL, Lesueur LC (2000) Phakic posterior chamber lenses for high myopia: functional and anatomical outcomes. J Cataract Refract Surg 26:369–374
8. Assetto V, Benedetti S, Pesando P (1996) Collamer intraocular contact lens to correct high myopia. J Cataract Refract Surg 22:551–556
9. Baikoff G (2000) Anterior chamber phakic intraocular lenses. In: Elander R (ed) Operative techniques in cataract and refractive surgery, vol. 3. WB Saunders, Philadelphia
10. Baikoff G (2004) Baikoff's foldable anterior chamber phakic intraocular lenses for myopia, hyperopia, and presbyopia. In: Hardten DR, Lindstrom RL, Davis EA (eds) Phakic intraocular lenses: principles and practice. Slack, Thorofare, NJ
11. Baikoff G, Joly P (1989) Surgical correction of severe myopia using an anterior chamber implant in the phakic eye. Concept-results. Bull Soc Belge Ophtalmol 233:109–125
12. Baikoff G, Arne JL, Bokobza Y, Colin J, George JL, Lagoutte F, Lesure P, Montard M, Saragoussi JJ, Secheyron P (1998) Angle-fixated anterior chamber phakic intraocular lens for myopia of -7 to -19 diopters. J Refract Surg 14:282–293
13. Barraquer J (1959) Anterior chamber plastic lenses. Results of and conclusions from five years' experience. Trans Ophthalmol Soc UK 79:393–424
14. Bleckmann H, Keuch RJ (2002) Implantation of spheric phakic posterior chamber intraocular lenses in astigmatic eyes. J Cataract Refract Surg 28:805–809
15. Bloomenstein MR, Dulaney DD, Barnet RW, Perkins SA (2002) Posterior chamber phakic intraocular lens for moderate myopia and hyperopia. Optometry 73:435–446

16. Budo C, Hessloehl JC, Izak M, Luyten GP, Menezo JL, Sener BA, Tassignon MJ, Termote H, Worst JG (2000) Multicenter study of the Artisan phakic intraocular lens. J Cataract Refract Surg 26:1163–1171

17. Carones F, Vigo L, Scandola E, Vacchini L (2002) Evaluation of the prophylactic use of mitomycin-C to inhibit haze formation after photorefractive keratectomy. J Cataract Refract Surg 28:2088–2095

18. Dejaco-Ruhswurm I, Scholz U, Pieh S, Hanselmayer G, Lackner B, Italon C, Ploner M, Skorpik C (2002) Long-term endothelial changes in phakic eyes with posterior chamber intraocular lenses. J Cataract Refract Surg 28:1589–1593

19. Dick HB, Alió J, Bianchetti M, Budo C, Christiaans BJ, El-Danasoury MA, Güell JL, Krumeich J, Landesz M, Loureiro F, Luyten GP, Marinho A, Rahhal MS, Schwenn O, Spirig R, Thomann U, Venter J (2003) Toric phakic intraocular lens: European multicenter study. Ophthalmology 110:150–162

20. El Danasoury MA, El Maghraby A, Gamali TO (2002) Comparison of iris-fixed Artisan lens implantation with excimer laser in situ keratomileusis in correcting myopia between −9.00 and −19.50 diopters: a randomized study. Ophthalmology 109:955–964

21. Fechner PU, van der Heijde GL, Worst JG (1988) Intraocular lens for the correction of myopia of the phakic eye. Klin Monatsbl Augenheilkd 193:29–34

22. Fink AM, Gore C, Rosen E (1999) Cataract development after implantation of the Staar Collamer posterior chamber phakic lens. J Cataract Refract Surg 25:278–282

23. Foss AJ, Rosen PH, Cooling RJ (1993) Retinal detachment following anterior chamber lens implantation for the correction of ultra-high myopia in phakic eyes. Br J Ophthalmol 77:212–213

24. Fyodorov SL, Zuyev VK, Aznabayev BM (1991) Intraocular correction of high myopia with negative posterior chamber lens. Ophthalmosurgery 3:57–58

25. Gonvers M, Othenin-Girard P, Bornet C, Sickenberg M (2001) Implantable contact lens for moderate to high myopia: short-term follow-up of 2 models. J Cataract Refract Surg 27:380–388

26. Hardten DR (2000) Phakic iris claw artisan intraocular lens for correction of high myopia and hyperopia. Int Ophthalmol Clin 40:209–221

27. Holladay JT, Piers PA, Koranyi G, van der Mooren M, Norrby NE (2002) A new intraocular lens design to reduce spherical aberration of pseudophakic eyes. J Refract Surg 18:683–691

28. Hoyos JE, Dementiev DD, Cigales M, Hoyos-Chacón J, Hoffer KJ (2002) Phakic refractive lens experience in Spain. J Cataract Refract Surg 28:1939–1946

29. Kohnen T, Baumeister M, Magdowski G (2000) Scanning electron microscopic characteristics of phakic intraocular lenses. Ophthalmology 107:934–939

30. Landesz M, Worst JG, van Rij G (2000) Long-term results of correction of high myopia with an iris claw phakic intraocular lens. J Refract Surg 16:310–316

31. Landesz M, van Rij G, Luyten G (2001) Iris-claw phakic intraocular lens for high myopia. J Refract Surg 17:634–640

32. Lombardo AJ (2004) Comparison of refractive outcomes and complications among current phakic intraocular lenses. In: Hardten DR, Lindstrom RL, Davis EA Phakic intraocular lenses: principles and practice. Slack, Thorofare, NJ, p 225

33. Malecaze FJ, Hulin H, Bierer P, Fournié P, Grandjean H, Thalamas C, Guell JL (2002) A randomized paired eye comparison of two techniques for treating moderately high myopia: LASIK and artisan phakic lens. Ophthalmology 109:1622–1630

34. Maloney RK, Nguyen LH, John ME (2002) Artisan phakic intraocular lens for myopia:short-term results of a prospective, multicenter study. Ophthalmology 109:1631–1641

35. Menezo JL, Cisneros A, Hueso JR, Harto M (1995) Long-term results of surgical treatment of high myopia with Worst-Fechner intraocular lenses. J Cataract Refract Surg 21:93–98

36. Menezo JL, Aviño JA, Cisneros A, Rodriguez-Salvador V, Martinez-Costa R (1997) Iris claw phakic intraocular lens for high myopia. J Refract Surg 13:545–555

37. Menezo JL, Cisneros AL, Rodriguez-Salvador V (1998) Endothelial study of iris-claw phakic lens: four year follow-up. J Cataract Refract Surg 24:1039–1049

38. Menezo JL, Peris-Martínez C, Cisneros A, Martínez-Costa R (2001) Posterior chamber phakic intraocular lenses to correct high myopia: a comparative study between Staar and Adatomed models. J Refract Surg 17:32–42

39. Mimouni F, Colin J, Koffi V, Bonnet P (1991) Damage to the corneal endothelium from anterior chamber intraocular lenses in phakic myopic eyes. Refract Corneal Surg 7:277–281

40. Moller-Pedersen T, Cavanagh HD, Petroll WM, Jester JV (2000) Stromal wound healing explains refractive instability and haze development after photorefractive keratectomy: a 1-year confocal microscopic study. Ophthalmology 107:1235–1245

41. Oshika T, Miyata K, Tokunaga T, Samejima T, Amano S, Tanaka S, Hirohara Y, Mihashi T, Maeda N, Fujikado T (2002) Higher order wavefront aberrations of cornea and magnitude of refractive correction in laser in situ keratomileusis. Ophthalmology 109:1154–1158

42. Pérez-Santonja JJ, Iradier MT, Sanz-Iglesias L, Serrano JM, Zato MA (1996) Endothelial changes in phakic eyes with anterior chamber intraocular lenses to correct high myopia. J Cataract Refract Surg 22:1017–1022

43. Pérez-Santonja JJ, Alio JL, Jimenez-Alfaro I, Zato MA (2000) Surgical correction of severe myopia with an angle-supported phakic intraocular lens. J Cataract Refract Surg 26:1288–1302

44. Pesando PM, Ghiringhello MP, Tagliavacche P (1999) Posterior chamber collamer phakic intraocular lens for myopia and hyperopia. J Refract Surg 15:415–423

45. Philipp WE, Speicher L, Göttinger W (2003) Histological and immunohistochemical findings after laser in situ keratomileusis in human corneas. J Cataract Refract Surg 29:808–820

46. Probst LE (2004) Comparison of phakic intraocular lenses with corneal refractive surgery. In: Hardten DR, Lindstrom RL, Davis EA (eds) Phakic intraocular lenses principles and practice. Slack, Thorofare, NJ

47. Purohit SJ, Angeles RT, Westeren AC et al. (2004) Angle-supported phakic intraocular lenses: the phakic 6H2. In: Hardten DR, Lindstrom RL, Davis EA (eds) Phakic intraocular lenses: principles and practice. Slack, Thorofare, NJ

48. Rao SN, Epstein RJ (2002) Early onset ectasia following laser in situ keratomileusus: case report and literature review. J Refract Surg 18:177–184

49. Rosen E, Gore C (1998) Staar Collamer posterior chamber phakic intraocular lens to correct myopia and hyperopia. J Cataract Refract Surg 24:596–606

50. Sanders DR, Vukich JA (2002) Incidence of lens opacities and clinically significant cataracts with the implantable contact lens: comparison of two lens designs. J Refract Surg 18:673–682

51. Sanders DR, Martin RG, Brown DC, Shepherd J, Deitz MR, DeLuca M (1999) Posterior chamber phakic intraocular lens for hyperopia. J Refract Surg 15:309–315

52. Sanders DR, Vukich JA, Doney K, Gaston M (2003) U.S. Food and Drug Administration clinical trial of the Implantable Contact Lens for moderate to high myopia. Ophthalmology 110:255–266

53. Schwartz GS, Lane SS (2004) CIBA vision phakic refractive lens. In: Hardten DR, Lindstrom RL, Davis EA (eds) Phakic intraocular lenses: principles and practice. Slack, Thorofare, NJ

54. Strampelli B (1954) Sopportabilita di lenti acriliche in camera anteriore nella afachia e nei vizi refrazione. Ann Ottamol Clin Oculist 80:75–82

55. Uusitalo RJ, Aine E, Sen NH, Laatikainen L (2002) Implantable contact lens for high myopia. J Cataract Refract Surg 28:29–36

56. Vukich J (2002) Phakic IOL's and LASIK: Comparison of Visual Outcomes in High Myopia. ISRS pre AAO Meeting. Orlando, FL

57. Werner L, Apple DJ, Izak AM, Pandey SK, Trivedi RH, Macky TA (2001) Phakic anterior chamber intraocular lenses. Int Ophthalmol Clin 41:133–152

58. Zaldivar R, Davidorf JM, Oscherow S (1998) Posterior chamber phakic intraocular lens for myopia of –8 to –19 diopters. J Refract Surg 14:294–305

59. Zaldivar R, Oscherow S, Ricur G (2000) The STAAR posterior chamber phakic intraocular lens. Int Ophthalmol Clin 40:237–244

60. Zaldivar R, Oscherow S, Piezzi V (2002) Bioptics in phakic and pseudophakic intraocular lens with the Nidek EC-5000 excimer laser. J Refract Surg 18:S336–339

Refractive Lens Exchange

Jose Luis Güell, Nancy Sandoval, Felicidad Manero, Oscar Gris

---

Core Messages

- Refractive Lens Exchange is possibly the best refractive surgical technique for the correction of high myopia and high hyperopia compared to the other possible surgical approaches in patients in the presbyopic age
- The surgical technique is similar to phacoemulsification for cataract extraction with Intraocular Lens implantation
- It is a safe and predictable technique. It provides refractive stability, rapid visual rehabilitation and better visual quality.
- Severe complications such as retinal detachment or endophthalmitis are rare
- It is open to possible refractive enhancements, using corneal refractive techniques

---

16.1
Introduction

Currently there are two general approaches to correct a refractive error: refractive corneal surgery and intraocular refractive surgery. In either case, the main goal of refractive surgery is to achieve the smallest residual refractive error preserving quality of vision with the same visual capacity. Surgical manipulation of the crystalline lens is one of our frequent refractive surgeries.

The correction of high myopia and high hyperopia is still a controversial topic. Refractive surgical procedures are usually performed at the cornea. Correction of myopia is relatively easier, but the correction of hyperopia by means of corneal surgery is used by few refractive surgeons due to its technical and conceptual complexity (it is clearly easier to flatten than to steepen the cornea), its lower predictability and more frequent unsatisfactory results [10, 11]. The correction of low to moderate myopia or hyperopia at the corneal plane provides acceptable quality of vision, but high corrections cause significant optical aberrations and poor quality of vision especially under dim light conditions [19, 25, 30, 42], such that intraocular refractive surgery becomes a valid alternative to correct cases of high ametropia.

Refractive lens extraction (RLE) is an intraocular refractive surgery consisting of the extraction of the natural lens and its substitution by an posterior chamber intraocular lens (IOL) of proper dioptric (D) power (Fig 16.1 and 16.2). When it is not associated with a cataract, others call it "clear or semi-clear lens extraction" or "refractive lensectomy" or "refractive lens exchange". This is a very ancient surgical technique; Fukala [13] first reported RLE in 1778. He is considered the pioneer of the refractive lensectomy concept. Later on, the increasing risk of retinal detachment (RD) with this procedure was reported, due to it this surgical technique was left of side and was finally abandoned.

Nowadays, RLE is a surgical technique that has been revived and is under constant investigation [38]. Theoretically, RLE is a surgical procedure with the same risks and complications as cataract extraction surgery. According to Werblin [47], in experienced hands, the incidence of permanent visual loss from an intraoperative or postoperative complication of IOL surgery is between 0.5% and 1.0%. In this regard, the procedures and materials have evolved promptly during the last 30 years, changing the

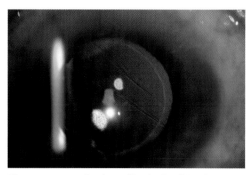

Fig. 16.1. Monofocal IOL "in the bag" implantation in a high myope. Note the oblique folds at the posterior capsule

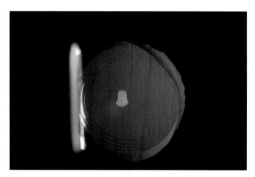

Fig. 16.2. Multifocal (refractive) IOL "in the bag" implantation in the other eye of the same patient as in Fig. 16.1 (non-dominant eye)

point of view of the ophthalmologists and the expectations of both, the professionals and the patients.

RLE might be considered today a surgical option for the correction of high myopia and, high hyperopia, in patients in presbyopic age. This procedure can provide rapid and predictable visual rehabilitation and refractive stability; moreover, the implant can be removed and replaced, usually easily and safely, in the rare case of "refractive surprise". In other cases, corneal refractive surgery may be used to adjust the final refraction. Furthermore, the visual quality and optical rehabilitation is superior than with other surgical modalities, especially with corneal techniques which are limited by both corneal thickness and corneal curvature. We limit our corneal intervention to expected post-operative corneal curvatures between 39.0 and 48.0 D in order to prevent optical aberrations, glare and other visual phenomena after the procedure.

Nevertheless controversy persists over whether RLE should be considered as "routine refractive surgery" since some questions about the risk : benefit ratio with this technique remain unanswered. Today, thanks to the phacoemulsification surgical technique, small incision surgery, viscoelastics materials, and foldable IOLs, the safety of the procedure and guarantee of the refractive results we have are better. We think that RLE is the best surgical technique for the correction of high myopia and high hyperopia, especially in patients older than 45 years since the majority of them, if not all, have some degree of degenerative changes in the natural lens. Under this conditions, corneal surgery induced aberrations might easily increase the total aberrations of the eye. As such, in order to optimise the results and provide refractive stability with visual quality, extracting an incipient cataract, in our opinion, is the first surgical option in this group of patients.

16.2
Myopia

16.2.1
Visual Results

Refractive lens exchange has been suggested for the treatment of high axial myopia. Lens removal could compensate the myopic refractive error. RLE fulfils satisfactorily the two main objectives of everything refractive surgery: predictability and safety. RLE for myopia, through phacoemulsification, **gives very good results**. All authors reported improvement in 100 % of the cases in UCVA and increase in BCVA in some cases (see Table 16.1).

Theoretically it would appear that there is a higher risk of Snellen VA loss with intraocular refractive surgery than with corneal refractive surgery. Nevertheless, we must remember that some studies showed a loss of BCVA with LASIK surgery up to 12 % of cases with high myopia (−7.00 D to −29.00 D) [16, 25]. Meanwhile, with

RLE the incidence of this complication, seems to be lower: between 0 and 4%. Colin and colleagues [4,5,6] reported 4% of patients (2/49) with a loss of BCVA of more than 2 lines, one after macular complication and one after retinal detachment (RD), at 7-years follow-up, and for this reason, it is not possible to clearly establish the relationship between the loss of BCVA and the surgical procedure.

The improvement in BCVA reported in the literature and also observed by us in daily practice is remarkable. The mean postoperative BCVA improved by an average of 1 line and other surgeons as Lee and Lee (27) report that 75% of patients gained tow or more Snellen lines of BCVA. However, Colin and colleagues [4, 5, 6] reported that this visual benefit is not constant in the time, they found that the improvement of BCVA from 0.57 pre-operatively to 0.61 post-operatively at 1 year, is identical to preoperative BCVA at 4-years, possibly due to the worsening of previously existing macular lesions. An explanation of this phenomenon remains to be found.

The results in predictability are variable. Chastang and colleagues (3) reported that in 87,9% of cases, the postoperative refraction was within ±2.00 D of emmetropia. In most recent report, Gabric and colleagues (14) reported 87,5% of cases within ±1,0 D and 95,8%, within ±2.0 D of emmetropia. On the other hand, Pucci (36) and Chastang (3) reported cases with 3.0 D and 3,5 D of biometric error, respectively.

Accuracy in the post-operative refraction depend on precise pre-operatory biometry The most frequent cause of imprecision in the IOL power calculation is due to an error in the axial length measurement; therefore, is necessary to realize an echographic exam in A and B modes, because this patients have frequently, posterior segment staphylomas. We use the SRK-T formula, which allows us to realize a IOL power calculation with sufficient precision. The post-operative target refraction is emmetropia or "monovision".

In our case series published recently [17], of 42 eyes with high myopia (mean of −15.8 D) that underwent phacoemulsification of clear or semi-clear lens; we found, 52.7% of the eyes had a manifest refraction within ±1.00 D and 94.1%

within ±2.00 D (−1.05 D on average) at 4 years after surgery. An improvement of BCVA of at least 1 line of Snellen visual acuity was seen in 72.5% of the eyes, while no eyes presented loss of BCVA. Obviously, predictability would be better if we included in the final results, eyes treated with corneal surgery for refractive residual error.

16.2.2
Complications

The most common significant complication in high myopic eyes is retinal detachment (RD). Perkins [34] has estimated the risk of RD in non-operated eyes with myopia ≥−10.0 D in 0.68% per year. Apparently, there is a linear correlation between the degree of myopia and the incidence of RD [15, 35, 48].

Likewise, in those eyes with high myopia which underwent RLE, the major risk for permanent visual loss is also secondary to RD. The main risk factors include: peripheral retinal degeneration, intra-operative posterior capsular rupture, absence of posterior chamber IOL, and Nd:YAG laser application after surgery [43, 31, 9].

Javitt [23] estimated an RD rate of 7.5% and assumes that 25% of RD are unsuccessfully reattached and that these cases have a 100% rate of severe visual loss. His conclusion is that 3.3% can expect severe visual loss due to RD following RLE. I think that Javitt overestimates the risk for visual loss due to RD, because Javitt's study is based on the rates of the case series presented by Barraquer (7.3%), Coonan (3.5%) and Lindstrom (9.6%) (1, 7, 28). Barraquer and colleagues, for example, included cases that underwent different surgical techniques: lens aspiration (59.4%), intracapsular extraction (3.0%) and manual extracapsular extraction (37.6%) with incisions larger than 140°. Only nine of the 165 (15%) cases received an IOL and the retina was reattached in 75% of cases. Obviously, these techniques are not comparable with the modern phacoemulsification and RD repair techniques.

The risk of severe visual loss due to RD in high myopic eyes that underwent RLE by phacoemulsification seems to be significantly low-

Table 16.1. Visual results and complications in myopic patients with RLE phacoemulsification

Reference (n)	Eyes (n)	Average age (years)	Average follow-up (range)	Average myopia (range)	Average post-operative SE (range)	UCVA (%) 20/40	Emmetropia (%) ±1.0 D (±2.0 D)	Number with loss of BCVA (%)	Number with RD (%)	Number with Nd:YAG (%)	Other complications
[24]	26	42.1	NR (12–24 months)	−20.85 (−12 to −33.75)		42	76.91 (96.16)	0	0		None
[29]c	31	45.5	21.7 months (5–57)	−12.0 (−8.0 to −20.0)	NR	77	68.0 (90.0)	NR	0		None
[27]	24	34.4	15 months (12–24)	−16.6 (−12.0 to −25.75)	NR	79.2	62.0 (91.7)	0	0	1 (2.4)	None
[4]	52	36.2	NR (1 year)	−16.9 (−12.0 to −23.75)	−0.86±0.8 (NR)	88.5		1 (2.0%)a	0		None
[5]	52	36.2	NR (4 years)	−16.9 (−12.0 to −23.75)	NR	NR		1 (2.0%)a	1 (1.9)		None
[6]	52	36.2	NR (7 years)	−16.9 (−12.0 to −23.75)	−1.01±0.94 (NR)	NR	59.1 (85.7)	1 (2.0%)a	4 (8.1)		None
[18]	46	38	NR (6–15 months)	−16.5 (NR)	−0.96±0.86		48.4 (92.5)	0	1 (2.2)		None
[36]	25	41.6	42.92 months (39–49)	−18.36 (−12.75 to −24.00)	NR	NR	NR	1 (4.0%)b	1 (4)		None
[17]	44	42.83	31.45 months (21–53)	−15.77 (−3.50 to −29.0)	−1.05 (+2.75 to −4.75)	NR	52.7 (94.1)	0	0	25 (56.8)	None
[46]	36	53.9	23.5 months (7–35)	−13.11 (NR)	−1.51±0.60 (NR)	69.4	NR	NR	0	NR (5.6)	None
[3]	33	31.04	27	−19.5 (−12.0 to −40.0)	−2.57±−1.84 (NR)	NR	NR (87.9)	NR	2 (6.1)	NR (30)	None
[2]	40		45.9 months (17–118)	−14.5 (NR)	NR	NR	NR	0	0	20 (50)	1 MCE
[39]e	4			NR (−14.0 to 28.0)	NR (−0.75 to +2.75)	NR	NR		0		1 VL

Table 16.1. Continued

Reference	Eyes (n)	Average age (years)	Average follow-up (range)	Average myopia (range)	Average post-operative SE (range)	UCVA (%) 20/40	Emmetropia (%) ±1.0 D (±2.0D)	Number with loss of BCVA (%)	Number with RD (%)	Number with Nd:YAG (%)	Other complications
[22]	284[d]		37.57 months (NR)	−15.96 (NR)	NR	NR	NR		0		None
[14]	72		48 months (5 months to 5 years)	NR	NR	58.3	87.5 (95.8)	NR	1 (7.2)	22 (30.5)	1 MCE
[45][c]	138	NR	NR	NR (−0.25 to −23.75)	NR	90	78.3 (93.5)	NR	NR (0.7)	NR (8.0)	None
[44]	736	NR	NR	NR (greater than −10.0)	NR	NR	NR	NR	6 (0.8)		None
Total	1411										

SE, spherical equivalent; UCVA, uncorrected visual acuity; BCVA, best corrected visual acuity; RD retinal detachment; NR, not registered; MCE, macular cystic oedema; VL, vitreous loss.
[a]Subretinal neovascularisation; [b]myopic degeneration; [c]inluding myopic and hyperopic patients; [d]4.57% with CLE; [e]patients with Marfan's syndrome.

er. Gris, Güell and colleagues (18) reported one RD (2,2%) that occurred 4 weeks after surgery in an eye with a posterior capsular tear. Likewise, Pucci and colleagues (36) in their study of 25 eyes with myopia higher than –12.0 D found 4,0% (one case) of postoperative RD. In other current clinical studies with follow-up of 4 years or less, tended to have excellent results: zero incidence of RD. In these reports, the incidence of RD may relate to degree of preoperative myopia, surgical technique and duration of follow-up.

In our last study [17], the incidence of retinal detachment was 0% in 44 eyes with a mean pre-operative spherical equivalent (SE) of –15.8 D. No eye required pre-operative peripheral retinal photocoagulation. Colin and colleagues [4,5,6] demonstrating an increased incidence with time, found an RD incidence of 8.1% over a follow-up of 7 years, versus 2.0% over a follow-up of 4 years. In patients whit Lattice degeneration retinal tear or hole, was performed argon laser before RLE.

Currently, it is not clear whether prophylaxis by means of laser onto the retina can reduce the RD incidence; in fact, many authors have reported that the prophylactic treatment not always avoids RD after RLE but might increase it. Ripandelli and colleagues [37] reported a study of 41 patients with high myopia (–14.00 to –29.00 D) who underwent surgery for RD after RLE; 26 of them received prophylactic laser retinopexy onto 360° of the retina, while RD occurred along the previous circumferential photocoagulation border in four patients. Only nine patients achieved BCVA ≥20/60 after retinopexy post-RLE. Although the authors did not report the RD incidence after RLE, they advised on the potential complications (27 of 41 eyes developed some degree of vitreo-retinal proliferation) able to produce visual loss, in spite of the prophylactic laser treatment. We only perform laser prophylaxis in those lesions where the vitreoretinal surgeon thinks there is a high risk of RD.

Visual acuity worsens after surgery due to the progression of posterior capsular opacification (PCO), Nd:YAG laser application becomes a mandatory procedure in these eyes. Nd:YAG laser capsulotomy has been associated with an additional risk factor for RD (31), especially in cases with high myopia, increasing the risk of permanent visual loss in patients with previous vitreo-retinal lesions. Both, RLE and Nd:YAG laser capsulotomy increase the incidence of posterior vitreous detachment (PVD). Javitt [23] have considered that the risk of RD in high myopia multiplies 3.9 times after laser YAG capsulotomy. For this reason it is usually recommended only in cases with a decrease of more than one line in BCVA and after a minimum of 6 months following surgery.

The reported PCO in the literature varies between 5.6% up to 61.2%. [2, 3, 14, 17, 27, 45, 46]. We have confirmed clinically significant PCO in 56.8% of the eyes, all of which required YAG laser capsulotomy [17]. Colin and colleagues [4–6] found an obvious increase of PCO with time, reporting a 36.4% incidence during the first 4-years versus 61.2% over 7-years of follow-up. Mean time for capsulotomy was 48.4 months after RLE. There were no reports of RD or other complications following laser YAG capsulotomy. It should be noted that the PCO variation could be mainly related to the design and type of material of the IOLs, as well as to the epithelial cells cleaning technique used during surgery, though PCO is not yet preventable.

Other important complication after RLE are the vitreo-retinal changes. More than the half of high myopic patients has a vitreal alteration previous to the surgery. Colin and colleagues (4,5,6) in their series reported 57,7% of pre-operatory vitro-retinal alterations, they found an incidence of post-operative PVD of 16,3% in overall at 7-years. Ripandelli and colleagues (37) suggested that RLE might play a major role in RD by precipitating vitreous changes that other wise would have occurred more slowly over time.

Macular complications are less frequent, but this complications might produce permanent visual loss. Colin and colleagues (6) reported one case of choroidal sub-foveal neovascularization, who decrease BCVA from 20/50 to 20/200 after this complication. We believe that by employing a careful surgical technique and preserving intraocular pressure (IOP) during the surgery, macular complications should be rare. On the other hand, a control group without RLE by myopia is required to an accurate evaluation of the incidence of macular complications attributable to RLE surgery. Other less frequent complications following RLE reported in the literature include: raised IOP [17], cystic macular oedema (CME) [2,14], and intra-operative vitreous loss [41]. (see Table 16.1)

In conclusion, patients with high myopia present several ocular abnormalities that progressively increase over time [15, 48] and the surgical options for refractive correction available to them might have some undesirable secondary effects. Any corneal surgery in high myopia induces visual aberrations and, combined with progressive lens opacification, significantly reduces the optical quality of the eye. This is one of the main reasons to select RLE as a refractive surgical procedure to correct high myopia in middle-age patients.

This does not mean that the procedure could then become broadly recommended. It should be performed in selected cases and following a complete examination to detect vitreo-retinal abnormalities. We offer RLE as the first option for patients older than 45 years or with presbyopic symptomatology, and with myopia greater than -6.0D that are out of the proper range for correction with other available refractive procedure. Finally, we consider a long and continuous follow-up of the outcomes of RLE for high myopia an absolute necessity before it can be practised routinely.

16.3
Hyperopia

Our ability to correct myopia has always been greater than our ability to correct hyperopia. In recent decades, several surgical techniques have been proposed for hyperopia correction with mildly encouraging results, although some of them are not currently used. RLE for hyperopia is an intraocular refractive procedure proposed initially by Osher in 1994 [32, 33]. With almost 10 years of experience, RLE with IOL implantation seems to be a safe and effective refractive technique, especially in patients around the presbyopic age.

Hyperopic individuals are totally dependent on optical correction, for both, near and distance vision, especially in presbyopic age, in contrast to myopic individuals which have, at least, some degree of near vision. According to Siganos and colleagues (40), hyperopes belonging to the age group of 35-years older will soon be needing presbyopic correction, adding more diopters to the already existing plus correction, translated, in turn, into more spherical and chromatic aberrations, more constricted visual field and further decrease in the image quality. These patients require a safe solution for their visual dependence and we believe that RLE is a satisfactory procedure for this intention.

16.3.1
Visual Results

Optional or elective surgery, as in most cases of refractive surgery, needs a safety level higher than the one related with surgery performed on the basis of medical indications. In an earlier prospective study, Siganos and colleagues (39) showed that RLE with subsequent implantation oh high power IOL in high hyperopia provided accuracy, high predictability, safety and rapid visual stability in a series of 10 eyes whit 18 months follow-up.

Likewise, Siganos and Pallikaris (40), in 17 normally sighted eyes, with spherical equivalent (SE) of +9.61 D (+6.75 D to +13.75 D) reported that postoperative SE was of +0.19 D and the mean UCVA improved from count fingers (CF) to 0.84 at three-years. In posterior report the same authors (41) reported similar results in 35 eyes whit hyperopia of +7.0 D to +14.0 D, they found a mean UCVA of 0.8 (0.5 to 1.0) after surgery. No eyes lost any lines of BCVA. Stability of refraction was noted from the second month after RLE.

A safe refractive procedure might at least maintain pre-operative BCVA. Theoretically, hyperopic eyes should loose BCVA after RLE, and in fact, some studies have confirmed this idea. Kolahdouz-Isfahani and colleagues [26], in a case series of 18 eyes, reported 11.1% deterioration of at least one line of Snellen BCVA. Similar findings were revealed by Fink and colleagues [12] when they reported a loss of one line of Snellen vision in 11.5% of the eyes with mean SE of +2.28 D (+1.25 to +4.0 D), and 29.00% in eyes with mean SE of +6.32 D (+4.75 to +10.25 D).

Table 16.2. Myopic patients with phacoemulsification with piggy-back or single implantation

Average myopia (range)	Post-operative SE Average (range)	UCVA (%) 20/40	Emmetropia (%) ±1.0 D (±2.0 D)	Number with loss of BCVA (%)	Number with RD (%)	Nd:YAG No (%)	Other complications
−20.85 (−12 to −33.75)		42	76.91 (96.16)	0	0		None
−12.0 (−8.0 to −20.0)	NR	77	68.0 (90.0)	NR	0		None
−16.6 (−12.0 to −25.75)	NR	79.2	62.0 (91.7)	0	0	1 (2.4)	None
−16.9 (−12.0 to −23.75)	−0.86±0.84 (NR)	88.5		1 (2.0%)[a]	0		None
−16.9 (−12.0 to −23.75)		NR	59.1 (85.7)	1 (2.0%)[a]	1 (1.9)		None
−16.9 (−12.0 to −23.75)	−1.01±0.94 (NR)	NR	48.4 (92.5)	1 (2.0%)[a]	4 (8.1)		None
−16.5 (NR)	−0.96±0.86 (NR)			0	1 (2.2)		None
−18.36 (−12.75 to −24.0)	NR	NR	NR	1 (4.0%)[b]	1 (4)		None
−15.77 (−3.50 to −29.0)	−1.05 (+2.75 to −4.75)	NR	52.7 (94.1)	0	0	25 (56.8)	None
−13.11 (NR)	−1.51±0.60 (NR)	69.4	NR	NR	0	NR (5.6)	None
−19.5 (−12.0 to −40.0)	−2.57±1.84 (NR)		NR (87.9)	NR	2 (6.1)	NR (30)	None
−14.5 (NR)	NR	NR	NR	0	0	20 (50)	1 EMC
NR (−14.0 to −28.0)	NR (−0.75 to +2.75)	NR	NR		0		1 PV
−15.96 (NR)	NR	NR	NR	NR	0		None
NR	NR	58.3	87.5 (95.8)	NR	1 (7.2)	22 (30.5)	1 EMC
NR (−0.25 to −23.75)	NR	90	78.3 (93.5)	NR	NR (0.7)	NR (8.0)	None
NR (greater than −10.0)	NR	NR	NR	NR	6 (0.8)		None

UCVA, uncorrected visual acuity; BCVA, best corrected visual acuity; RD retinal detachment; NR, not registered.

Nevertheless, Fink and colleagues(12) found that 80.7% and 70.9% of eyes, had no change or gained a line in BCV in 26 eyes with low hyperopia (up to +4.0 D) and in 24 patients with highest hyperopia (up to +10.25), respectively. These results could be due to the extraction of a highly positive natural lens with magnifying effect that causes spherical aberrations and retinal defocusing in an eye with high hyperopia and some degree of opacification lens, although the cause of these outcomes is not completely understood.

The final refraction is possibly more important in hyperopic that in myopic individuals. Any error is very badly tolerated by this kind of patient. Apparently, the most important single limiting factor for the success of RLE in hyperopia is the inaccuracy of the formulas used for the IOL power calculation. Different formulas have been used (SRK-II, SRK-T, Hoffer-Q y Holladay-II), and there is still a debate regarding which is the most adequate formula. The Holladay-II formula takes into account different variables such as anterior chamber depth, axial length, lens thickness, white-to-white distance, pre-operative manifest refraction and age. All these variables enable a calculation of the accurate IOL position following surgery. This aspect is very important in short eyes because a displacement of 1 mm produces an error of ±1.0 D for each 10.0D of IOL power.

Fink and colleagues [12] reported good predictability in low hyperopic eyes, (mean SE of +2.28 D); 88,5% of the cases were within ±1.0 D of the intended refraction using the Holladay II formula, comparable with other low hyperopia studies; Lyle and Jean (29), recorded 75% of eyes within ±1.0 D of intented refraction, using various formulas. Furthermore, Fink (12) found that with higher refractive errors, predictability was less accurate, only 58.3% of eyes within ±1.0 D of emmetropia. Koladouz-Isfahani and colleagues [26], in their study with 18 eyes with SE of +6.17 D (+4.25 to +9.25 D) reported a mean IOL calculation error of +0.81 D. Only 39% of the eyes achieved a post-operative manifest refraction within ±1.0 D. Biometric calculation was performed using the Hoffer-Q formula in 16 eyes, and Holladay-II, in two nanophthalmic eyes.

However, Siganos and colleagues [41] achieved good predictability with a previous generation

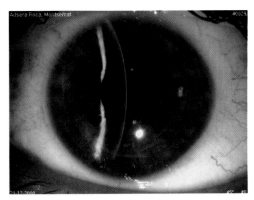

Fig. 16.3. LASIK for the final enhancement after clear lens extraction and IOL implantation for high hyperopia

formula: They reported 100% and 83% within ±1.0 D of emmetropia using the SRK-II and SRK-T formula, respectively, in hyperopic eyes of +7.0 to +14.0 D. In contrast, Hoffer [20] found an error greater than 2.0 D, in 11% of cases using the SRK-II formula in short eyes. There is still much unresolved debate about which is the best formula to use for short eyes. It would appear that a lot depends on the accuracy of the biometrist and on the experience or preference of the surgeon in the selection of the formula to be used.

In any case, it is possible to adjust the final manifest refraction by means of a corneal refractive procedure (Fig. 16.3). With regard to this point, in our experience, is easier to correct a myopic residual refraction in the corneal plane because is more predictable than a hyperopic residual refraction.

In agreement with Fink and colleagues (12), the incidence of secondary enhancement procedures depends not just on the degree of accuracy of the initial surgery, but also on the subjective satisfaction of the patient. Each additional refractive procedure carries additional risk, both specific to the procedure and also to the potential interaction with optical sequel from the primary surgery. The surgical technique chosen depends on the preferences of the surgeon, on the available technology and the magnitude of change required. In the majority of cases, the surgeon is able to improve the situation with a small refinement, but the predictability of this second procedure might be re-

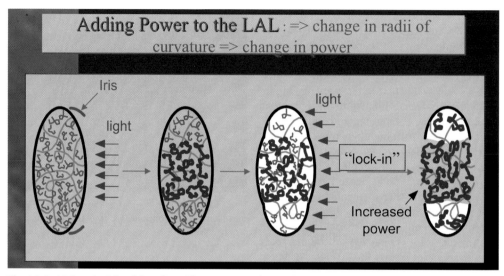

Fig. 16.4. Main principle of the adjustable IOL project from Calhoun Vision. Note the capability of refractive refinement once the IOL is already in the eye

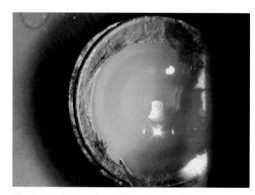

Fig. 16.5. "Piggy back" "in the bag" implantation. The anterior IOL is a multifocal implant (diffractive)

duced compared with the same procedure on a virgin eye.

We preferred to try the mono-vision in hyperopic patients initially, leaving a final residual myopia of –0.50 D to –1.0 D or a myopic astigmatism in the non-dominant eye, deliberately; to facilitate nearby vision without glasses. The ideal solution to perfect predictability in the future seems to be new polymers (Calhoun Vision Project) that enable the refractive power to be adjusted once the IOL is implanted in the eye. (Fig 16.4)

In many cases, hyperopic eyes require IOL powers higher than 30 D, making IOL insertion difficult in relatively small eyes due to the central thickness of the optical part of the IOL. Furthermore, the high spherical aberrations in IOLs of more than 35.00 D limit fabrication and suggest that in very high hyperopic eyes, piggyback IOL implantation might be recommended. Holladay and colleagues [21] recommend the use of two biconvex IOLs with proper alignment of the optical centre into the capsular bag, nonetheless this is difficult to achieve in hyperopic small eyes and it is more an optical than a biological concept; therefore, one IOL placement into the bag and other onto the sulcus can be a proper and more adequate surgical approach, and is in fact, the technique recommended by most surgeons and practiced by us. (Fig.16.5)

According to Holladay and colleagues [21] a double lens implantation provides better optical quality because it induces less spherical aberration. Nonetheless, studies have reported several related complications such as the formation of Elsching pearls between the IOLs, inducing an increase in hyperopia as a consequence of IOL separation. On the other hand, the new IOL designs and the larger optical zones used have improved the optical quality and, therefore, piggy-back implantation is not so commonly used today.

16.3.2
Complications

RLE has the same related complications as cataract extraction in hyperopic eyes, including PCO, intra-operative posterior capsular rupture or vitreous loss, RD, choroidal haemorrhage, glaucoma, CME, and endophthalmitis. However, RD has not been as well associated with hyperopia as myopia.

Following RLE, a frequent and expected complication is PCO, and the necessary ND:YAG laser capsulotomy (in the same way as intra-operative posterior capsular rupture) predisposes to PVD and, as a result, possibly facilitates CME and RD (9, 43). Siganos and colleagues [41] reported a PCO frequency of 54% of cases (19/35 eyes) that were uneventfully treated with Nd:YAG laser capsulotomy. Theoretically, the wider IOL adhesion to the posterior capsule in hyperopic eyes would have an inhibitory effect in the formation of Elsching pearls. On the other hand, this surgery is performed in younger eyes with a more compact vitreous, and PVD would be less frequent than in patients with myopia. Therefore, we believe that PCO is a complication that can be successfully treated and without the expected vitreo-retinal complications in hyperopic eyes as in myopic eyes.

In our surgical experience, up to 10% of the hyperopic eyes are nanophthalmic with axial lengths of less than 21 mm. The possibilities of the following intraocular surgery complications are increased in these eyes: choroidal haemorrhage and RD during surgery and malignant glaucoma following surgery. For this reason it is still highly recommended to perform a peripheral iridotomy in eyes with an axial length of <21 mm and corneal diameter <11.0 mm, to diminish the malignant glaucoma risk in the postoperative period.

Of the posterior segment complications, CME can lead to transient or permanent loss of BCVA, Fink and colleagues [12] reported a case of symptomatic CME with complete recovery, reducing the BCVA first to 20/25 but improving following treatment to 20/15. It must be pointed out that corneal refractive surgery in hyperopia, is not exempt of retinal complications (10, 11).

There have been cases of bilateral macular haemorrhage and injury to the optical nerve fibres reported, probably secondary to an increase in IOP during the suction and corneal flap procedure, commonly more difficult is these small and deep eyes.

In conclusion, even though there is some resistance from a number of refractive surgeons to perform an intraocular procedure in a "healthy" eye, RLE is a good alternative for the correction of moderate or high hyperopia, especially in presbyopic eyes where natural accommodative power of the lens tends to decrease at a younger age than in the general population. We prefer to use intraocular refractive surgery for hyperopic correction s higher than +3.0 D; if the patients are in the presbyopic age, our preferred procedure is RLE, including patients with lower hyperopia; if not, phakic IOL implantation is our procedure of choice.

16.3.3
Multifocal IOLs

Although presbyopia correction with multifocal and accommodative IOLs at the time of crystalline lens surgery is just starting, several types of this IOL are have been investigated in recent years [8].The collateral effects of the multifocal IOL include: undesirable optical phenomena and loss of contrast sensitivity, for this reason it must be properly defined and evaluated preoperatively. On the other hand, the accommoda-

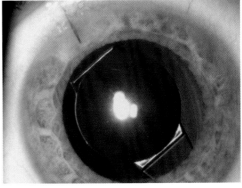

Fig. 16.6. Crystalens (AT.45) "accommodative" style pseudophakic IOL

tive range of these IOLs, is still **in** debate. Our clinical experience with the use of this type of IOL is limited. Currently, the visual effects of this type of IOL regarding visual function and patient satisfaction are being studied. (Fig. 16.6)

16.4
Surgical Technique: Phaco-rolling

There are almost as many surgical technique as there are surgeons. We will discuss some of our own techniques in greater depth. We regularly use the surgical technique named phaco-rolling (presented at the ASCRS in 2001 and pending publication at the JCRS): After hydrodissection, the phaco-tip is introduced in the periphery of the lens and with high aspiration pressure and low to medium ultrasound power, the lens "rotates" into the phaco-tip. The position of the lens is controlled during aspiration with an additional instrument through a lateral paracentesis. (Fig. 16.7)

We generally use a foldable acrylic IOL and prefer introducing it with an injector system, thus avoiding a large corneal incision. With our standard corneal incision of 2.75 mm, the induced astigmatism is near to zero. For the calculation of the IOL power, we used the SRK-II formula and Holladay-II formula in high hyperopia. The target refraction is emmetropia with an attempted residual refractive defect of −0.50 D to −1.0 D in the non-dominant eye. The Nd:YAG laser capsulotomy for PCO is generally indicated after a minimum time of 6-months from the surgery. We like to do a large one, close to the edge of the IOL (almost 5 mm diameter). With this surgical technique we have been very successful in our surgery of RLE and we have not had serious intra or post-operative complications.

Summary for the Clinician

- Refractive lens exchange is a well established technique in myopic patients and is an increasingly used option for the correction of moderate or high hyperopia in the presbyope age group.
- Quality of vision, surgical simplicity and easy adjustability with many forms of corneal refractive surgery are its main advantages.
- A long-term study on safety and its comparison with an appropriately designed control group is still needed.

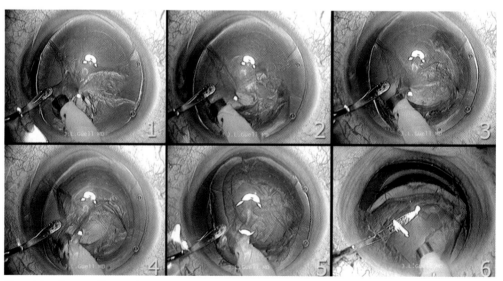

Fig. 16.7. Phaco –rolling Technique: Note the rotatory movement of the nucleus an epinucleus "against" the phaco-tip. High vacuum and low aspiration pressure (Venturi) are used with low ultrasonic power.

References

1. Barraquer C, Cavelier C, Mejía LF (1994) Incidence of retinal detachment following clear lens extraction in myopic patients; retrospective analysis. Arch Ophthalmol 112:336–9
2. Ceschi GP, Artaria LG (1998) Clear lens extraction (CLE) zur Korrektur der hochgradigen myopie. Klin Monatsbl Augenheilkd (5) 212:280–282 (article in German)
3. Chastang P, Ruellan YM, Rozenbaum JP, et al. (1998) Phakoémulsification à visée réfractive sur cristallin clair . A propos de 33 yeux myopes forts. J Fr Ophthalmol 21:560–566 (article in French)
4. Colin J, Robinet A (1994) Clear lensectomy and implantation of low-power posterior chamber intraocular lens for the correction of high myopia. Ophthalmology 101:107–112
5. Colin J, Robinet A, Cochener B (1997) Clear lensectomy and implantation of low-power posterior chamber intraocular lens for the correction of high myopia. Ophthalmology 104:73–77 (discussion by RC Drews, 77–78)
6. Colin J, Robinet A, Cochener B (1999) Retinal detachment after clear lens extraction for high myopia; a seven-year follow-up. Ophthalmology 106:2281–2284 (discussion by M Stirpe, 2285)
7. Coonan P, Fung WE, Webster RG Jr et al. (1985) The incidence of retinal detachment following extra capsular cataract extraction; ten year study. Ophthalmology 92:1096–1101
8. Cumming JS, Slade SG, Chayet A (2001) Clinical evaluation of the model AT-45 silicone accommodation intraocular lens: results of feasibility and the initial phase of a Food and Drug Administration clinical trial. Ophthalmology 108:2005–2009
9. Dardenne MU, Gerten GJ, Kokkas K, Kermani O (1989) Retrospective study of retinal detachment following Nd:Yag laser posterior capsulotomy. J Cataract Refract Surg 15:676–680
10. Dausch D, Smecka Z, Klein R et al. (1997) Excimer laser photorefractive keratectomy for hyperopia. J Cataract Refract Surg 23:169–176
11. Ditzen K, Huschka H, Pieger S (1998) Laser in situ keratomileusis for hyperopia. J Cataract Refract Surg 24:42–47
12. Fink A, Gore C and Rosen E. (2000) Refractive lensectomy for hyperopia. Ophthalmology 107:1540–1548
13. Fukala V (1890) Operative Behandlung der hochstgradigen Myopie durch Aphakie. Albrecht von Graefes Arch Ophthalmol 36:230–244
14. Gabric N, Dekaris I, Karaman Z (2002) Refractive lens exchange for correction of high myopia. Eur J Ophthalmol 12:384–387
15. Goldschmidt E, Fledelius HC (1998) Clinical features in high myopia: a 30 years follow-up a representative sample. In Tokoro T (ed) Myopia updates, proceedings of the 6th international Conference on Myopia, Tokyo, Springer Verlag, pp 101–105
16. Guell JL, Muller A (1996) Láser in situ keratomileusis (LASIK) for myopia from −7 to −18 diopters. J Cataract Refract Surg 12:222–228
17. Güell JL, Rodriguez Arenas A et al. (2003) Phacoemulsification of the crystalline lens and implantation of an intraocular lens for the correction of moderate and high myopia: four years follow-up. J Cataract Refract Surg 29:34–38
18. Gris O, Guell JL, Manero F, Müller A (1996) Clear lens extraction to correct high myopia. J Cataract Refract Surg 22:686–689
19. Hersh PS, Brint SF, Maloney RK et al. (1998) Photorefractive keratectomy versus laser in situ keratomileusis for moderate to high myopia. Ophthalmology 105:1512–1523
20. Hoffer KT (1993) The Hoffer Q formula: a comparison of theoretic and regression formulas. J Cataract Refract Surg 19:700–712
21. Holladay JT, Hills JP, Leidlein J, Cherchio M (1996) Achieving emmetropia in extremely short eyes with tow piggyback posterior chamber intraocular lenses. Ophthalmology 103:1119–1123
22. Izák M, Oslanec J, Gáfricová J, Nikel J (1996) Extraction of a clear lens – cataract as refractive surgery in severe myopia. Cesk Slov Oftalmol 52:82–87 (article in Czechoslovakian)
23. Javitt JC (1994) Clear lens extraction for high myopia is this an idea whose time has come? Arch Ophthalmol 112:321–323 (editorial)
24. Jiménez-Alfaro I, Mígueles S, Bueno JL, Puy P (1998) Clear lens extraction and intraocular lens implantation of negative-power posterior chamber intraocular lenses to corrct extreme myopia. J Cataract Refract Surg 24:1310–1316
25. Knooz MC, Liermann A, Seiberth V et al. (1996) Laser in situ keratomileusis to correct myopia of −6.0 to −29.0 diopters. J Cataract Refract Surg 12:575–584
26. Kolahdouz-Isfahani AH et al. (1999) CLE with IOL implantation for hyperopia. J Refract Surg 15:316–323
27. Lee KH, Lee JH (1996) Long term results of clear lens extraction for severe myopia. J Cataract Refract Surg 22:1411–1415
28. Lindstrom RL, Lindquist TD, Huldin J, Rubenstein JB (1998) Retinal detachment in axial myopia following extracapsular cataract surgery. In: Cadwell DR (ed) Cataracts: transactions of the New Orleans Academy of Ophthalmology: New York, NY, Raven Press, pp 253–60 (discussion, 260–268)

29. Lyle WA, Jin GJC (1994) Clear lens extraction for the correction of high refractive error. J Cataract Refract Surg 20:273–276

30. Manche EE, Maloney RK (1996) Keratomileusis in situ for high myopia. J Cataract Refract Surg 22:1443–1450

31. Ober RR, Wilkinson CP, Fiore JV Jr, Maggiano JM (1986) Rhegmatogenous retinal detachment after Nd:Yag laser capsulotomy in phakic and pseudophakic eyes. Am J Ophthalmol 101:81–89

32. Osher RH (1994) Clear lens extraction J Cataract Refract Surg 20:674

33. Osher RH (1994) Comments on CLE and IOL implantation in normally sighted hyperopic eyes. J Cataract Refract Surg 19:122

34. Perkins ES (1979) Morbidity from myopia. Sight Saving Rew 49:11–19

35. Praeger DL (1979) Five years follow-up in the surgical management of cataract in high myopia treated with the Kelman phakoemulsification technique. Ophthalmology 86:2024–2033

36. Pucci V, Morselli S, Romanelly F et al. (2001) Clear lens phacoemulsification for correction of high myopia. J Cataract Refract Surg 27:896–900

37. Ripandelli G, Billi B, Fedeli R, Stirpe M (1996) Retinal detachment after clear lens extraction in 41 eyes with axial myopia. Retina. 16:3–6

38. Séller T (1999) Clear lens extraction in the 19th century – an early demonstration of premature dissemination. J Cataract Refract Surg 15:70–3

39. Siganos DS, Siganos CS, Pallikaris IG. (1994) Clear lens exchange for high hiperopia in normally sighted eyes. J Cataract Refract Surg 10:117–24

40. Siganos DS, Pallikaris IG, Siganos CS (1995) Clear lensectomy and IOL implantation in normally sighted highly hyperopic eyes. Three-year follow-up. Eur J Implant Ref Surg 7:128–133

41. Siganos DS, Pallikaris (1998) Clear lensectomy and IOL implantation for hyperopia from +7. to +14 diopters J Cataract Refract Surg 14:105–13

42. Steinert RF, Bafna S (1998) Surgical correction of moderate myopia: which method would you chose? II. PRK and LASIK are the treatments of choice. Surv Ophthalmol 43:157–179

43. Steinert RF, Puliuafito CA, Kumar SR et al. (1991) Cystoid macular oedema, retinal detachment following Nd:Yag laser posterior capsulotomy. Am J Ophthalmol 112:373–380

44. Verzella F (1990) Refractive microsurgery of the lens in high myopia. Refract Corneal Surg 6:273–275

45. Vicary D, Sun XY (1999) Refractive lensectomy to correct ametropia. J Cataract Refract Surg 25:943–948

46. Wang J, Shi Y (2001) Clear lens extraction with phacoemulsification and posterior chamber intraocular lens implantation for treatment of high myopia. Chun Hua Yen Ko Tsa Chich 37:350–354 (Chinese)

47. Werblin TP (1992) Should we consider clear lens extraction for routine refractive surgery? Refract Corneal Surg 8:480–481

48. Younan C, Mitchell P, Cuming RG et al. (2002) Myopia and incident cataract and cataract surgery: the blue mountains eye study. Invest Ophthalmol Vis Sci 43:3625–3632

LI WANG, DOUGLAS D. KOCH

Core Messages

- Wavefront-guided corneal surgery has become a reality. Although visual performance is limited by optical, cone anatomical and neural factors, correction of optical aberrations increases retinal image resolution and contrast
- Wavefront aberrations measured using various techniques are mathematically reconstructed, typically using Zernike polynomials, and then displayed in a number of formats, including aberration maps and various indices
- Accuracy and repeatability of current wavefront systems for measuring refractive errors is generally excellent. However, clinically large variations in higher-order aberration measurements can occur, and further work is needed to improve reproducibility

- Several platforms are undergoing clinical trials to investigate the effectiveness of the wavefront-guided ablation. Currently, three laser systems have been approved by the FDA for wavefront-guided LASIK in the US: Alcon CustomCornea, VISX CustomVue system, and Bausch & Lomb Zyoptix system
- Reported outcomes of wavefront-guided ablation are excellent. In contrast to standard ablation, mean contrast sensitivity levels and patient satisfaction scores are improved; mean increases in higher-order aberrations are much smaller than the aberrations induced by standard LASIK or PRK
- Although limitations of wavefront-guided corneal surgery exist, on average wavefront-guided correction provides improved quality of vision both objectively and subjectively

17.1
Principle of Wavefront Technology

17.1.1
Basics of Wavefront Aberration

Wavefront technology was original developed for two non-medical applications: (1) to enhance telescopic images by minimising the wavefront distortions that occur as light from a distant star travels through the earth's turbulent atmosphere, and (2) to track incoming warheads as part of a missile defence program. The human eye is not a perfect optical system, and a flat planar wave of light deviates when it travels through the eye. In 1962, Smirnov [25], an early pioneer in the characterisation of the eye's higher-order aberrations, suggested that it would be possible with customised lenses to compensate for aberrations in individual eyes. Recently, more rapid and accurate instruments for measuring the ocular aberrations have emerged, and wavefront-guided corneal surgery has become a reality.

Deviations of the actual wavefront from an ideal wavefront define aberration. Higher-order aberrations are the aberrations that cannot be corrected by simple spherocylindrical systems, such as spectacles, contact lens or traditional refractive surgery.

17.1.2
Visual Benefit
of Higher-Order Aberration Correction

17.1.2.1
Factors Limiting Visual Performance

The finest details we can see are limited by optical, cone anatomical and neural factors.

Optical Limitation

A standard measure of optical quality in the optical industry is optical transfer function (OTF), which has two components: modulation (contrast) transfer function (MTF) and phase transfer function (PTF). In a perfect optical system, increasing aperture size (pupil in the eye) increases the diffraction-limited (no blur) MTF, and there are no phase shifts from object to image. However, in an optically aberrated system, optical performance decreases with increasing pupil diameter, reducing MTF and producing phase reversals of images [1].

The human eye is an imperfect optical system. Studies based on large populations have revealed that the wavefront aberrations vary widely among subjects and increase slightly with ageing [22, 29]. In 532 eyes measured with a Hartmann-Shack sensor (WaveScan, VISX, Inc., Santa Clara, CA) across a 6-mm pupil, the mean root-mean-square (RMS) value of total higher-order aberrations from 3rd–6th order was 0.305 ± 0.095 (SD) μm. For individual terms, the highest mean absolute values were for 4th-order SA and the 3rd-order coma and trefoil terms. With the exception of the 4th order spherical aberration term, the absolute values, standard deviations and ranges were highest for the 3rd order terms and tended to progressively decrease up to the 6th order [29].

Cone Mosaic Limitation

The ability of the cone photoreceptors to sample the retinal image is the fundamental retinal limitation to visual performance. Cones in the foveola are approximately 2 μm in diameter. To differentiate a letter, for example "E", the components of the letter "E" must be distributed over an adequate number of receptors to allow each to be detected. Independent of the quality of the optics, the coarseness of the foveolar photoreceptor mosaic limits letter acuity to between 20/8 and 20/10 [33].

Neural Limitation

By producing interference fringes on the retina to eliminate the influence of diffraction and most aberrations in the eye, Williams et al. demonstrated that the neural contrast sensitivity function monotonically decreases with increasing higher spatial frequencies, indicating that the post-receptoral visual system also blurs the neural image, just as the optics blur the retinal image [32].

17.1.2.2
Visual Benefit
of Optical Aberration Correction

Theoretically, any deviation from a perfect plane wavefront will lead to a corresponding defect in the resulting image. Interventions that reduce the optical aberrations of the eye will increase retinal image resolution and contrast, which in turn should allow one to see the world with finer detail and higher contrast. This benefit has been demonstrated by laboratory study using adaptive optics [9].

In 109 normal subjects and four keratoconic patients, Guirao et al. [6] evaluated the visual benefit theoretically by calculating the ratio of the modulation transfer function (MTF) in white light when the monochromatic higher-order aberrations are corrected to the MTF corresponding to the best correction of defocus and astigmatism. The average visual benefit for normal eyes at 16 c/deg was approximately 2.5 times for a 5.7-mm pupil but was negligible for small pupils (1.25 for a 3-mm pupil). The benefit varied greatly among eyes, with some normal eyes showing almost no benefit and others a benefit higher than four times at 16 c/deg across a 5.7-mm pupil. The benefit for the keratoconic eyes was much larger.

Summary for the Clinician

- Visual performance is limited by optical, cone anatomical and neural factors
- Optical aberration correction increases retinal image resolution and contrast
- The visual benefit of optical aberration correction varies among eyes; the benefit for the keratoconic eyes or highly aberrated eyes is much larger

17.1.3
Principles
of Measuring Wavefront Aberration

Several principles have been used to measure the wavefront aberrations of the eye and will be discussed below. Currently available wavefront aberrometers and their laser system linkage status are shown in Table 17.1.

17.1.3.1
Hartmann-Shack Wavefront Sensor

The most widely used method is the Hartmann-Shack sensor. Wavefront analysers utilising this principle include: WaveScan (VISX Inc. Santa Clara, CA), Zywave Aberrometer (Bausch & Lomb, Claremont, CA), Complete Ophthalmic Analysis System (COAS) (WaveFront Sciences, Albuquerque, NM), and LADARWave aberrometer (Alcon Laboratories, Fort Worth, TX). A small spot of laser light is projected onto the retina and then reflected back through the pupil. The reflected light exiting from the eye is imaged by a micro-lenslet array, and the array of spot images is captured by a video sensor. The location of each spot gathered from the video sensor is compared to the theoretical ideal locations, and the wavefront aberrations are computed (Fig. 17.1) [27].

Table 17.1. Summary of currently available wavefront systems

Name	Principle	Company	Linked laser system
WaveScan	Hartmann-Shack	VISX Inc. (Santa Clara, CA)	VISX Star S4 excimer laser
Zywave	Hartmann-Shack	Bausch & Lomb (Claremont, CA)	Bausch & Lomb Technolas 217 excimer laser
COAS G-200 COAS™-HD	Hartmann-Shack	WaveFront Sciences (Albuquerque, NM)	Asclepion-Meditec Inc. MEL-70 laser
CustomCornea	Hartmann-Shack	Alcon Laboratories Inc. (Fort Worth, TX)	LADARVision 4000 excimer laser
WaveLight Analyzer	Tscherning	WaveLight Laser Technologie AG, Erlangen, Germany	ALLEGRETTO WAVE Excimer Laser
OPD-Scan	dynamic retinoscopy	Nidek Co., Ltd., Gamagori, Japan	Nidek EC-5000 excimer laser
Tracey VFA	Retinal ray-tracing	Tracey Technologies, (Houston, TX)	Pending
Spatially resolved refractometer	Psychophysical ray-tracing approach	Unknown	Unknown

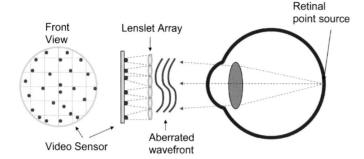

Fig. 17.1. Principle of Hartmann-Shack sensor. A point of light (typically infrared) is reflected off of the retina and is refracted as it exits the eye. The light is focused by lenslets onto a CCD array, and the deviation of the beams is used to calculate the shape of the wavefront

17.1.3.2
Tscherning Sensor

The WaveLight Analyzer is based on the Tscherning sensor, in which a grid or equidistant spot pattern of lights is projected onto the retina through the pupil. The image of the grid or spot pattern formed on the retina is photographed by means of a closed-circuit-device (CCD) camera using the principle of indirect ophthalmoscopy. Each real spot position taken from the retinal image is compared to its corresponding ideal spot position. From the resulting deviations, the wavefront aberrations are mathematically reconstructed [15].

17.1.3.3
Dynamic Skiascopy

The optical path difference scanning system (OPD-Scan) uses the principle of dynamic skiascopy by measuring the time it takes a given ray to traverse the entire optical system (time-based aberrometry). The retina is scanned with an infrared light (880 nm) slit beam in 0.4 s, and the reflected light is captured by an array of rotating photodetectors over a 360° area. The photodetectors are excited at different times by the reflecting slit light, and the time differences between the centre of the cornea and each of the photodetectors are measured. This difference is proportional to the refractive power. Wavefront aberrations and auto-refraction data for the 2.5-mm, 3.0-mm and 5.0-mm zones are generated [10].

17.1.3.4
Retina Ray-Tracing Technology

The Tracey visual function analyser (Tracey VFA) uses a single-beam scanner based on retina laser ray-tracing technology. In an interval of less than 50 ms, the Tracey VFA sends a series of tiny parallel light beams sequentially through the entrance pupil of the eye. Semiconductor photodetectors measure where each light ray strikes the retina and provide raw data that measures the (x-y) error distance from the ideal conjugate focal point (Fig. 17.2) [14]. From these data the wavefront aberrations can be mathematically reconstructed.

17.1.3.5
Psychophysical Ray-Tracing Approach

The spatially resolved refractometer (SRR) uses a psychophysical ray-tracing approach, which is similar to the principle used in Scheiner's disc. With Scheiner's disc, if light is allowed into the pupil from two small apertures, one at the top of the pupil and the other one in the centre of the pupil, the emmetropic subject would see only one spot; the myopic or hyperopic subject, however, would see two points. The amount and the direction of the displacement of the retinal location from the ideal is a measure of the ray deviation for that point in the pupil. The ray deviation, in turn, is proportional to the slope of the wavefront aberration function for that pupil location.

In the SRR system, the holes on a wheel are scanned across the pupil in 1-mm steps. The subject is asked to align a spot (viewed in ran-

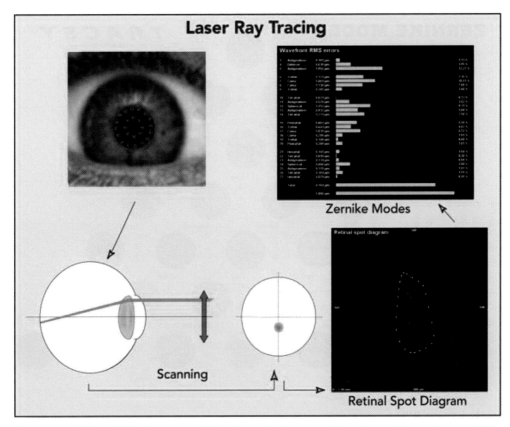

Fig. 17.2. Principle of the Tracey visual function analyser. The device sends a series of tiny parallel light beams sequentially through the entrance pupil of the eye. It measures the position of each ray as it ex- its the eye and therefore calculates where each light ray strikes the retina. The distance between this site and the ideal conjugate focal point is determined, and from this the wavefront aberrations are calculated

dom order, one at a time through each pupil location) to a cross (always viewed through the centre of the pupil). The angle required to null the aberrations at each pupil position represents the slope of the wavefront at that location. The slope measurements are then fitted to reconstruct the wavefront errors and calculate the Zernike polynomials [31].

Summary for the Clinician

Several principles of measuring wavefront aberration are available:
- Hartmann-Shack wavefront sensor
- Tscherning sensor
- Dynamic skiascopy
- Retina ray-tracing technology
- Psychophysical ray-tracing approach

17.1.4
Quantifying Wavefront Aberrations

Currently, wavefront aberrations measured using various techniques are mathematically reconstructed, typically using Zernike polynomials, and then displayed in a number of formats, including aberration maps at the pupil plane, the retinal images in the image plane and various metrics (indices) at the pupil and image planes [3].

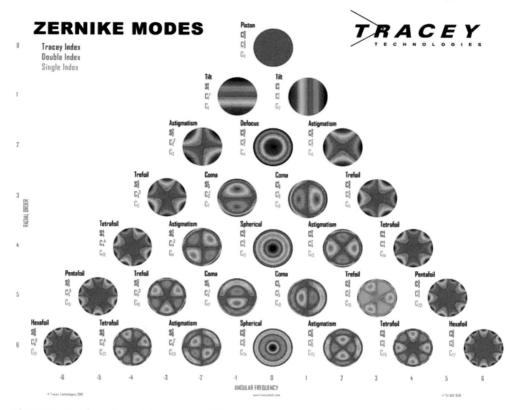

Fig. 17.3. Zernike polynomial terms up to 6th order

17.1.4.1
Wavefront Aberration Fitting

Zernike polynomials, named after the Dutch physicist Frits Zernike (1888–1966) [34], have been in use since 1934 to mathematically describe the aberrations in an optical system. The compelling feature of this analysis is that the wavefront can be broken into independent components that represent specific aberrations, such as spherical aberration, coma and trefoil (Fig. 17.3). The set of Zernike polynomials can be easily modified so that each polynomial is mathematically independent of the others. This has several advantages: (1) statistical analysis can be performed for each Zernike term independently; (2) the total variance in a wavefront can be calculated as the sum of the variances in the individual components; (3) relative magnitudes of Zernike coefficients in a normalised Zernike expansion can be easily compared; and (4) by simply scanning the values of the coefficients, one can quickly identify the term or terms having the greatest impact on the total RMS wavefront error of the eye [28].

Despite these advantages of Zernike polynomials, it has been shown that they limit the data resolution in eyes with high amounts of irregular astigmatism [26]. Fourier analysis can decompose the image into spatial frequency components and may provide a more accurate wavefront reconstruction, especially in more highly aberrated eyes.

17.1.4.2
Aberration and Retinal Image Maps

Wavefront analysers present wavefront aberrations in colour-coded maps similar to topography maps.

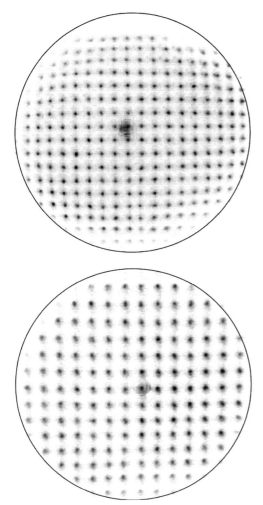

Fig. 17.4. *Above,* high quality Hartman Shack image. *Below,* image with poor quality of the lenslet images

Total Aberration and Higher-Order Aberration Maps

All wavefront devices display two-dimensional colour maps for the total aberration and higher-order aberrations (3rd order and higher), which facilitate qualitative assessment of the aberrations (Fig. 17.5, upper left and lower left).

Point Spread Function

The point spread function (PSF) is a graphical representation of the image when a small dot of light or a point is projected on the retina. If the eye is a perfect optical system, the image of this point will be the same as the original. Otherwise, the image will be somewhat blurred or distorted (Fig. 17.5, upper right). Moreover, the PSF should qualitatively reflect the patient's perception when viewing a point source of light. Clinically, this can often be seen to occur, but the PSF does not always reflect the patient's perception, especially in more highly aberrated eyes, due to the above mentioned (see Sect. 17.1.4.1) limitations of Zernike polynomials.

17.1.4.3 Wavefront Aberration Metrics

Although colour-coded two-dimensional wavefront aberration maps are useful, indices for quantitative analysis are necessary.

Root-Mean-Square (RMS) Values

The RMS values represent the variation in height of the wavefront aberration from the reference plane. Lower RMS values indicate a flatter wavefront and higher optical quality. However, in the human eye, Applegate et al. demonstrated that, for low levels of aberration, the overall RMS wavefront error is not a good predictor of quality of vision [2]. For a total wavefront error RMS of 0.25 µm (6.0 mm pupil), the investigators found that the visual acuity varied significantly depending on which aberrations were present and their relative contribution. Zernike terms that were two radial orders apart and had the same sign and angular frequency tended to combine to increase visual

Hartmann-Shack Image

Some devices display the Hartmann-Shack images (Fig. 17.4), which is useful for evaluating the quality of the raw data. The presence of blurred spots may indicate disrupted tear film or a highly aberrated area, such as in keratonic eye.

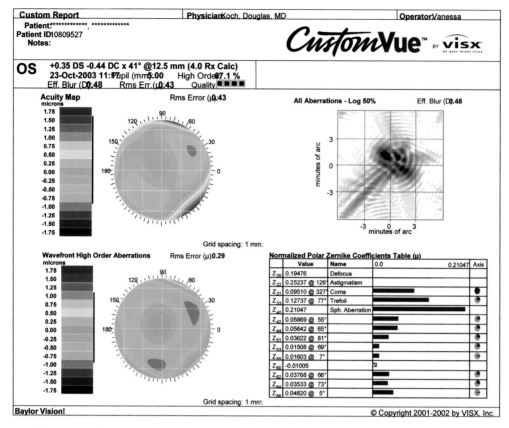

Fig. 17.5. Overall display provided by the WaveScan. *Upper left*, acuity map in microns with the total aberration RMS value displayed. *Lower left*, wavefront higher order aberration map with higher-order aberration RMS value presented. *Upper right*, point-spread function map. *Lower right*, normalised polar Zernike coefficients table

acuity, whereas modes within the same radial order tended to combine to decrease acuity.

Point-Spread Function (PSF) Metrics

A high-quality PSF is characterised by high contrast and compact form. One popular metric that quantitatively describes the PSF is the *Strehl ratio*, defined as the maximum intensity in the PSF divided by the maximum intensity for an optically perfect PSF limited only by diffraction at the pupil. Other metrics include "light-in-the-bucket", "equivalent width", and "half-width-at-half-height" [3].

Optical Transfer Function (OTF) Metrics

The OTF is the combination of "modulation transfer function" (MTF) and "phase transfer function" (PTF), which represent the amount of contrast attenuation and the amount of phase shift as a function of the grating's spatial frequency. A high-quality OTF is indicated by high MTF values and low PTF values. Metrics include the cut-off frequency and the volume under the MTF or PTF.

These metrics quantify the optical quality of the eye only. Visual quality of the eye also depends on the function of photoreceptors and the neural processing. Researchers are focusing on the development of better metrics that accurately and precisely quantify visual performance based on wavefront measurements of the optical quality.

Summary for the Clinician

- Methods of reconstructing wavefront aberrations:
  - Zernike polynomials: numerical advantages, but limit the data resolution in highly aberrated eyes
  - Fourier analysis: may provide more accurate wavefront data
- Presentation of wavefront aberrations:
  - Hartmann-Shack image
  - Colour-coded maps: total aberration and higher-order aberration maps
  - Point spread function
  - Numerical indices: root-mean-square (RMS) values, point-spread function (PSF) metrics and optical transfer function (OTF) metrics

17.2
Accuracy and Repeatability of Wavefront Aberrometers

Several peer-reviewed articles have investigated the accuracy and repeatability of the wavefront aberrometers (Tables 17.2 and 17.3). In general, using manifest refraction as the standard,

lower-order aberrations (refractive errors) measured by these aberrometers are reliable and reproducible, although discrepancy over 1 D does occasionally occur. For the repeatability of higher-order aberration measurements, the instruments have small but clinically important variability. Sources of variance include instrument factors and, perhaps more importantly, micro-fluctuations of the eye (e.g. changes in tear film and accommodation). Detailed data for some aberrometers are shown in Tables 17.2 and 17.3 and will be discussed briefly below.

17.2.1
WaveScan

In a previous study, we evaluated the accuracy and repeatability of the WaveScan system for measuring refractive errors in 28 virgin eyes and 41 eyes that had undergone corneal refractive surgery [30]. The mean differences, standard deviation and ranges in spherical equivalent (SE), sphere and cylinder between manifest refraction (MR) and WaveScan (MR-WaveScan) were -0.26 ± 0.41 D (range -1.20 to 1.05 D), -0.12 ± 0.51 D (range -1.30 to 1.40 D), and -0.28 ± 0.34 D (range -1.30 to 0.45 D), respectively; the repeatability (standard deviation, SD) for SE, sphere and cylinder were 0.13 D, 0.14 D and 0.08 D, respectively.

Table 17.2. Accuracy of wavefront aberrometers (manifest refraction – wavefront refraction) (D)

Wavefront aberrometer	Study	Number of eyes	Spherical equivalent Mean±SD (range)	Sphere Mean±SD (range)	Cylinder Mean±SD (range)
WaveScan	Wang et al. 2003 [30]	69 (28 virgin eyes and 41 post-surgery eyes)	-0.26 ± 0.41 (-1.20 to 1.05)	-0.12 ± 0.51 (-1.30 to 1.40)	-0.28 ± 0.34 (-1.30 to 0.45)
Zywave	Hament et al. 2002 [7]	20 virgin eyes	-0.55 ± 0.48 (NR)	-0.50 ± 0.49 (NR)	-0.27 ± 0.49 (NR)
COAS	Cheng et al. 2003 [4]	6 model eyes	NR	(-0.25 to $+0.25$)	(-0.10 to $+0.10$)
Tracey VFA	Wang et al. 2003 [30]	48 (22 virgin eyes and 26 post-surgery eyes)	-0.21 ± 0.58 (-1.02 to 1.66)	-0.01 ± 0.63 (-0.80 to 2.23)	-0.40 ± 0.35 (-1.15 to 0.25)

NR, not reported.

Table 17.3. Repeatability (standard deviation) of wavefront aberrometers for lower-order and higher-order aberration measurements

Wavefront aberrometer	Study	Number of eyes (repeated measurements)	Lower-order aberrations (D)			Total higher-order RMS (µm)
			SE	Sphere	Cylinder	
WaveScan	Wang et al. 2003 [30]	35 Virgin and post-surgery eyes (3)	0.13	0.14	0.08	NR
	Unpublished data	24 Virgin eyes (9)	NR	0.17	0.09	0.028 (3rd–6th)
Zywave	Hament et al. 2002 [7]	20 Virgin eyes (3)	0.13	0.15	0.15	NR
	Mirshahi et al. 2003 [13]	2 Test models (6)	NR	0.04	0.05	0.017 (3rd–5th)
		40 Virgin eyes (6)	NR	0.15	0.16	0.097 (3rd–5th)
COAS	Cheng et al. 2003 [4]	1 Model eye (5)	NR	NR	NR	0.0024 (3rd–4th)
	Cheng et al. 2004 [5]	4 Eyes (5)	NR	NR	NR	0.018 (3rd–4th)
Tscherning	Mrochen et al. 2000 [15]	300 Virgin eyes (5)	NR	0.08	0.08	0.02 (3rd–8th)
Tracey VFA	Wang et al. 2003 [30]	48 Virgin and post-surgery eyes (3)	0.15	0.18	0.16	NR
	Pallikaris et al. 2000 [19]	7 Pseudophakic eyes (30)	NR	NR	0.14	NR

NR, not reported.

In a recent study, we investigated the repeatability of wavefront measurements with the WaveScan system in 24 virgin eyes (unpublished data). Three measurements were taken at each of the time points (8 am, 12 noon and 4 pm) by the same examiner. The values of SD were 0.17 D and 0.09 D for sphere and cylinder, respectively; the SD for total higher-order RMS was 0.028 µm.

To study the reproducibility of measuring total higher-order RMS values (3rd–5th order), Mirshahi et al. used both test model eyes and human subjects and repositioned the Zywave before each repeated measurement. The SDs were 0.017 µm and 0.097 µm for the test model eye and human subjects, respectively; the coefficients of variation (ratio of SD to mean in percentage) were 13.3 % and 13.4 %, respectively [13].

17.2.2
Zywave

In a study of 20 virgin eyes, the mean differences between MR and Zywave refraction with a 3.5-mm pupil (MR-Zywave) were –0.55±0.48 D for SE, –0.50±0.49 D for sphere, and –0.27 ±0.49 D for cylinder; the repeatability (SD) for SE, sphere and cylinder were 0.13 D, 0.15 D and 0.15 D, respectively [7].

17.2.3
COAS

In measuring 40 eyes of 20 myopic subjects, taking MR as the standard, the COAS had mean power vector errors of 0.3–0.4 D [24]. Using six model eyes, Cheng and colleagues [4] evaluated the accuracy and repeatability of the COAS system. When comparing the COAS-measured defocus and astigmatism with the refraction errors introduced into the model eye, the instrument was accurate to within 0.25 D over a range of –6.50 to +3.00 D, and the accuracy declined with further increases in refractive error. The amplitude of measured astigmatism was accurate to within ±0.10 D over the range –3.00 to +3.00 D, and estimates of astigmatic axis were accurate to within ±2°.

Cheng et al. [4] also investigated the accuracy of spherical aberration and coma by comparing ray-tracing predictions with measured values. The average absolute error was 0.007 µm for both 4th order spherical aberration and 3rd order coma. Without realignment between each measurement of the model eye, the SD of higher-order RMS (3rd and 4th order) was 0.001 µm, which was 0.45 % of the mean higher-order RMS. When the operator realigned the instrument between measurements, the SD increased to 0.0024 µm (1.2 % of the mean), indicating that the instrument has very little fluctuation and that the major source of measurement variance appears to be alignment noise. In four normal eyes, the SD of higher-order RMS (3rd and 4th order) with five repeated measurements taken within 1 h was 0.018 µm [5].

17.2.4
Tscherning Aberrometer

In a study of more than 300 eyes with large range of refractive errors, five measurements of each eye were measured across a 7-mm pupil with the Tscherning aberrometer; the absolute reproducibility for the sphere and cylinder was reported to be ±0.08 D [15]. The reproducibility for the total RMS and higher-order RMS values was 0.04 µm and 0.02 µm, respectively.

17.2.5
Tracey VFA

In 22 virgin eyes and 26 eyes that had undergone corneal refractive surgery, the mean differences in SE, sphere and cylinder between MR and Tracey (MR-Tracey) were –0.21±0.58 D (range –1.02 to 1.66 D), –0.01±0.63 D (range –0.80 to 2.23 D), and –0.40±0.35 D (range –1.15 to 0.25 D),

respectively; the repeatability (SD) for SE, sphere and cylinder were 0.15 D, 0.18 D and 0.16 D, respectively [30]. Using an early prototype of the Tracey device, Pallikaris and colleagues [19] evaluated the reproducibility by performing 30 consecutive measurements in each of seven pseudophakic eyes; the SD for measurement of cylinder was found to be 0.14 D.

Summary for the Clinician

- Accuracy is good, although discrepancy over 1 D occurs with reported differences between MR and wavefront refraction as high as 1.66 D
- Repeatability for lower-order aberration measurements is excellent; however, clinically large variations in higher-order aberration measurements can occur, and further work is needed to improve reproducibility

17.3
Clinical Outcome
of Wavefront-Guided Corneal Surgery

Theoretical and experimental demonstrations of the visual benefit of correction of higher-order aberrations have stimulated the emergence of wavefront-guided corneal surgery, which is designed to correct the traditional sphere and cylindrical error of the eye and reduce the eye's higher-order aberrations (Fig. 17.6). However, we are unaware of any peer-reviewed studies that have directly compared the outcomes of wavefront-guided LASIK/PRK with the standard LASIK/PRK.

17.3.1
Methods

The wavefront aberration data measured using wavefront analyser are linked to the laser system. The laser system then determines what adjustments must be made to the subject's corneal surface in order to produce a crisply focused image on the patient's retina, and wavefront-guided ablation is then delivered onto the cornea through LASIK or PRK.

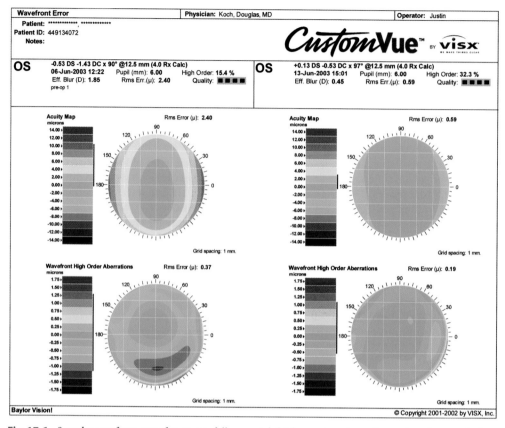

Fig. 17.6. Sample wavefront map for an eye following CustomVue LASIK. The total wavefront aberrations decreased from 2.40 µm pre-operatively (*upper left*) to 0.59 µm post-operatively (*upper right*). The to-tal higher-order aberrations also decreased from 0.37 µm pre-operatively (*lower left*) to 0.19 µm post-operatively (*lower right*)

Currently, several platforms are undergoing clinical trials to investigate the effectiveness of the wavefront-guided ablation for correcting a range of refractive errors. At the time of writing this article, three laser systems have been approved by the FDA for wavefront-guided LASIK in the USA: (1) LADARVision 4000 excimer laser for treatment of myopia up to –7.00 D with less than –0.50 D of astigmatism; (2) VISX CustomVue system for correction of myopia up to –6 D with up to 3.0 D of astigmatism; and (3) Bausch & Lomb Zyoptix system for treatment of myopia with sphere up to –7.00 D, cylinder up to –3.00 D, and spherical equivalent up to –7.5 D. Several more are available internationally.

There are some important variations in approaches among the three systems. With the VISX WaveScan, measurements are obtained without pupil dilation, whereas dilated pupils are used for the Alcon and Bausch & Lomb systems. In the Bausch & Lomb Zyoptix system, the Zylink software combines the Zywave aberrometer data and the data from the Orbscan corneal topography to determine ablation parameters. In the VISX system, one option is to ablate a PreVue lens, using the wavefront aberration obtained pre-operatively. The PreVue lens is then fitted in a trial frame so that the patient can preview his or her potential vision. This provides an estimate of the potential outcome and is particularly helpful when treating more highly aberrated eyes.

17.3.2
Summary of Results

17.3.2.1
Refractive Outcome

Myopic LASIK

The FDA clinical trial data from Alcon, VISX and Bausch & Lomb demonstrated excellent visual results for wavefront-guided LASIK in correcting myopia and myopic astigmatism (Table 17.4). Overall, 74.8%–100% of eyes were within ±0.50 D, and 95.7%–100% were within ±1.0 D of attempted correction; 34%–74% of eyes had UCVA of 20/16 and 91.5%–100% had UCVA of 20/20. Loss of one line of BSCVA occurred in 0%–8.6% of eyes.

Myopic PRK

Using the Asclepion wavefront-supported customised ablation (WASCA) workstation, wavefront-guided myopic PRK produced excellent refractive outcomes [16]. With 6 months follow-up, 98.5% of eyes were within ±0.50 D, and 100% were within ±1.0 D of attempted correction; 80.7% of eyes had UCVA of 20/20. Loss of one line of BSCVA occurred in 0.7% of eyes.

Hyperopic PRK

Nagy et al. [17] first reported the results of WASCA in hyperopic PRK in 40 eyes with the Asclepion-Meditec MEL 70 flying-spot excimer laser. At 6 months post-operatively, 85% of eyes were within ±0.50 D, and 100% were within ±1.0 D of target refraction; 70% of eyes had UCVA of 20/20, and 12.5% (five of 40 eyes) lost two Snellen lines of BSCVA.

17.3.2.2
Contrast Sensitivity

In addition to improved BSCVA and UCVA, wavefront-guided corneal surgery also improves the low-contrast acuity, which is a parameter most sensitive to optical quality of the eye.

In the VISX FDA clinical trial, at 6 months, contract sensitivity at bright light without glare significantly increased than pre-operative contract sensitivity. In the Alcon CustomCornea FDA clinical trial, under mesopic conditions, 15.2% of eyes experienced an increase of >2 levels (>0.3 Log) on CSV-1000 at two or more spatial frequencies at 6-month follow-up, while 5.8% of eyes experienced a decrease of >2 levels at two or more spatial frequencies.

17.3.2.3
Patient Satisfaction

In the VISX FDA clinical trial, patient satisfaction with their vision at night improved significantly after wavefront-guided LASIK. At 6 months post-operatively, 44% of the respondents said they were "very satisfied" with their vision at night, compared with 12% pre-operatively; 35% reported they were "very satisfied" with their vision at night with glare, in contrast with 8% pre-operatively. The incidence of glare and halos around lights was also decreased after surgery.

17.3.2.4
Higher-Order Aberrations

Unfortunately, the creation of a LASIK flap alone produces changes in the higher-order aberrations of the eye. In two separate studies [20, 23], authors have demonstrated a range of induced aberrations, and these were not consistent for flaps produced with any given microkeratome. In 15 eyes, Pallikaris and colleagues [20] found a higher-order RMS increase of 0.096 µm for a 6-mm pupil with a nasally hinged corneal flap (Flapmaker microkeratome, Refractive Technologies, Cleveland, OH); 3rd order horizontal coma (Z_3^{-1}) and 4th order spherical aberration (Z_4^0) also increased significantly. In 17 eyes, Porter et al. [23] reported an increase in higher-order RMS (0.128 µm, 6-mm pupil) after the flap creation with a superior hinge (Hansatome microkeratome); 3rd order trefoil (Z_3^3) had small but significant negative shift when compared with the control eyes. The magnitude of these changes tended to be small, but they certainly could impact the quality of the post-operative vision.

Table 17.4. Results of wavefront-guided ablation

Custom ablation system	Treatment	Follow-up in months (eyes available)	Range of pre-operative myopia (D) (astigmatism)	Mean pre-operative refraction (D) (astigmatism)	Mean post-operative refraction (D) (astigmatism)	Percent within ±0.5 D/ ±1.0 D SE (cylinder)	Post-operative UCVA ≥20/16 (%)	Post-op UCVA ≥20/20 (%)	Loss of ≥1 line BSCVA (%)
LADARVision 4000 excimer laser[a]	Myopic LASIK	6 (139)	Up to −7	−3.0±1.16	−0.2±0.34	74.8/95.7	NR	80	8.6
VISX CustomVue[a]	Myopic LASIK	6 (277)	−0.6 to −6.0 (0 to 3)	−3.2±1.3 (0.7±0.7)	−0.2	90/99	74	94	3
Zyoptix system[b]	Myopic LASIK	6 (340)	NR	NR	NR	75.9/93.8	NR	91.5	0.6
WASCA Asclepion Workstation [16,17]	Myopic PRK	6 (150)	−1.5 to −6.5 (0 to −2.5)	−4.02±1.04	−0.12	98.5/100	2	80.7	0.7
	Hyperopic PRK	6 (40)	+1.5 to +4.0 (0 to 1.0)	+2.9±0.8	−0.10±0.25	85/100	15	70	12.5 (≥2 lines)
Nidek EC-5000 excimer laser [21]	Myopic LASIK	3–6 (10)	NR	−7.09±3.32	0.08±0.32	100/100	NR	100	0

NR, not reported.
[a] FDA clinical trial data (www.fda.org).
[b] FDA clinical trial data (www.bausch.com).

Fortunately, the aberrations induced by making a LASIK flap typically are much smaller than the aberrations produced in the eye by performing standard LASIK or PRK. Therefore, although they may in many instances reduce the efficacy of wavefront-correction, they by no means negate the positive impact of this approach on quality of vision.

Studies are needed to better understand the role of epithelial wound healing following PRK and LASEK in the creation of corneal aberrations. We are unaware of any reports that have directly compared wavefront-guided LASIK versus PRK.

Summary for the Clinician

- Several platforms are undergoing clinical trials, and three laser systems have been approved by the FDA (LADARVision 4000 excimer laser, VISX CustomVue system, and Bausch & Lomb Zyoptix system)
- Refractive and contrast sensitivity outcomes are promising
- Increased higher-order aberrations are much smaller than the aberrations induced by standard LASIK or PRK

17.4
Limitations of Wavefront-Guided Corneal Surgery

There are several limitations with the wavefront-guided corneal surgery:
- We are currently only measuring and treating monochromatic aberrations. However, we are living in a polychromatic world. Chromatic aberration reduces the visual benefit when only monochromatic aberrations are corrected. In addition, there is some evidence that chromatic aberration would be unacceptably high if monochromatic aberrations were fully corrected [12].
- Some degree of optical aberrations in the human visual system might be beneficial for vision and therefore should probably not been corrected. There is much yet to be learned about which aberrations and combinations of aberrations provide optimal visual quality. For example, complete elimination of all

aberrations might result in decreased depth of focus, which could be disturbing for patients who are presbyopic. More subtle symptoms of this nature might also occur in pre-presbyopic patients. It is conceivable that we will learn that other aberrations in fact provide enhanced visual performance in certain settings. Extensive further study is required to better understand these issues.
- Aberrations also change with age and accommodation [8, 11, 18, 29]. Therefore, correction of aberrations is in part temporary due to the ongoing changes that occur in both the cornea and especially the crystalline lens.
- Finally, the effect of flap creation and wound healing on the wavefront aberrations is not controllable.

Despite these limitations, data are convincing in demonstrating that wavefront-guided correction provides better quality of vision both objectively and subjectively. The current level of technology tends to minimise the induction of aberrations rather than reducing aberrations; this benefit alone represents a major advance in corneal refractive surgery.

Summary for the Clinician

- Limitations of wavefront-guided corneal surgery include treatment of only monochromatic aberrations, changes in ocular aberrations with ageing, and unpredictable changes induced by the flap and wound healing
- Despite these limitations, on average wavefront-guided correction provides better quality of vision both objectively and subjectively

17.5
Future of Wavefront-Guided Corneal Surgery

For current technology, aberrometers objectively measure the eye's aberrations, and patients' subjective preferences are not included in this assessment. In the near future, it is hoped that adaptive optics will permit patients to experience the type of correction that might be achieved and to adjust it in order to optimise the visual outcome to best address their individual needs.

For some patients, it may be more beneficial to provide more complete correction of aberrations for the eye in an accommodated state. One example might be monovision, in which one eye is corrected for distance and the other for near. Wavefront customisation to maximise near vision may become available and would potentially benefit these patients.

A major goal in wavefront-guided corneal ablation is to improve accuracy and reproducibility of key steps of the procedure, including data acquisition, corneal ablation, and aspects of wound healing. Refinements in aberrometers are needed to improve reproducibility, and work is required to better understand factors that result in fluctuations in aberrometry measurements. Improved algorithms are needed to overcome the limitations of Zernike polynomials in reconstructing the wavefront from the raw data. A better understanding of excimer laser–corneal interaction will improve reproducibility of the corneal ablation. Finally, work is needed to better understand flap mechanics and the role of corneal wound healing in modifying aberrations postoperatively. With these combinations of factors, corrections of greater predictability and accuracy will ensue.

Perhaps the greatest hurdle is the tendency of the eye to change over time. New technology and procedures are required to provide a mechanism for adjusting the wavefront correction as the eye ages and its aberrations change. The holy grail of wavefront-guided correction is an approach that permits ongoing refinement of patients' vision throughout their lifetime.

References

1. Applegate RA, Thibos LN, Hilmantel G (2001) Optics of aberroscopy and super vision. J Cataract Refract Surg 27:1093–1107
2. Applegate RA, Marsack JD, Ramos R, Sarver EJ (2003) Interaction between aberrations to improve or reduce visual performance. J Cataract Refract Surg 29:1487–1495
3. Cheng X, Thibos LN (2003) The ultimate challenge: converting wavefront aberration maps to visual quality. Review of refractive surgery, pp 15–18
4. Cheng X, Himebaugh NL, Kollbaum PS, Thibos LN, Bradley A (2003) Validation of a clinical Shack-Hartmann aberrometer. Optom Vis Sci 80:587–595
5. Cheng X, Himebaugh NL, Kollbaum PS, Thibos LN, Bradley A (2004) Test-retest reliability of clinical Shack-Hartmann measurements. Invest Ophthalmol Vis Sci 45:351–360
6. Guirao A, Porter J, Williams DR, Cox IG (2002) Calculated impact of higher-order monochromatic aberrations on retinal image quality in a population of human eyes. J Opt Soc Am A Opt Image Sci Vis 19:620–628
7. Hament WJ, Nabar VA, Nuijts RM (2002) Repeatability and validity of Zywave aberrometer measurements. J Cataract Refract Surg 28:2135–2141
8. He JC, Burns SA, Marcos S (2000) Monochromatic aberrations in the accommodated human eye. Vision Res 40:41–48
9. Liang J, Williams DR, Miller DT (1997) Supernormal vision and high-resolution retinal imaging through adaptive optics. J Opt Soc Am A 14:2884–2892
10. MacRae S, Fujieda M (2000) Slit skiascopic-guided ablation using the Nidek laser. J Refract Surg 16: S576–580
11. McLellan JS, Marcos S, Burns SA (2001) Age-related changes in monochromatic wave aberrations of the human eye. Invest Ophthalmol Vis Sci 42:1390–1395
12. McLellan JS, Marcos S, Prieto PM, Burns SA (2002) Imperfect optics may be the eye's defence against chromatic blur. Nature 417:174–176
13. Mirshahi A, Bühren J, Gerhardt D, Kohnen T (2003) In-vivo and in-vitro repeatability of Hartmann-Shack aberrometry. J Cataract Refract Surg 29:2295–2301
14. Molebny VV, Panagopoulou SI, Molebny SV, Wakil YS, Pallikaris IG (2000) Principles of ray tracing aberrometry. J Refract Surg 16:S572–575
15. Mrochen M, Kaemmerer M, Mierdel P, Krinke HE, Seiler T (2000) Principles of Tscherning aberrometry. J Refract Surg 16:S570–571

16. Nagy ZZ, Palagyi-Deak I, Kelemen E, Kovacs A (2002) Wavefront-guided photorefractive keratectomy for myopia and myopic astigmatism. J Refract Surg 18:S615–619

17. Nagy ZZ, Palagyi-Deak I, Kovacs A, Kelemen E, Forster W (2002) First results with wavefront-guided photorefractive keratectomy for hyperopia. J Refract Surg 18:S620–623

18. Ninomiya S, Fujikado T, Kuroda T, Maeda N, Tano Y, Oshika T, Hirohara Y, Mihashi T (2002) Changes of ocular aberration with accommodation. Am J Ophthalmol 134:924–926

19. Pallikaris IG, Panagopoulou SI, Molebny VV (2000) Clinical experience with the Tracey technology wavefront device. J Refract Surg 16:S588–591

20. Pallikaris IG, Kymionis GD, Panagopoulou SI, Siganos CS, Theodorakis MA, Pallikaris AI (2002) Induced optical aberrations following formation of a laser in situ keratomileusis flap. J Cataract Refract Surg 28:1737–1741

21. Phusitphoykai N, Tungsiripat T, Siriboonkoom J, Vongthongsri A (2003) Comparison of conventional versus wavefront-guided laser in situ keratomileusis in the same patient. J Refract Surg 19[Suppl 2]:S217–220

22. Porter J, Guirao A, Cox IG, Williams DR (2001) Monochromatic aberrations of the human eye in a large population. J Opt Soc Am A Opt Image Sci Vis 18:1793–1803

23. Porter J, MacRae S, Yoon G, Roberts C, Cox IG, Williams DR (2003) Separate effects of the microkeratome incision and laser ablation on the eye's wave aberration. Am J Ophthalmol 136: 327–337

24. Salmon TO, West RW, Gasser W, Kenmore T (2003) Measurement of refractive errors in young myopes using the COAS Shack-Hartmann aberrometer. Optom Vis Sci 80:6–14

25. Smirnov MS (1962) Measurement of the wave aberration of the human eye. Biophysics 7:766–795

26. Smolek MK, Klyce SD (2003) Zernike polynomial fitting fails to represent all visually significant corneal aberrations. Invest Ophthalmol Vis Sci 44:4676–4681

27. Thibos LN (2000) Principles of Hartmann-Shack aberrometry. J Refract Surg 16:S563–565

28. Thibos LN, Applegate RA, Schwiegerling JT, Webb R et al. (2001) Standards for reporting the optical aberrations of eyes. In: MacRae SM, Krueger RR, Applegate RA (eds) Customized corneal ablation, the quest for supervision. Slack Inc., Thorofare, NJ, pp 348–361

29. Wang L, Koch DD (2003) Ocular higher-order aberrations in individuals screened for refractive surgery. J Cataract Refract Surg 29:1896–1903

30. Wang L, Wang N, Koch DD (2003) Evaluation of refractive error measurements of the Wavescan Wavefront system and the Tracey Wavefront aberrometer. J Cataract Refract Surg 29:970–979

31. Webb RH, Penney CM, Thompson KP (1992) Measurement of ocular wavefront distortion with a spatially resolved refractometer. Applied Optics 31:3678–3686

32. Williams DR (1985) Visibility of interference fringes near the resolution limit. J Opt Soc Am A 2:1087–1093

33. Williams DR, Coletta NJ (1987) Cone spacing and the visual resolution limit. J Opt Soc Am A 14:1514–1523

34. Zernike F (1934) Beugungstheorie des Schneidenverfahrens und seiner verbesserten Form, der Phasenkontrastmethode. Physica I:689–704

The Pupil and Refractive Surgery

Emanuel Rosen

The author acknowledges no financial interest in the subject matter of this chapter.

Core Messages

- The eye is an imperfect optical instrument; the quality of vision it yields is limited by diffraction when the pupil is small and by aberrations when the pupil is large
- The cornea has an aspheric design to limit spherical aberration in particular as the pupil enlarges
- Corneal laser refractive surgery by its nature alters the asphericity of the cornea reversing the natural order. The whole cornea is not altered, just the central zone through which the most important rays of light pass to be focussed onto the fovea
- If the pupil is large and the effective optical zone of the cornea is small, then the potential for aberrant rays to reduce the quality of vision exists
- Similarly if treatments are decentred or the cornea is irregular then image quality will suffer
- The principal of any surgical intervention is to gather pre-operative data so that treatment planning can be as exact as possible. For corneal refractive surgery it is necessary to gather a great deal of data such as refraction, keratometry, pachymetry and topography
- Many surgeons believe that accurate pupil data is also required for correct treatment planning
- This chapter is concerned with the theoretical and practical issues posed by corneal laser surgery in the face of a large pupil. The methodology of accurate and precise pupillometry is described.

18.1
Introduction

In 1979 I.E. Loewenfeld [7] stated:
- "Pupils are never entirely at rest but undergo continuous oscillations".
- "A single 'snapshot' estimate of the pupil size cannot, therefore, be accepted as a reliable predictor of true mean size."
- "Instead, the pupil should be monitored continuously for a suitable period to enable a confident measurement".

Many observers have concluded that simple anisocoria and pupil unrest does exist and varies in individuals depending on illumination and accommodation. Other factors that influence the size of our pupils include; state of adaptation, iris colour/pigmentation, the level of alertness or correspondingly levels of fatigue, medications, diurnal rhythms, alcohol, caffeine etc. [6, 8, 11, 13]. Wide variations in anisocoria also depends on factors such as the observer and the use of non-objective pupillometry.

18.2
Pupillometry and Refractive Surgery

Why measure pupil diameters? An analogy with the early days of biometry for pseudophakia is appropriate. Many practitioners averred that use of a 20-D IOL would suit most eyes, but there were many unhappy patients because of induced ametropia and anisometropia. So with pupillometry. Why do we need it? Ignoring pupillometry may not bother the majority but there will be a very unhappy minority of pa-

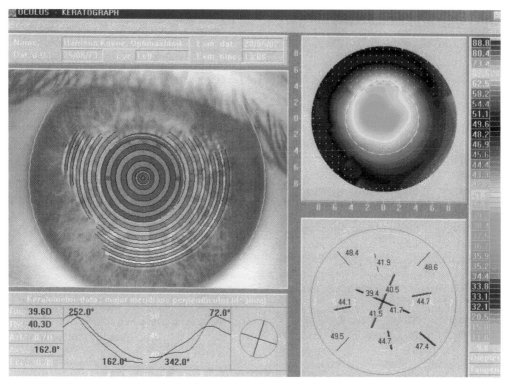

Fig. 18.1. Left eye topography indicates that in spite of a wide ablation diameter the effective optical zone is no more than 3–4 mm. The gradient of the oblate central cornea profile through 6 mm is over 10 D

tients who are very easily identified. The following example illustrates the issue of a large pupil and an effective optical zone that caused significant visual symptoms. Patient KH had a preoperative refraction of –7.0 DS in each eye. His keratometry was 42.5 D. Treatment using the Nidek laser platform utilised an ablation zone of 6.5 mm with a transition zone extending to 7.5 mm. Post-operative accurate pupillometry using the procyon pupillometer revealed a peak scotopic pupil of 7.96 mm (mean 7.92 mm) and a low mesopic diameter of 6.61 mm (mean 6.26 mm). Values similar for each eye. Following surgery the patient complained bitterly of night vision disturbances in particular (halos and starburst effects from each eye) and image ghosting in general.

As can be seen in Fig. 18.1, the left eye topography indicates that in spite of a wide ablation diameter the effective optical zone is no more than 3–4 mm. The gradient of the oblate central cornea profile through 6 mm is over 10 D which, even allowing for the mitigating prospect of the Stiles-Crawford effect, surely explains why an eye with a scotopic pupil of nearly 8 mm is symptomatic.

In the Tracey technologies aberrometry summary given in Fig. 18.2 poor point spread function is illustrated, an objective expression of the patient's complaints.

18.2.1
The Pupil and the Cornea

Measurement of the diameter of the human pupil of each eye is an important parameter in the planning of laser refractive surgery. As the excimer laser is used to change corneal curvature over an area of the cornea (the optical zone) it is obvious that this optical zone should be large enough to include all rays entering the

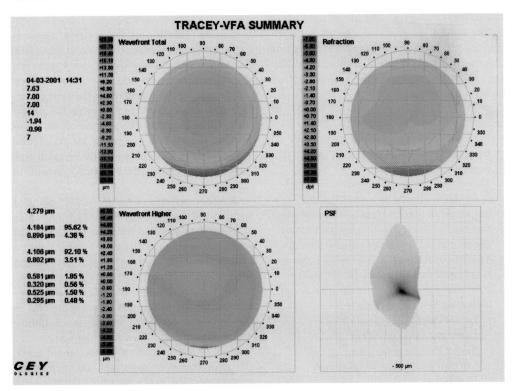

Fig. 18.2. Tracey aberrometry of left eye seen in Fig. 18.1

eye that will eventually pass through the pupil. In the past pupil measurement involved visual comparison of the pupil to a calibrated card or ruler. More recently video-pupillometry systems image the pupil using CCD video cameras.

Infrared video-pupillometry is the most efficient modality for pupil measurement and involves viewing the pupil through the cornea and so actually measures the diameter of the virtual image of the pupil produced by the dioptric power of the cornea. The reported pupil diameter is therefore slightly larger than the physical diameter of the pupil. Because of this corneal magnification, some practitioners use a correction factor to adjust the measured pupil diameter to correspond to its actual physical diameter. Most clinicians believe that for paraxial rays, the diameter of the bundle of rays entering the cornea is equal to the diameter of the magnified image of the pupil. This means that the diameter of the corneal *effective* optical zone treated should be considered relative to the diameter of

the magnified pupil. If the latter exceeds the former, then theoretically there is a greater risk of producing post-operative halos and glare, although further studies are required to better define this issue. Use of a correction factor is not appropriate as, on a balance of probabilities, this will result in an underestimation of the required optical zone size [9, 12].

In their paper "Is selection of a minimum ablation zone size for refractive surgery based on dark-adapted pupil diameter substantiated by geometric optical analysis?" Freedman et al. [4] utilise an optical model of the anterior segment to calculate the effective corneal optical zone, i.e. the diameter of the area of cornea that refracts all incident light rays arising from objects along the line of sight though the entrance pupil. They found that, for a given entrance pupil size, the effective optical zone was significantly influenced by keratometry values but slightly influenced by the distance from the cornea to the actual or physical pupil. They concluded that for objects in the line of sight, the effective optical zone was smaller than the entrance pupil in all cases. However, for rays from objects in the periphery, the effective optical zone expanded rapidly as the angle of oblique incidence increased.

Summary for the Clinician

- Off axis objects may form images away from the fovea which will result in parafoveal halos and flare
- Therefore, the functional/effective optical zone ideally should be larger than the largest pupil (peak scotopic pupil, although this may not be achievable without removing excessive amounts of corneal tissue)
- The area over which correction is achieved is invariably smaller than the planned ablation zone due to many constant factors including:
  - Initial keratometry
  - Laser ablation algorithm
  - Tissue healing responses
  - Corneal biomechanical response to ablation
  - Magnitude of correction

18.3
Planning Corneal Refractive Surgery

"Pupils are dynamic and often asymmetric a factor found to increase with reduced illumination" [7]. Ophthalmologists performing refractive surgery require extensive data from their patients to enable an informed decision regarding the correct modality of treatment. Pupil data have been largely ignored in the quantitative sense, with most surgeons relying on qualitative assessment or ignoring the role of the pupil in refractive surgical calculations. In our increasingly litigious society, an awareness of the need to fully document the pre-operative physical and dynamic aspects of eyes is logical.. Bilateral simultaneous dynamic infra-red pupillometry provides both data and a record of the examination under varied lighting conditions.

By measuring the pupils' responses to different levels of illuminance, the surgeon is able to plan treatment, knowing that wider ablations

are deeper ablations, whichever laser platform is utilised. Titration of the ablation diameter against the central corneal thickness, especially in myopia treatments, will verify whether or not the safety parameters that are generally agreed will be transgressed. If they are, then either surface ablation or an alternative refractive procedure will be required. The ablation profile is important; prolate being more natural than oblate is less likely to be associated with visual disturbances, as will the degree and gradient of change imposed.

Another example of LASIK surgery planned without reference to pupillometry is shown in Fig. 18.3. The planned ablation of 5.5 mm (to avoid too deep an ablation in a cornea with a central thickness <500 nm) measures 3.3 mm on topographic analysis. A quantitative judgement would have precluded this unfortunate intervention, for the patient has severe symptoms in mesopic and scotopic conditions of illuminance. Figure 18.4ab illustrates the issue by ray tracing. LASIK practitioners who would argue that pupil size is not important in refractive surgery, neglect the ease with which pupillometry is accomplished with modern instrumentation. Better to plan surgical intervention with all the facts than leave an element of chance in the outcome. Better to know than to guess! Better to avoid errors of omission before committing errors of commission.

Some investigators (Schallhorn [10], Brint (AAO 2003)[2] and Pop [8]) concluded that there is no relationship between pupil size and post-LASIK symptoms, especially night vision disturbances. Their conclusions are based on inadequate pupillometry, for unless pupils are measured correctly, (bilateral dynamic digital infra-red pupillometry under controlled conditions of illuminance) then no such conclusion should be reached. It is true that some patients with large pupils and demonstrably smaller effective ablated optical zones, are symptom free, whilst others will have unacceptable symptoms, which confirms the issue is complex. The equation is simple: if the effective optical zone on the cornea (especially if it is *oblate* and embraces a dioptric range of more than 2–3 D; or is irregular) is smaller than the entrance pupil, then a blur circle of defocused light may cause unwant-

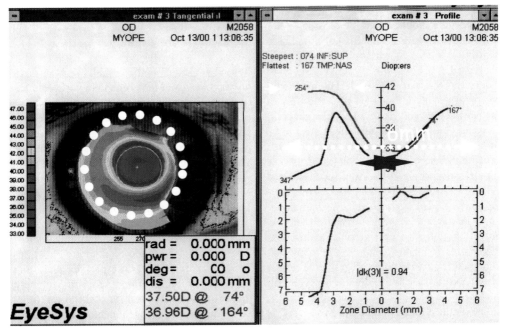

Fig. 18.3. Corneal topographic map following LASIK performed to correct –7 D. A 5.5-mm ablation using a NIDEK laser was utilised in order to protect a "thin" cornea, planning nevertheless a residual corneal stromal thickness of only 200 μm. The consequential functional optical zone (base of corneal refractive profile map) is no more than 2–3 mm. As the eye had a scotopic pupil of 6.8 mm it is easy to comprehend why the patient suffered visual disturbances, especially at night. The main focussed image is surrounded by a halo of defocused light

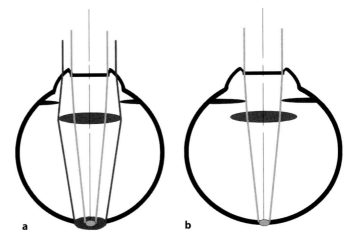

Fig. 18.4 a,b. Why is pupil size important? **a** Pupil size is unsatisfactory when the pupil is larger than the ablated zone. Aberrations and halos are caused by transition zone and untreated cornea. **b** Pupil size is ideal when the pupil is smaller than the functional optical zone

ed imagery (see Fig. 18.1). There seems to be no doubt that cerebral image processing may filter out unwanted effects in some patients whereas others are ultra-sensitive to minor aberrations.

Time also does seem to be a healer as Pop reported in the dramatic reduction of symptoms over a 12-month period [8]. A similar phenomenon occurs regularly amongst contact lens wearers who happen to have large pupils. Such data of course should always be recorded prior to corneal laser surgery. As it is not possible to identify an individual patient's sensitivities in this regard, it behoves the refractive surgeon to understand the issue and undertake preventative measures as far is possible. The aim of corneal laser surgery is to adjust the shape of the cornea and hence its refractive power to be compatible with the other elements of the eye's focusing system, namely the length of the eye globe. As the whole cornea cannot be treated and as the central zone of the cornea is most relevant, attention has to be paid to the diameter of the treated area and, more importantly, the nature of the effective optical zone within that treated area, to ensure as far as is possible that unfocussed light rays do not degrade the retinal image. The problem magnifies as the correction increases.

The dictum "understand before you treat" is particularly relevant to corneal refractive surgery because failures cannot be hidden. Pupillometry is therefore desirable as a component of refractive surgery pre-operative data collection. Most refractive surgeons are aware of patients with glare disability and large pupils post-operatively; they will also recall patients with large pupils but no night vision disturbances, as well as those with small pupils and multiple glare complaints. The indefinite correlation of pupil size to night vision disturbances may be due to the difficulties of definition, as well as many other variables in the equation.

Summary for the Clinician

- Pupils are measured to identify disparities between:
  - Corneal ablated zone
  - Corneal effective "optical" zone (EOZ)
  - Entrance pupil diameter
  - Theoretically a disparity between the EOZ and the entrance pupil could cause unfocussed rays to create a halo of blurred imagery

18.4
Pupils and Night Vision

Refractive surgery embraces interventions in or on the cornea and replacement or supplementation of the crystalline lens. Whichever modality is used, the refracting element must cover the entrance pupil or defocused light rays will impinge on the fovea and induce visual confusion. The criticality of the effect of pupil size on night vision and visual acuity is discussed in the work of Holladay et al. [5] and Boxer Wachler et al. [1]. The subjective manifestations of a disparity between the effective optical zone on the cornea (or the diameter of the optic of an intra-ocular lens – phakic or pseudo-phakic) are ghost images, blurred vision, and especially glare and haloes at low illumination levels. Unfortunately, there is no standard test for night vision functional disturbances which includes methods for measuring glare disability and contrast sensitivity. The lack of standardisation, and therefore scientific validity, confuses consistent correlation with symptoms. The aspheric design of the cornea serves to limit spherical aberration which is nevertheless pupil-dependent. It follows from this perspective alone that refractive surgeons must be cautious when treating patients with large pupils. It behoves the surgeon to understand through dynamic pupillometry both the dimension of the pupils as well as the briskness of their response to the light stimulus for this too will be a factor in the prospect of dim light, i.e. night visual disturbances.

Summary for the Clinician

- Large pupils enhance:
  - Spherical aberration
  - Other aberrations
- If a normal aspheric cornea is present this may:
  - Render the cornea oblate
  - Add a steep gradient
- If a small effective optical zone is created then:
  - Visual problems may multiply

18.5
Pupillary Unrest, Anisocoria and Measurement

Every refractive surgical procedure should take cognisance of the pupil in each eye, its peak diameter in dim light conditions and anisocoria, which is usual. Pupils are constantly in motion (known as pupillary unrest or Hippus). This means that single measurements cannot be reliable. Furthermore, because pupils are invariably unequal, measuring one pupil is not sufficient to determine the peak size of each pupil. Controlled levels of illuminance plus multiple measurements are required in order to establish the peak scotopic pupil on the basis of which the planned ablation zone for LASIK should be calculated. [9]. The aim is to create an effective optical zone of the cornea at least equal to the peak scotopic pupil in order to reduce or eliminate that potential component of post-corneal laser surgery, namely unwanted image degradation.

Anisocoria is usual though its degree varies in every individual and is not easily observed. Use of gauges, rulers and monocular measuring devices, especially without total control of illuminance, is not compatible with accurate measurement and therefore not compatible with the sophisticated and precise process of corneal laser surgery, where microns rather than millimetres are important! A dynamic binocular, the digital infrared pupillometer provides accurate data which is saved as documents which complement other aspects of the patient record. The images of the pupil are acquired by means of infrared imaging, followed by computerised determination of the pupil size through multiple images utilising customised software. The print out of the data in graphic and/or tabulated format is then instantly available for efficient pre-operative assessment, planning of treatment and archiving.

Subjective measurement of pupil diameters under varied lighting conditions is inaccurate. In their comparisons of inter-observer grading of anisocoria, Ettinger and co-authors [3] report high variability. Simple devices such as rulers and comparison charts can give approximate data, but are unreliable because of the inherent difficulty of measuring a moving object, especially without controlled illuminance.

The need for reliable data has driven the development of electronic pupillometers during the past 50 years. Now computerised infrared video pupillometers are accepted as industry benchmarks by ophthalmologists and scientists whose research involves the pupil. Single measurements using a graduated scale are not repeatable or reliable because pupils are highly motile and subject to considerable unrest. Use of corneal topographers and or aberrometers are monocular and reduce pupil diameters due to their intrinsic illumination systems.

Summary for the Clinician

Pupil reactions
- Never at rest
- Anisocoria is usual
- Subject to light and accommodation reflexes
- Dark adaptation
- Affected by:
  - Age
  - Iris pigmentation
  - Fatigue
  - Medications
  - Diurnal rhythm
  - Caffeine
  - Alcohol

Pupillometry at its most refined level includes:
- Bilateral simultaneous study
- Multiple measurements
- Controlled illuminance
- Infrared detection
- Relaxed accommodation (distant target)
- Computerised record and data presentation
- Permanent record of the data collected
- Avoiding gauges and monocular devices

18.6
How Should Pupils Be Measured?

The dynamic and asymmetric nature of pupil activity demands a dynamic, bilateral simultaneous system for measurement, and one in which the levels of illuminance to which the eyes are exposed are strictly controlled and documented. Accommodation must be relaxed with the subject viewing a distant target. Multiple images of the moving pupil then require a rapid computerised measure of the pupil diameter of each rapid sequence image to then be translated into a clinically useful table or graph from which the clinical decisions will be made.

18.6.1
Data Acquisition and Processing System

With the Procyon Pupillometer (Figs. 18.5–18.7) at each level of illumination, ten images are acquired by the system at five images per second, providing a measurement period of 2 s. The optical system is fixed magnification. Circles are automatically fitted to image data derived from the pupil–iris borders, allowing many occlusions (corneal reflections, eyelashes, eyelid partial closures) to be ignored. The diameters of the fitted circles are stored as the results. The operator receives feedback concerning the quality of the resulting data (check focus, goodness

of fit, and rejection of blinks). The two eyes are imaged at the same time, with a spatial resolution of 0.03 mm per pixel. Random errors introduced by the pupillometer are typically 1 pixel (± 0.03 mm) from image to image, which is an order of magnitude less than the variation seen in the measurements themselves. The software re-analyses the same image with identical results. Figure 18.5 shows a typical image from a sequence with circles fitted (dotted lines around the pupil border). Figure 18.6 shows an output example of a typical measurement sequence in which pupillary unrest and anisocoria are present. The mean and standard error of each 2-s measurement set are also presented for each eye at each light level in graphic or tabular format.

18.6.2
Illumination

The fixation targets presented to the two eyes are identical white opal disks subtending an angle of 8° in the central visual field. The virtual image of a black dot in the middle of each disk is positioned at a distance of at least 10 m using a convex lens. The non-illuminated part of the visual field is well occluded with rubber eyecups. The accepted thresholds for the CIE (International Commission on Illumination) curve for vision are as follows: scotopic, illuminance levels below 0.05 lux; photopic, illuminance levels above 50 lux (National Physical Laboratory,

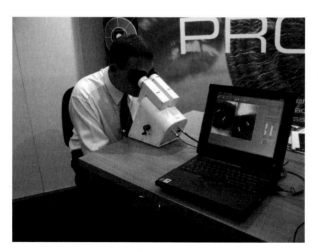

Fig. 18.5. Bilateral pupillometry utilising the Procyon bilateral simultaneous infra-red digital pupillometer. Patient's eyes fixed onto rubber cups to exclude external light

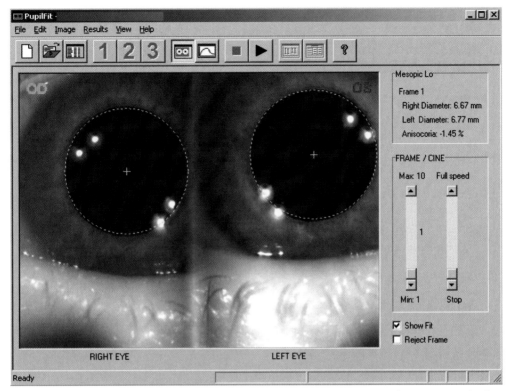

Fig. 18.6. Bilateral simultaneous images of the pupils. One image out of a sequence of ten taken in 2 s. Note firstly, anisocoria and secondly, *dotted circles* which conform to pupil size for computerised calculation of pupil diameters of each image set

London, UK). Table 18.1 gives some examples of illuminance in real life.

The study by Rosen et al. [9] (Tables 18.2 and 18.3) revealed an appreciable degree of pupillary motility during measurement at all illumination levels. The motion was greatest under low mesopic illumination. In addition, the two

Table 18.1. Illuminance in real life

Scotopic illuminance = <0.05 lux
    Dark night
    No moon
    Highway
Low mesopic illuminance = 0.05 lux
    Dark night oncoming car
    Dim lit room
High mesopic illuminance = 49 lux
    Night driving road illuminated (in town)

Table 18.2. Pupillary unrest is significant and large at all levels of illumination in more than 50% of patients

Scotopic (0 lux)
    Median = 0.13 mm, maximum = 1.01 mm
Mesopic (1 lux)
    Median = 0.34 mm, maximum = 1.57 mm

Table 18.3. Anisocoria is also significant and large in some patients at all levels of illumination in more than 50% of patients

Scotopic (0 lux)
    Median = 0.29 mm, maximum = 1.47 mm
Mesopic (1 lux)
    Median = 0.34 mm, maximum = 1.99 mm

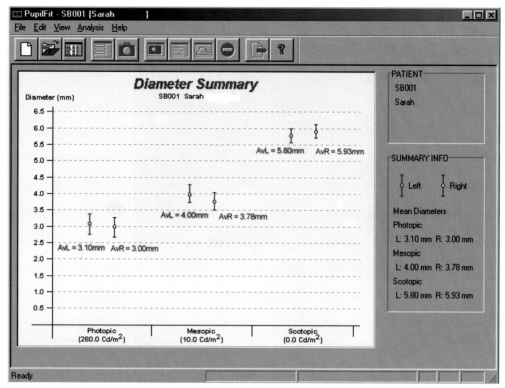

Fig. 18.7. Procyon data graph: photopic (>50 lux), low mesopic (0.05 lux), high mesopic (49 lux) and scotopic pupil measurements(<0.05 lux), mean and range of ten taken in a 2-s period

pupils were rarely identical. The results suggest there was a dynamic range of pupillary motion, characterised by maximum-amplitude unrest under high and low mesopic illuminations. There was significant unrest (maximum 1.01 mm) under scotopic conditions, although pupil size was closer to the saturation level.

The degree of absolute anisocoria varied among individuals. It was as high as 1.99 mm, with median values of 0.16 mm (high mesopic), 0.32 mm (low mesopic) and 0.28 mm (scotopic).

18.7
Pupillometry Studies

Pupil data is non-parametric and skewed. In any measurement system there are two types of error at play: Systematic errors (accuracy, bias, calibration) and random errors (precision and repeatability).

18.7.1
Precision

Since the pupil is always moving single measurements amount to little more than guesswork. This was alluded to by Winn [12] and demonstrated by Rosen et al. [9], while Kohnen et al. [6] demonstrated that single measurements using simple hand-held instruments are highly variable. The inter-operator repeatability was substantially better with the Procyon than the Colvard; 0.64 mm (Procyon), 1.16 mm (Colvard), i.e. a 95 % chance that two consecutive readings with the Colvard on the same patient will be up to 1.16 mm apart. Schmitz et al. [11] showed that only multiple measurements using simple hand-held devices could attempt to match more sophisticated dynamic devices concluding that the Colvard matched the Procyon's performance but only if nine measurements were taken and averaged, which was very time consuming! They also found that the WASCA aberrometer's pupil measuring function did not measure the same thing as the Procyon because of its bright illumination.

The argument is relatively simple: because the pupil is changing in size all the time, only multiple measurements will give statistical confidence in the resulting measurement. A single measurement has an infinitely wide confidence interval which is not much good when it is necessary to know a dimension as precisely as possible. It is probable that the Stiles Crawford effect only mitigates partially against visual disturbances such as halos and glare because generally the shape of the cornea changes from prolate to oblate post-operatively, thus negating the effect.

Illumination during pupillometry is also critically important. Because pupil size is dependent on illumination, pupillometry should also be done at controlled levels of illumination, and that illumination should be binocular [9], otherwise there is a danger of over-estimating pupil size and taking off more tissue than is necessary. Some practitioners report that "Device A" which controls illumination internally consistently over- or under-measures pupil size compared to "Device B" which relies on ambient illumination. No real attempt is made to ensure that both devices bring about identical illumination conditions and therefore such statements are meaningless until it can be shown that the lighting is identical for both methods. Devices A and B might well reverse their apparent over- or under-reading if the ambient conditions change. Devices that bring about controlled illumination will be consistent under a wide range of ambient illumination conditions.

18.7.2
Accuracy

Illumination levels (and accommodation) will affect the accuracy or bias of the measurement system. A shift in light level will cause a shift in bias.

There is a need to compare the repeatability of different pupillometers and to standardise measurement conditions for illumination and accommodation as a first step towards getting better agreement between studies.

Measurement requires recognition of the dynamic nature of pupil activity, its asymmetry and the effects of internal and external factors. By simply observing a patient at consultation in the usually dimmed lighting of the consulting room, large pupils will be immediately apparent. Increasing the room's illuminance and the pupils will respond by constriction, some briskly, others hardly at all. In other words, our responses in this regard are very individual. Pupils respond to light and accommodation reflexes but are also subject to many other internal and external factors (see "Summary for the Clinician" below). Therefore it is pertinent to ask when should pupillometry be conducted and on how many occasions should their peak values be established? How can the science of pupil measurement be combined with the practicalities of the clinical situation? It is impractical for example to expect a patient to attend for pupil measurements in the morning as well as in the evening. There obviously has to be a compromise in this regard recognising that *one set of measurements performed as well as possible is better than guesswork.*

Summary for the Clinician

Two types of error occur with any measurement system:

- Systematic errors:
  - Accuracy
  - Bias
  - Calibration errors
- Random errors:
  - Precision
  - Repeatability

Useful Definitions

- **Aberrometry** The measurement of aberrations.
- **Aberration** Deviation from what is normal, expected or usual.
- **Aberrations (optical)** Aberrations cause exiting wavefronts to be distorted from their initial spherical shape and cause light rays to depart from their ideal paths.
- **Anisocoria** Pupils which are not equal, i.e. physiological asymmetry. Often a sign of pathology. It is necessary to study the dynamic characteristics of the anisocoria, i.e. how it increases and decreases during different pupillary movements, in order to learn the location of the responsible defect.
- **Average** Numerical averages take several forms: mean, median and mode.
  - **Mean average (arithmetic mean)** Divide the total by the number of components to yield the mean
  - **Median average** The mid-point, half the number of variables above and half below, the "median"
  - **Mode average** The value which occurs most frequently, the usual, the mode average
    A symmetrical unimodal bell curve its peak value is the average and because of it symmetry the peak value is the median, the mean and the mode. In an asymmetric unimodal bell curve the peak will be the mode average, the median the half way house and the mean average the lower value.
    A symmetrical bimodal bell curve would have 2 peak values the mode averages 1 and2 whereas the median and mean averages would have the same value i.e. between the 2 modes.
- **Contrast sensitivity** A glare source can also reduce *contrast sensitivity*.
- **corneal magnification coefficient** The coefficient of correlation between real pupil size and refraction is only –0.104 (158 Loewenfeld), e.g. average diameter of real pupil 4.23 mm, 4.38 mm for –5 D myopia and 4.08 mm for 5D hyperopia. Approximately 1 % of variability in real pupil size is associated with ametropia.
- **Defocus** Focussing is not usually exact and therefore in any imaging system, there is some residual defocus. A reason for this focus error is that there is always a range of positions of the "image" plane within which the image appears to be correctly focussed. Defocus spreads light out.
- **Diffraction** Not refraction.
- **Effective/functional optic zone (EOZ)** That central zone of the cornea which after corneal laser ablation, provides the major refracting surface of the eye. In a normal eye with a prolate profile in the absence of astigmatism there is a range of limited dioptric power in this zone, e.g. 2–3 D. Following a laser ablation which renders the cornea oblate, the dioptric range beyond 2–3 D will define the limit of the effective or functional optical zone of the cornea.
- **Glare** A physical term that refers to a light source, bright and intense.
- **Glare disability** The term used to describe the subjective reduction of visual performance due to a glare source scattered by the ocular media.
- **Image degradations** Halos and starburst represent an alteration in the object shape or size.
- **Irreducibly minimal latent period** Depends on properties of iris smooth muscle (180 ms) but increases with age.
- **Mesopic** There are two types of receptors on the retina of the eye: rods and cones. The rods operate at low light levels, the cones operate at high light levels, and both operate over a range at intermediate light levels. Rod vision does not provide colour response or high visual acuity. In fact, there is no rod vision along the line of sight; in looking for a very faint signal light on a dark night, one must look about 15 degrees to the side of it. The cones are responsible for colour vision and the high acuity necessary for reading and seeing small details.
  In the mesopic region as the light level decreases from photopic to scotopic vision, the spectral response gradually changes from the photopic to the scotopic curve. There is a

continuous range of mesopic curves changing in both shape and maximum sensitivity, and the appropriate curve depends on such factors as the light level and the distribution of light in the field of view. Because of this and a range of other problems, there is no agreement, either within the United States or internationally, on a standard method for computing lumens in the mesopic region.

- **Mesopic vision** *(term of* physiology
  Mesopic vision is the scientific term for a combination between *photopic vision* and *scotopic vision* in low but not quite dark lighting situations. The human eye uses pure *scotopic vision* in the range below 0.05 LUX, and pure *photopic vision* in the range above 49 LUX
  Mesopic vision involves complex interactions between rod and cone receptor signals that are not fully understood. The variation in receptor class density with retinal location, the differences in spatial summation properties of rod and cone receptors and the diminishing contribution of chromatic signals to target conspicuity as the illumination level is reduced makes it difficult to model and predict visual performance in the mesopic range.
- Night vision disturbances (NVD) Glare disability, reduced contrast sensitivity, and image degradation are all examples.
- **Oblate** Adjective; describing an object with an equatorial diameter of greater length than the polar diameter
- **Peak** Top of the curve. Highest value
- **Prolate** Adjective; describing an object with a polar diameter of greater length than the equatorial diameter.
- **Pupil and dark adaptation** After the acute "light off" response, pupils continue to enlarge at decelerating rates until their full dark adapted state is recovered. The speed and extent of the enlargement is dependent upon preceding conditions which have to be defined to be meaningful, e.g. partially dark adapted prior to "light off".

- **Pupil latent period** The reaction of a pupil to a light stimulus is delayed, the delay being known as the latent period. This is not a simple phenomenon but is composed of two separate mechanisms; first, the *irreducibly minimal latent* period built into the motor system of the iris; and a second, a variable *additional delay* due mainly to properties of the retinal discharges and their brain processing.
- **Photopic** Normal adaptation of the eye to day (light) vision.
  The level of light adaptation of the retina.
- **Illuminance** The luminous flux incident on unit area of a surface. Measured in lux. Also known as illumination.
- **Illumination** Another term for illuminance (physics); a source of light (adjective).
- **Lux** The derived SI of illumination equal to a luminous flux of 1 lumen per square metre. 1 lux is equivalent to 0.0929 foot candles. Symbol, lx.
- **Parametric** Data measurable on interval or ratio scales, so that arithmetic operations are applicable, enabling parameters such as the mean of the distribution to be defined (PUPIL data is non-parametric)
- **Pupil** The central dark aperture within the iris diaphragm from the 14th century French *pupille*, Latin *pupilla*, literally meaning little doll, from *pupa* so called from the tiny image seen when observing an eye.
- **Pupillary unrest (hippus)** Normal papillary oscillations brought on by steady light and absent in darkness.
- **Pupillometry** The science of measuring pupil diameters.
- **Skewed data** Pupil data is skewed ; Not having equal probabilities above and below the mean

References

1. Boxer Wachler BS (2003) Effect of pupil size on visual function under monocular and binocular conditions in LASIK and non-LASIK patients. J Cataract Refract Surg 29:275–279
2. Brint S (2003) The effect of pupil size on night visual disturbances after LASIK. Presentation at the AAO Anaheim, November
3. Ettinger ER, Wyatt HJ, London R (1991) Anisocoria. Variation and clinical observation with different conditions of illumination and accommodation. Invest Ophthalmol Vis Sci 32:501–509
4. Freedman KA, Brown SM, Mathews SM, Young RS (2003) Pupil size and the ablation zone in laser refractive surgery: considerations based on geometric optics. J Cataract Refract Surg 29:1924–1931
5. Holladay JT, Janes JA (2002) Topographic changes in. corneal asphericity and effective optical zone after laser in situ keratomileusis. J Cataract Refract Surg 28:942–947
6. Kohnen T, Terzi E, Buhren J, Kohnen EM (2003) Comparison of a digital and a handheld infrared pupillometer for determining scotopic pupil diameter. J Cataract Refract Surg 29:112-117
7. Loewenfeld IE (1999) The pupil. Butterworth Heinemann, Oxford, UK
8. Pop M, Payette Y (2004) Risk factors for night vision disturbances after LASIK for myopia. Ophthalmology 111:3–10
9. Rosen ES, Gore CL, Taylor D, Chitkara D, Howes F, Kowalewski E (2002) Use of a digital infrared pupillometer to assess patient suitability for refractive surgery. J Cataract Refract Surg 288:1433–1438
10. Schallhorn SC, Kaupp SE, Tanzer DJ, Tidwell J, Laurent J, Bourque LB (2003) Pupil size and quality of vision after LASIK. Ophthalmology 1108: 1606–1614
11. Schmitz S, Krummenauer F, Henn S, Dick HB (2003) Comparison of three different technologies for pupil diameter measurement. Graefes Arch Clin Exp Ophthalmol 241:472–477 (Epub 2003 May 09)
12. Winn B, Whitaker D, Elliott DB, Phillips NJ (1994) Factors affecting light-adapted pupil size in normal human subjects. Invest Ophthalmol Vis Sci 35:1132–1137

Quality of Vision After Refractive Surgery

Thomas Kohnen, Jens Bühren, Thomas Kasper, Evdoxia Terzi

The authors have no proprietary interest in any of the devices used in this study.

Core Messages

- After inventing, evaluating and perfecting refractive surgical procedures in recent years, one of the current efforts is to focus on "quality of vision" after various refractive surgical interventions
- Quality of vision is acceptable if a refractive surgical procedure results in retinal image quality that does not produce a subjective or objective decrease in vision
- Quality of vision after refractive surgery is a complex topic with many variables
- Measuring quality of vision involves four major parameters: patient's sensation, functional, optical and anatomical features
- For corneal surgery, optical zone, pupil size and ablation depth, for lens procedures, centration and optic design play a major role
- The overall improvement of the quality of vision after refractive surgical interventions will be a major step for the success of refractive surgery

19.1
Introduction

After inventing, evaluating and perfecting refractive surgical procedures in recent years, one of the current efforts is to focus on "quality of vision" after various surgical interventions. The number of surgical procedures to correct refractive errors is steadily increasing, old procedures are replaced by newer, mostly better ones, the complication rate is decreasing, and the results of each of the established procedures are im-proving with more experience, better technology and scientific evaluation. Success or failure of refractive procedures, defined by criteria like safety, efficacy, stability and predictability [13] is based on Snellen acuity. However, some patients present with anatomically perfect results and excellent visual outcome with respect to these criteria measured in Snellen acuity, but complain of visual disturbances like decreased contrast, different colour perception, glare, halos or simply "bad vision". In some cases the problem can be explained, e.g. by residual astigmatism or a decentred ablation zone in excimer surgery or the optic diameter of a phakic intraocular lens implant on halo perception, in other cases an immediate answer is not found. On the contrary, in retrospect there should have been problems (6-mm ablation zone for LASIK with 7-mm scotopic pupil size diameter) that fortunately have never occurred. Therefore determining the outcome seems to be more complex. Why do only some patients complain? Are some complaints associated with simple residual refractive error or are there other much more sophisticated reasons for visual disturbances yet unknown to the patients [14]? The present chapter gives an overview of how quality of vision could be defined and determined and summarises typical disturbances which are known to date.

19.2
Defining Quality of Vision

Although "quality of vision" seems to be a major concern in modern refractive surgery there is no systematic approach to define quality of vision as yet. Certainly, quality of vision is not a

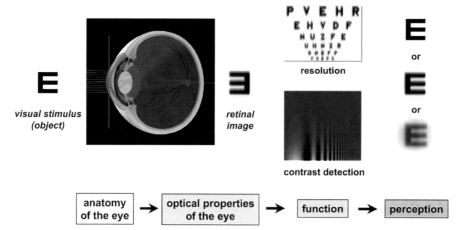

Fig. 19.1. Overview of the different levels of factors affecting quality of vision

metric which can be determined in a straight line, e.g. like the objective refraction or the axial length of the eye. Therefore, operationalisation is necessary to access the somewhat vague concept of "quality of vision". Vision is a complex process and the perception of a visual stimulus is affected by many factors which are illustrated in a simplified way in Fig. 19.1. Primarily, anatomic features such as characteristics of the corneal surface, corneal curvature, clearness of the optical media and axial length of the eye determine the quality of the retinal image. The quality of the retinal image influences basic visual tasks like resolution and contrast detection. Finally, the image is processed by the visual system. A variety of subtle mechanisms (e.g. the Stiles-Crawford effect) provide compensation for errors of the optical system of the eye. This leads to a specific perception of the initial visual stimulus. The final valuation of the overall image quality by the viewer depends on many intrinsic factors and situations. Given the same retinal image, the letter "E" as shown in Fig. 19.1, might appear crisp to one and blurry to the other observer. Therefore, when defining "quality of vision", one should start with the patient's assessment of his quality of vision. This is crucial, because it is the patient who ultimately decides if his vision is "good" or "bad". Conversely, the changes made by refractive surgery are changes of anatomy. For an operational definition of

"quality of vision", typical features of "good" or "bad" vision have to be catalogued. At the next step, factors of the underlying pathway in Fig. 19.1 and their association with "good" or "bad" vision should be identified. This would enable one to establish evidenced-based approaches to improve quality of vision after refractive surgery or to forestall bad outcomes and patient dissatisfaction.

19.2.1
Subjective Symptoms

It is important to mention that for most patients their visual impression with a particular correction (glasses or contact lenses) before undergoing refractive surgery is their reference for the post-operative situation. Obviously, some unwanted visual phenomena are familiar to all refractive surgical patients, e.g. blurry vision because of residual refractive error. Other symptoms, like haloes, starbursts, ghosting and loss of contrast sensitivity may be new to the patient and cause certain alarm. The patient's expectations and tolerance to possible side effects play a key role for the outcome. Some patients definitely report starbursts and haloes, but they nevertheless are comfortable with the result. Connecting the same eye to another brain could possibly result in an extremely unhappy patient.

Thus, it is both important to know what side-effects have to be expected performing a certain treatment and how the patient's assessment of his quality of vision would be influenced by these symptoms. In a clinical environment, a careful anamnesis would address the patient's subjective symptoms, whereas in clinical trials standardised questionnaires should be used to quantify symptoms. There is a range of questionnaires on vision and daily activities, some set up for cataract patients, some recently created to assess refractive procedures (see Sect. 19.3). These questionnaires are very important for understanding and defining quality of vision, because they are the link between the patient's sensations and all other measurements [20].

19.2.2
Visual Function

Most patient complaints regarding refractive surgery concern some type of decrease in visual function. Blurriness or fuzziness of sight can become evident in reduction of the contrast sensitivity function with diminishing maximum contrast sensitivity on the one hand and decreasing maximum resolution on the other hand. There is a large variety of psychophysical tests to determine visual function, ranging from standard Snellen acuity charts to contrast sensitivity or low-contrast acuity tests up to sophisticated procedures to assess haloes, glare disability and stray light (see Sect. 19.3). Up to now, the main outcome measure in assessment of refractive-surgical procedures was "Snellen acuity", the angular visual acuity determined by high-contrast optotypes. As many activities in daily life do not take place under optimal lighting conditions, Snellen acuity reflects only one element of visual function and gives only partial insight into the quality of vision. Thus, contrast sensitivity or low-contrast visual acuity testing will play a major role besides Snellen acuity testing to determine quality of vision. For the definition of quality of vision, the psychophysical tests act as a standardised representation of single visual tasks that may be more or less affected in daily life by a refractive surgical procedure. Correlation of functional results with subjective symptoms on the one hand and with objective measurements on the other hand will establish connections between the patient's complaints and the quantitative measurements performed in clinical practice and trials.

19.2.3
Optical Image Quality

An ideal optical system would depict an object without loss of contrast or resolution, i.e. a point will be imaged as a point. In fact, the eye is not a perfect optical system. There are three major reasons for degradation of the retinal image: diffraction, aberrations and scatter. Diffraction is only clinically relevant for small pupil sizes (<3 mm), whereas aberrations and scatter (stray light) are important factors which influence quality of vision, particularly at larger pupil sizes. All three conditions affect the retinal image by transforming a point-shaped object into a more or less fuzzy dot. Lower-order aberrations, known as prismatic, spherical and cylindrical error [tilt, defocus and astigmatism in terms of Zernike polynomials, (see Chap. 17)] are dominant in many eyes and have tremendous impact on image quality. Besides the lower-order aberrations, other irregularities, known as higher-order aberrations (HOA) have been described. Coma and spherical aberration are two aberrations leading to characteristic image degradation and have been well-known for quite some time. They have been included in the set of Zernike polynomials, which can be used to describe the wavefront error of a certain optical system in a systematic way [3, 28]. From the wavefront error of an eye, several metrics as the point spread function (PSF; the distribution of light intensity at the retinal focal plane when a point-shaped light source is imaged) or the modulation transfer function (MTF, the degree of contrast transfer of a sinusoidal grating as a function of spatial frequency) can be derived (see Chap. 17). These metrics, which could be obtained easily by objective measurements (wavefront sensing or double-pass measurements) reflect the retinal image quality of the eye considering the eye as an optical instrument and ignoring the role of neural image transfer and processing. This is of high value when assessing the plain optical effect of a certain refractive procedure or comparing different techniques, because these metrics are objective.

19.2.4
The Role of Anatomy

The anatomy of the eye plays a major role for quality of vision, because the effects achieved by refractive surgery, side effects included, are exclusively anatomical. Therefore, anatomy is the "input" level of the pathway in Fig. 19.1, in contrast to the subjective symptoms, which represent the "output" level. This is very important because all other changes are consequences of the anatomical change induced by surgery. Examining anatomy does not provide direct conclusions on quality of vision, but it gives perhaps the most objective feedback on the precise effect of the treatment. Establishing correlations between anatomy, function and subjective symptoms enables further improvements in the field of refractive surgery and safer treatments to provide good quality of vision.

Summary for the Clinician

- Quality of vision after refractive surgery is a complex topic with many variables which are influenced by many factors, both extrinsic and intrinsic
- Thus, for a working definition it could be stated that a good quality of vision is given if a refractive surgical procedure does not affect the retinal image quality in the way that vision is experienced worse than before surgery

19.3
Measuring Quality of Vision

From the operational definition for quality of vision given above, it can be concluded that several parameters could be assessed to determine optical quality before and after refractive surgery. However, many of the tests are not part of clinical routine and therefore uncommon to both patient and examiner. Some of the tests could be added easily to a clinical setting, others will be reserved for investigational purposes.

Before describing the tests in detail, some initial comments on desirable testing conditions should be made: First, visual testing, particularly in myopes, needs to be performed under the same conditions pre- and post-operatively. Only the best pre-operative measurement (often better with contact lenses than with spectacles) should be compared to the post-operative outcome, because the patient will always compare the result to the optimal pre-operative situation. Second, at least in the clinical setting, there should be internal standards on how to test. Up to now there have only been few standards for a common procedure like testing visual acuity, mostly applied in cases of medico-legal issues. Interestingly, no guidelines for determining Snellen acuity or contrast sensitivity in refractive surgery have as yet been established. In different studies, or in daily practice, different investigators and devices may be involved and produce biased results, making these results less comparable. It is important to point out that testing visual acuity or contrast sensitivity means determining psychophysical thresholds. It is desirable that all these thresholds are tested pre- and post-operatively under comparable and reproducible conditions which means, to name only some, similar optotypes and lightening conditions, forced-choice testing, no feedback by the investigator and low probability of guessing [14]. When the threshold is defined as the steepest point of the psychometric function and rigorous forced-choice is applied, acuity values can be around 20/10 even without "super normal correction" [32].

The following sections give an overview of common tests which test parameters that are relevant for quality of vision. In a clinical environment not all of the test types could be used, but it is helpful to have a range of routine examinations such as standardised anamnesis, visual acuity (VA), contrast sensitivity (CS), corneal topography and aberrometry to assess the outcome of the procedures carried out in the clinical setting.

19.3.1
Subjective: Questionnaires

Quality of vision can be measured objectively (high- or low-contrast visual acuity, contrast sensitivity, glare disability, wavefront aberrations, corneal topographical changes) or subjectively by questionnaires. Functional measurements of contrast sensitivity or glare disability, measurements of optical parameters like wavefront error, and anatomical observations by corneal topography or biomicroscopy can be correlated to the patients' subjective judgement on the surgical outcome with questionnaires. Thus, quality of vision can be approached systematically.

There are questionnaires described in the literature that have been especially developed for post-operative evaluation of refractive patients [5, 11, 16, 26]. However, until now, none of them has been established for general use. For use in a daily clinical environment, a careful anamnesis with standardised questions (Do you see haloes? How is your night vision?) or a small selection of questions is a helpful tool to evaluate the outcome of subsequent procedures.

19.3.2
Functional

19.3.2.1
High-Contrast VA (Snellen Acuity)

High-contrast testing is the first way to assess visual acuity in clinical praxis. The common test principle is to present optotypes of decreasing size, at a constant contrast level of approximately 100%. High-contrast visual acuity is measured either with letters (e.g. Snellen chart, Bailey-Lovie chart or the ETDRS chart) or Landolt-C rings. Optotypes can be presented as charts or on a computer screen. Computer tests such as the Freiburg Visual Acuity and Contrast Test (FrACT) [4] use sophisticated algorithms to determine psychophysical thresholds.

19.3.2.2
Low-Contrast VA

Low-contrast visual acuity can be measured, as high-contrast visual acuity, by optotypes of a constant low contrast and of varying, decreasing size. Letter charts applying this principle are the Reagan charts, the Bailey-Lovie charts and the low-contrast ETDRS charts, that are provided at different low contrast levels. Landolt-C rings are used by the FrACT.

19.3.2.3
Contrast Sensitivity

Contrast sensitivity (CS, the reciprocal value of the minimal contrast which is recognised by the patient) can be measured with optotypes (letters or Landolt-C rings) or sine-wave gratings [9].

Common optotype tests are the Pelli-Robson charts (Fig. 19.2a) and the Small Letter Contrast Test [24]. These charts use letters of constant size but progressively decreasing contrast levels. Landolt-Cs are used for CS measurements by the computer-based FrACT. Based on the concept of different channels for detection of different spatial frequencies, sine-wave gratings have been used for contrast sensitivity testing for a long time. Gratings of different spatial frequencies with decreasing contrast are provided on each chart. Commonly used sine-wave tests are the Vistech charts, the F.A.C.T. chart (Fig. 19.2b), the Contrast Sensitivity Tester 1800 (Vision Sciences Research Corporation, San Ramon, CA) (Fig. 19.2c) and the CSV 1000E. The Vistech charts and their modification, the F.A.C.T. chart, are wall charts. Five spatial frequencies, each with nine different contrast levels are present. The Contrast Sensitivity Tester 1800 integrates a F.A.C.T. chart and provides testing under controllable illuminance levels. The CSV 1000E provides gratings at four spatial frequencies, each with eight different contrast levels, at 85 cd·m^{-2}.

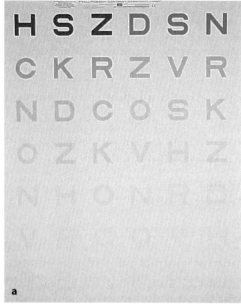

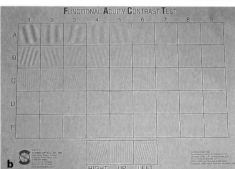

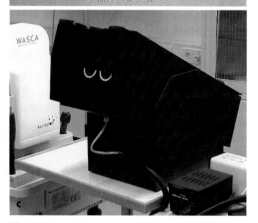

Fig. 19.2 a–c. Contrast sensitivity tests. **a** Pelli-Robson chart. **b** F.A.C.T. **c** Contrast Sensitivity Tester 1800

19.3.2.4
Glare, Scatter and Halo Testing

Glare disability can be measured when a glare source is added to a contrast sensitivity test. For testing with letter (Pelli-Robson charts) or gratings (Vistech charts, F.A.C.T. charts) wall charts, a hand-held device, the Brightness Acuity Tester (BAT) can be used to induce a glare effect. In the Contrast Sensitivity Tester 1800, a glare source of varying luminance is integrated in the test system. Landolt-C based glare tests are the Miller-Nadler Glare Tester and the Frankfurt-Freiburg Contrast and Acuity Test System (FF-CATS). The first one uses Landolt-Cs of different contrast levels at a constant spatial frequency, which are surrounded by a glare source of unchanged luminance. The latter is based on the FrACT computer program that displays Landolt-C rings on a monitor which is surrounded by a glare source of constant luminance created by a circle of eight white light-emitting diodes (LED) in 3° to the centre of the Landolt ring. Devices for testing scotopic vision like the Rodenstock Nyktometer (Rodenstock) or the Mesoptometer (Oculus) test CS at a very low luminance level of 0.032 cd·m^{-2} and are equipped with an integrated glare source for glare testing.

For scientific use, devices to objectively determine forward scatter (van den Berg stray light meter [30]) and haloes (Tomey Glare and Halo software [17]) have been designed.

19.3.3
Optical: Wavefront Sensing, MTF, PSF

Changes in the optical properties of the eye lead to changes in the quality of the retinal image and thus to changes in quality of vision. Wavefront deformation describes changes in the optical system, and it can be quantified by metrics as the modulation transfer function (MTF) or the point spread function (PSF) (see Fig. 19.3 and Chap. 17).

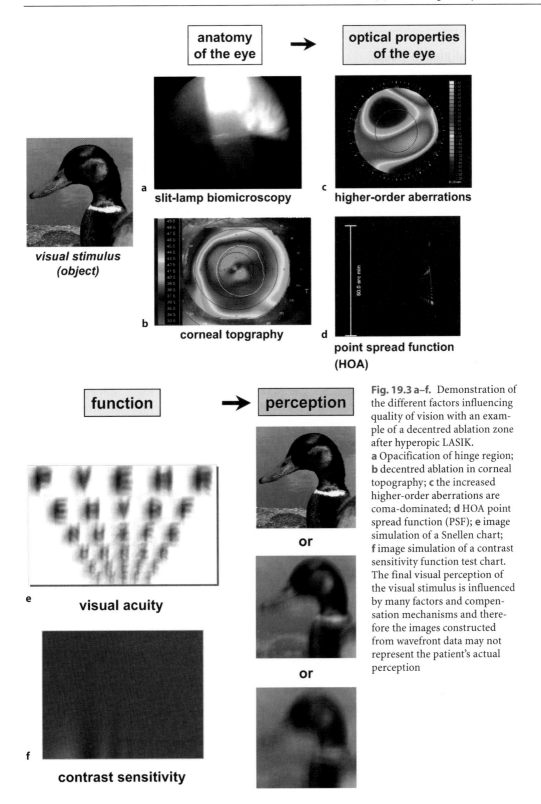

Fig. 19.3 a–f. Demonstration of the different factors influencing quality of vision with an example of a decentred ablation zone after hyperopic LASIK. **a** Opacification of hinge region; **b** decentred ablation in corneal topography; **c** the increased higher-order aberrations are coma-dominated; **d** HOA point spread function (PSF); **e** image simulation of a Snellen chart; **f** image simulation of a contrast sensitivity function test chart. The final visual perception of the visual stimulus is influenced by many factors and compensation mechanisms and therefore the images constructed from wavefront data may not represent the patient's actual perception

19.3.4
Anatomical: Biomicroscopy, Corneal Topography

Slit-lamp biomicroscopy, corneal topography and confocal microscopy reveal anatomical changes resulting from refractive procedures. Wanted (corneal flattening or steepening) or unwanted (haze, snowflakes, folds, decentration, surface irregularities; Fig. 19.3) effects on the ocular anatomy directly affect quality of vision. Therefore, anatomical observations in post-operative patient care are essential in describing quality of vision as morphological correlates of functional, optical and subjective parameters.

In Fig. 19.3 an example case of hyperopic LASIK with a decentred ablation zone and the impact of the decentration on different dimensions of quality of vision is shown. At the slit-lamp (Fig. 19.3a) an opacification at the hinge region could be seen. Corneal topography (Fig. 19.3b) reveals a decentred ablation with eccentric steepening. Wavefront analysis of higher-order aberrations (HOA) (Fig. 19.3c) shows the coma-dominated wavefront deformation. From the HOA, an HOA point spread function (PSF) (Fig. 19.3d) could be derived which represents the theoretical retinal image which could be obtained after total correction of defocus and astigmatism. From the PSF, images (Fig. 19.3e, f) could been constructed by convolution to simulate image distortion. For the particular case, the typical coma-induced ghosting could be visualised. It has to be said, that the final visual perception is influenced by many factors and compensation mechanisms and therefore the images constructed from wavefront data may not represent the patient's actual perception.

Summary for the Clinician

- Measuring quality of vision involves four major parameters: patient's sensation, functional, optical and anatomical features
- Correlation of all four parameters may lead to a complete understanding of the visual function and quality of vision after refractive surgery

- For reporting refractive surgery data, standardised tests under standardised conditions need to be established

19.4
Specific Changes in Quality of Vision After Refractive Surgery

19.4.1
Incisional Surgery

The complaints frequently described after *radial keratotomy* (RK) are glare disability, decreased contrast sensitivity and image degradations [1, 8]. The incidence of glare disability and changes in contrast sensitivity is highest immediately after surgery and decreases in most cases after 6 and 12 months.

It has been shown that this negative effect on visual performance arises with increasing pupil diameter because of increased higher order aberrations [2]. Regarding this, the diameter of the optical clear zone plays the most important role in creating such higher order aberrations and the appearance of night vision disturbances after radial incisional surgery. Grimmett et al. showed that an optical clear zone smaller than 3 mm can provoke such severe glare disability that patients become unable to drive a car at night or even lose employment [10]. Because of that, it is necessary to create an optical clear zone which is greater than the scotopic or mesopic pupil diameter to reach glare-free vision at night [29]. However, this limits the corrective range of RK because the correction of higher refractive errors causes a smaller optical clear zone.

Another problem after RK is the variation of the refraction from morning to evening (diurnal shift) which also leads to subjective image degradations. This phenomenon could be persistent over years. A possible reason for this is the corneal instability due to the radial incisions which causes variable corneal steepening or/and irregular astigmatism.

Because of these severe disadvantages, today, RK has been abandoned and is not a standard method to correct high myopia.

19.4.2
Excimer Surgery

19.4.2.1
Surface Ablation

After photorefractive keratectomy (PRK), patients often report decreased contrast sensitivity [8, 31]. Mostly, these complaints change with time: immediately after surgery, contrast sensitivity is worse than after 6 months or 1 year. Although most patients' complaints decrease with time, there are some who still have severe contrast sensitivity loss after 12 months or more. These patients often received treatment of myopia higher than 6 dioptres (D) [31]. Also monocular diplopia (ghosting), glare and halos may occur after PRK [11].

An important factor for the end result of PRK treatment is the pupil diameter, especially at night. Seiler et al. showed that spherical aberrations after PRK treatment rose markedly with increasing pupil diameter [27]. Because spherical aberrations lead to blur of the retinal image, patients with large pupils at night could develop night vision disturbances like glare, haloes, starbursts and loss of contrast sensitivity.

Of equal importance to pupil size is the diameter of the ablation zone. It has been shown that larger diameters of ablation reduce night halos, initial hyperopic shift, wound haze and higher order aberrations [6, 22]. With optical computer analysis, Roberts et al. simulated that ablation zones had to be at least as large as pupil aperture at night to preclude glare at the fovea [25].

Also important for a good visual outcome is a well-centred ablation (Fig. 19.3). As a result of decentred ablation patients complain about halos, glare, monocular diplopia and ghost images (Fig. 19.3) [18]. Even subclinical decentrations may lead to increasing higher-order aberrations with image degradation. In this context, it seems important to centre the ablation to the line of sight because it is possible that the geometric centre of the pupil moves as the pupil diameter changes [7].

Apart from sufficient ablation diameter and well-centred ablation, the amount of ablation correlates with a higher incidence of vision problems after PRK. This is attributed to larger refractive differentials between the ablated and untouched cornea as well as more haze due to wound healing [21].

19.4.2.2
Laser In Situ Keratomileusis (LASIK)

Just as for surface ablation also after LASIK, pupil size, ablation diameter, centration of the ablation and the amount of ablation depth play important factors in visual outcome and in the appearance of visual complaints like monocular diplopia, glare, halos, starbursts and decreased contrast sensitivity. These optical phenomena appear especially at mesopic or scotopic lighting conditions. LASIK specific problems may occur due to striae in the flap, epithelial ingrowth and misalignment of the flap. Fortunately, similar to PRK, most complaints improve or resolve with time.

Hersh et al. found that compared to the pre-operative situation with glasses or contact lenses, more patients report decreasing rather than worsening of glare symptoms 6 months after LASIK [11]. In the same study, the patients described a mild increase in halo symptoms and monocular diplopia. Lee et al. found a correlation between halo symptoms and the amount of attempted correction of the spherical equivalent (SE) [16]. They also found a decrease in contrast sensitivity under mesopic and partially under photopic lighting conditions, although without any correlation to pupil size (patients' pupil diameter was not larger than 7 mm) or amount of ablation. Schallhorn et al. and Pop et al. did not find a significant correlation between pupil size and night vision complaints in patients with moderate myopia [23, 26]. Schallhorn et al. found increase of glare reports in patients with larger pupil diameters only within the first 3 months. Also, haze and halo reports were more frequent, but this for all pupil diameters and only in the first 3 months. After a period of 6 months, they could not find significantly increased glare, haze and halo reports compared to pre-operative reports with contact lenses. Like Lee et al., they suspect the amount of treated spherical equivalent and residual cylinder to be the cause of patients' complaints. They hold remodelling effects of the cornea and adaptation mechanisms of the patient responsible for this recovery.

19.4.3
Intraocular Lens Procedures

19.4.3.1
Phakic Intraocular Lenses (pIOL)

The most frequently described visual complaints after phakic IOL implantations are glare and halos in mesopic and scotopic lighting conditions. Maroccos et al. showed that patients report glare regardless of whether anterior or posterior chamber phakic IOLs were implanted [19]. However, they showed that patients with 6.0 mm optical diameter irisclaw lenses are significantly better than posterior chamber IOLs with smaller optical diameter. Moreover, they showed an increase in the halo area, for posterior chamber IOLs more than for anterior chamber iris-claw lenses. This main reason for this is stray light due to the IOL edges. At daylight conditions, this stray light causes no complaints, but with increasing pupil diameter at night, it enters the pupil's aperture and leads to the described complaints, and even more so in eyes with large pupil diameter.

19.4.3.2
Refractive Lens Exchange (RLE)

After refractive lens exchange (RLE) with implantation of an IOL, patient complaints such as glare disability, halos, light streaks, arcs or circles and loss of contrast sensitivity by night may occur. This can be the result of corneal irregularities and astigmatism, as well as IOL-dependent. For IOL-dependent problems several possible reasons exist such as decentration, tilt, anterior or posterior capsule opacifications (PCO), stretch-folds in the posterior capsule or the lens design itself. Many of the currently used IOLs have squared, sharp-edged design to prevent PCO. The edges of the IOL may cause photopic phenomena, like light arcs or circles and glare, particularly if the pupil diameter is greater than the optical diameter of the IOL or

due to decentration. Modified rounded or non-reflective edges reduce this potential for edge glare phenomena [15]. Another problem currently discussed is decreased mesopic contrast sensitivity. Holladay et al. named high spherical aberrations as a possible reason [12]. They propose increasing contrast sensitivity via implantation of aspherical IOLs, which reduce spherical aberration to the level found in young people's eyes. However, full-scale comparative clinical studies have not yet convincingly proved these theoretical beginnings.

Summary for the Clinician

- A large diameter of the optical clear zone for RK plays the most important role in avoiding night vision disturbances and glare
- For surface ablation and LASIK, a well-centred ablation zone is important for myopic and particularly for hyperopic treatments
- Larger ablation zones seem to reduce unwanted visual symptoms
- Higher corrections with deep ablation zones seem to correlate with halo reports
- In eyes with larger pupils, small optical diameter or decentred phakic IOLs may lead to glare and halos symptoms
- Stray light due to decentration of the IOL or opacification of the posterior capsule can provoke light phenomena and glare disability
- Modern posterior chamber lenses with squared, truncated optic edges to prevent PCO may also lead to glare

19.5
Future Approaches to Improve Quality of Vision After Refractive Surgery

After quality of vision has been recognised as an important factor for refractive surgical interventions, the evaluation of current procedures is necessary.

The advent of wavefront technology enables the quantification of higher-order ocular aberrations (HOA). Experience with adaptive optics from astronomy led to the concept of correcting ocular HOA by excimer laser surgery (wave-front-guided ablation), which should improve the image quality of the eye and therefore improve visual outcome. Recent studies demonstrate that, on average, wavefront-guided corrections can provide objectively and subjectively better quality of vision than standard ablation profiles.

The concept of customised corneal treatments was proposed to improve eyes with poor optical quality due to corneal abnormalities (e.g. irregular astigmatism and decentred or small excimer laser zones). A combination of wavefront sensing and corneal topography may be the future for customised ablation, because optical and biomechanical factors are taken into account.

The idea of customised corneal procedures may also be transferable to lens surgery, which means that after lens removal, customised IOLs could compensate for residual ocular aberrations. The average cornea has a positive spherical aberration, which could be reduced or eliminated by implanting an IOL with negative spherical aberration (aspheric IOL). All current studies have shown that ocular aberrations could be reduced with aspheric IOLs compared to standard IOLs, but the improvement of visual quality is still under investigation.

The optic edge design of the IOL after refractive lens exchange can affect optical and mechanical performance. The reported optical effects are glare, halos, peripheral arcs of light and other unwanted optical images. Modified IOL designs are necessary to improve the optical quality of the eye.

Studies to prove all these concepts are necessary. The overall improvement in quality of vision after refractive surgical interventions will be a major step for the success of refractive surgery.

References

1. Applegate RA, Gansel KA (1990) The importance of pupil size in optical quality measurements following radial keratotomy. Refract Corneal Surg 6:47–54
2. Applegate RA, Howland HC, Sharp RP et al (1998) Corneal aberrations and visual performance after radial keratotomy. J Refract Surg 14:397–407
3. Applegate RA, Thibos LN, Hilmantel G (2001) Optics of aberroscopy and super vision. J Cataract Refract Surg 27:1093–1107
4. Bach M (1996) The Freiburg Visual Acuity test – automatic measurement of visual acuity. Optom Vis Sci 73:49–53
5. Brunette I, Gresset J, Boivin JF et al (2000) Functional outcome and satisfaction after photorefractive keratectomy. Part 2: survey of 690 patients. Ophthalmology 107:1790–1796
6. Endl MJ, Martinez CE, Klyce SD et al (2001) Effect of larger ablation zone and transition zone on corneal optical aberrations after photorefractive keratectomy. Arch Ophthalmol 119:1159–1164
7. Fay AM, Trokel SL, Myers JA (1992) Pupil diameter and the principal ray. J Cataract Refract Surg 18:348–351
8. Ghaith AA, Daniel J, Stulting RD et al (1998) Contrast sensitivity and glare disability after radial keratotomy and photorefractive keratectomy. Arch Ophthalmol 116:12–18
9. Ginsburg AP (1996) Next generation contrast sensitivity testing. In: Rosenthal B, Cole R (eds) Functional assessment of low vision. Mosby-Year Book, St. Louis, pp 77–88
10. Grimmett MR, Holland EJ (1996) Complications of small clear-zone radial keratotomy. Ophthalmology 103:1348–1356
11. Hersh PS, Steinert RF, Brint SF (2000) Photorefractive keratectomy versus laser in situ keratomileusis: comparison of optical side effects. Summit PRK-LASIK Study Group. Ophthalmology 107:925–933
12. Holladay JT, Piers PA, Koranyi G et al (2002) A new intraocular lens design to reduce spherical aberration of pseudophakic eyes. J Refract Surg 18:683–691
13. Koch DD, Kohnen T, Obstbaum SA et al (1998) Format for reporting refractive surgical data (editorial). J Cataract Refract Surg 24:285–287
14. Kohnen T (2001) Measuring vision in refractive surgery (editorial). J Cataract Refract Surg 27:1897–1898
15. Kohnen T (2001) The squared, sharp-edged optic intraocular lens design (editorial). J Catataract Refract Surg 27:485

16. Lee YC, Hu FR, Wang IJ (2003) Quality of vision after laser in situ keratomileusis: influence of dioptric correction and pupil size on visual function. J Cataract Refract Surg 29:769–777

17. Lohmann CP, Fitzke F, O'Brart D et al (1993) Corneal light scattering and visual performance in myopic individuals with spectacles, contact lenses, or excimer laser photorefractive keratectomy. Am J Ophthalmol 115:444–453

18. Maloney RK (1990) Corneal topography and optical zone location in photorefractive keratotomy. Refract Corneal Surg 6:363–371

19. Maroccos R, Vaz F, Marinho A et al (2001) Glare and halos after "phakic IOL". Surgery for the correction of high myopia. Ophthalmologe 98:1055–1059

20. McLeod SD (2001) Beyond Snellen acuity. The assessment of visual function after refractive surgery (editorial). Arch Ophthalmol 119:1371–1373

21. Møller-Pedersen T, Cavanagh HD, Petroll WM et al (1998) Corneal haze development after PRK is regulated by volume of stromal tissue removal. Cornea 17:627–639

22. O'Brart DP, Corbett MC, Verma S et al (1996) Effects of ablation diameter, depth, and edge contour on the outcome of photorefractive keratectomy. J Refract Surg 12:50–60

23. Pop M, Payette Y (2004) Risk factors for night vision complaints after LASIK for myopia. Ophthalmology 111:3–10

24. Rabin J, Wicks J (1996) Measuring resolution in the contrast domain: the small letter contrast test. Optom Vis Sci 73:398–403

25. Roberts CW, Koester CJ (1993) Optical zone diameters for photorefractive corneal surgery. Invest Ophthalmol Vis Sci 34:2275–2281

26. Schallhorn SC, Kaupp SE, Tanzer DJ et al (2003) Pupil size and quality of vision after LASIK. Ophthalmology 110:1606–1614

27. Seiler T, Reckmann W, Maloney RK (1993) Effective spherical aberration of the cornea as a quantitative descriptor in corneal topography. J Catataract Refract Surg 19[Suppl]:155-165

28. Thibos LN, Applegate RA, Schwiegerling JT et al (2002) Standards for reporting the optical aberrations of eyes. J Refract Surg 18:S652–660

29. Uozato H, Guyton DL (1987) Centering corneal surgical procedures. Am J of Ophthalmol 103:264–275

30. Van den Berg TJTP, Ijspeert JK (1992) Clinical assessment of intraocular stray light. Applied Optics 31:3694–3966

31. Vetrugno M, Quaranta GM, Maino A et al (2000) Contrast sensitivity measured by 2 methods after photorefractive keratectomy. J Cataract Refract Surg 26:847–852

32. Wesemann W (2002) Visual acuity measured via the Freiburg visual acuity test (FVT), Bailey Lovie chart and Landolt Ring chart. Klin Monatsbl Augenheilkd 219:660–667

Subject Index